Optimal Health With
Multiple Sclerosis

Also by Allen C. Bowling, MD, PhD

Complementary and Alternative Medicine and Multiple Sclerosis, Second Edition

Dietary Supplements and Multiple Sclerosis: A Health Professional's Guide
with Thomas M. Stewart, JD, PA-C, MS

Multiple Sclerosis: The Guide to Treatment and Management, Sixth Edition
with Chris Polman, MD, PhD; Alan Thompson, MD, FRCP, FRCPI; T. Jock Murray, MS,
and John Noseworthy, MD

Optimal Health With Multiple Sclerosis

A Guide to Integrating Lifestyle, Alternative, and Conventional Medicine

Allen C. Bowling, MD, PhD
Physician Associate
Colorado Neurological Institute
Englewood, Colorado
and
Clinical Professor of Neurology
University of Colorado
Aurora, Colorado

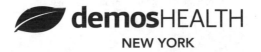

NEW YORK

Visit our website at www.demoshealth.com

ISBN: 978-1-936303-70-0
e-book ISBN: 978-1-61705-208-8

Acquisitions Editor: Julia Pastore
Compositor: diacriTech

Medical information provided by Demos Health, in the absence of a visit with a health care professional, must be considered as an educational service only. This book is not designed to replace a physician's independent judgment about the appropriateness or risks of a procedure or therapy for a given patient. Our purpose is to provide you with information that will help you make your own health care decisions.

The information and opinions provided here are believed to be accurate and sound, based on the best judgment available to the authors, editors, and publisher, but readers who fail to consult appropriate health authorities assume the risk of injuries. The publisher is not responsible for errors or omissions. The editors and publisher welcome any reader to report to the publisher any discrepancies or inaccuracies noticed.

Library of Congress Cataloging-in-Publication Data

Bowling, Allen C.
    Optimal health with multiple sclerosis : a guide to integrating lifestyle, alternative, and conventional medicine / Allen C. Bowling, MD, PhD, Physician Associate, Colorado Neurological Institute, Englewood, Colorado and Clinical Professor of Neurology, University of Colorado, Aurora, Colorado.
        pages cm
    Includes bibliographical references and index.
    ISBN 978-1-936303-70-0 (alk. paper)
    1. Multiple sclerosis—Alternative treatment. 2. Multiple sclerosis—Treatment. I. Title.

    RC377.B69 2014
    616.8'34—dc23

                    2014027383

Special discounts on bulk quantities of Demos Health books are available to corporations, professional associations, pharmaceutical companies, health care organizations, and other qualifying groups. For details, please contact:

Special Sales Department
Demos Medical Publishing, LLC
11 West 42nd Street, 15th Floor
New York, NY 10036
Phone: 800-532-8663 or 212-683-0072
Fax: 212-941-7842
E-mail: specialsales@demosmedical.com

Printed in the United States of America by McNaughton & Gunn.
15 16 17 18 / 5 4 3 2

To my wife, Diana

Contents

Part 3: Types of Lifestyle and Unconventional Medicine

Foreword

Let me start by sharing my personal bias. As a psychologist providing individual, group and family therapy for people living with MS, I always recommended Dr. Bowling's previous, very valuable book, *Complementary and Alternative Medicine and Multiple Sclerosis* to my patients as the go-to, comprehensive and objective resource for their questions about the role of complementary and alternative strategies in managing their multiple sclerosis (MS). And when my husband and I recently down-sized to a new home, Dr. Bowling's book was one that I was determined to make room for on my MS shelf.

With this new book, Dr. Bowling has gone far beyond his earlier effort to explain what is known and not known about the wide variety of treatment strategies that lie outside the realm of conventional medicine. He provides an evidence-based roadmap for fully integrating lifestyle and unconventional medicine strategies into MS management so that readers can knowledgeably attend to their physical, emotional, and spiritual well-being while utilizing a comprehensive approach to disease and symptom management.

The layout of the book allows readers to delve deeply into the current knowledge about more than 50 different lifestyle and unconventional approaches and hundreds of dietary supplements and herbs, while also providing quick-reference summaries—complete with helpful icons—indicating approaches that are safe and effective for use by everyone, those for which we have insufficient data regarding their safety and effectiveness, and those for which the risks clearly outweigh any possible benefits. If only all our roadmaps could be this clear!

To live fully and well with a chronic, unpredictable disease like MS requires a comprehensive and integrated approach to managing the "whole you." I can think of no better reference tool to guide you. Dr. Bowling brings to bear his years of training and experience as an MS specialist neurologist, his passion for promoting health and well-being, his determination to support informed and collaborative decision-making by people with MS and their health care providers, and his endless curiosity about the potential benefits and risks of the wide range of conventional and unconventional approaches to disease and symptom management. Keep this book handy just as I do.

Rosalind Kalb, PhD
Vice President, Clinical Care
Advocacy, Services and Research Department
National Multiple Sclerosis Society

Preface

This book provides objective and practical information and guidance about using lifestyle approaches, unconventional medicine, and conventional medicine to optimize health in those with MS. Medical care of MS typically involves the use of conventional medical approaches to slow down the disease course and treat the symptoms of MS. In its most narrowed form, MS care focuses exclusively on administering and monitoring the safety and effectiveness of FDA-approved disease-modifying medications. However, there is much evidence that many other treatment strategies, which generally are not components of MS care, have significant health effects on those with MS. For example, lifestyle approaches, such as nutrition, tobacco smoking, and physical activity, may have beneficial, as well as harmful, effects on MS. Similarly, among unconventional medical approaches, some may be beneficial and others may be harmful. This book aims to fill these gaps in MS care by providing information and guidance on incorporating lifestyle and unconventional medicine into a broad-based treatment plan for people with MS.

Objective information about conventional MS therapies is readily available. However, it is difficult to find evidence-based information about the safety and effectiveness of lifestyle strategies and unconventional medicine approaches in MS. Also, there are currently no objective, comprehensive guides on how to use these lifestyle and unconventional approaches in combination with conventional medicine in treating MS. To address these needs, this book provides objective, MS-specific information about more than 50 different lifestyle and unconventional medicine approaches and hundreds of dietary supplements and herbs. This information is based on reviews of dozens of books and thousands of scientific and clinical research studies. These books and studies are referenced throughout the text and are also provided as Additional Readings at the end of each chapter. In addition to providing objective information about specific lifestyle and unconventional strategies, this book transforms this information into a practical treatment approach. The Seven-Step Approach that is presented integrates lifestyle and unconventional medicine with conventional medicine to provide a multidimensional treatment strategy that is designed to optimize health in those with MS.

How to Use This Book

This book was written so that it would be accessible and useful for nearly everyone in the MS community. It is written in lay language, but, for those who are interested, references are provided to the relevant studies in the scientific and medical literature. Thus, this book may be used by people with MS and their family and friends as well as by health professionals. Indeed, a goal for this book is to have it serve as a common ground for people with MS and health professionals to explore and use treatment approaches that may be beneficial but are underutilized and also to avoid approaches that are ineffective or harmful.

This book is divided into five main sections, each of which has a specific purpose:

- Part 1: Introduction

    This section lays the foundation for the remainder of the book by providing broad overviews of MS, lifestyle and unconventional medicine, placebos, and precautions about using lifestyle and unconventional medicine.

- Part 2: Optimal Health With Multiple Sclerosis: A Seven-Step Guide to Integrating Lifestyle, Alternative, and Conventional Medicine

    In many ways, this is the heart of the book. It distills the vast information about MS and lifestyle, unconventional, and conventional medicine. The Seven-Step Approach that is provided may be used as a practical treatment guide for people with MS and health professionals.

- Part 3: Types of Lifestyle and Unconventional Medicine

    This part of the book is an A-to-Z compendium of MS-relevant information about more than 50 different lifestyle and unconventional medicine approaches. This section may be used to find detailed information about a specific approach, including a general overview, details of the treatment method, relevant studies in MS and other conditions, side effects, practical information about using the therapy, a concise MS-relevant conclusion about the therapy, and additional readings.

- Appendices

  Appendix 1 provides a listing of the overall ratings of the effectiveness and safety (see below) of all of the lifestyle and unconventional approaches that are discussed in Part 3. Appendix 2 provides an alphabetical listing of dietary supplements and herbs that may produce MS-relevant side effects or drug interactions. These two appendices serve as quick references to therapies that may be helpful and those that may be harmful.

- Index

  The index of this book is extremely detailed because it may not be apparent from the Table of Contents where to find information on particular therapies, such as uncommon dietary supplements and herbs. Like the Appendices, the Index may be used to quickly find information on specific therapies.

Icons are used throughout this book to indicate the relative effectiveness and safety of specific lifestyle and unconventional approaches. The use of any of the therapies that are in this book, even those with the highest rating, should be discussed with health professionals. The icons in this book are designed to provide a visual indicator of the overall rating of specific strategies:

★

"Essential"—This is the "highest rating" and indicates that these approaches have benefits that far outweigh risks. With rare exceptions, approaches in this category should be used by everyone with MS.

✓

"Worth Considering"—These approaches have some indication of beneficial effects in MS and have little or no risk. These approaches may be worth consideration by many people with MS.

?

"Uncertainties"—A question mark indicates that there are uncertainties about safety or effectiveness. If these therapies are considered, one should be aware of the uncertainties and carefully weigh the risks and benefits.

!

"Caution"—Therapies in this category have significant safety concerns or the risks significantly outweigh the benefits. These approaches should be avoided or used with caution.

Acknowledgments

Many individuals and organizations made this book possible. First, I would like to thank my wife, Diana, who is a clinical psychologist. Much of her clinical acumen and life wisdom is woven into this book. She provided valuable thoughts about challenging topics as well as formatting and design features. Also, she tolerated the ridiculously early morning risings that allowed me to have writing time in my daily schedule. Our two daughters, Elizabeth and Sarah, provided much inspiration—they continually motivate me to search for what constitutes a healthy, happy, and meaningful life.

I am thankful for the thousands of people with MS who, over the past few decades, have had the openness and courage to share their personal experiences and perspectives with me. These interactions have shaped me as a clinician and greatly influenced the general approach of this book as well as many of its specific details.

Several decades ago, Dr. David Jenkins was kind enough to take me in and mentor me in ways that still influence my career, including some of the underlying concepts of this book. More recently, Dr. Rosalind Kalb provided a critical "push" that motivated me to undertake this project. Nola Nielsen made it possible for me to have "protected" time to write. Sharon Martin, Nancy Peterson, and the Dorsey Medical Library provided efficient and high quality library services that were essential.

I am grateful for my ongoing involvement with the Colorado Neurological Institute (CNI) and appreciate the support for this project by Tami Lack, MA, Executive Director of CNI. Hugh"Monty"Loud and his family provided financial support and inspiration.

Finally, I am thankful for my long-term relationship with Demos Medical Publishing. In the past, Dr. Diana M. Schneider heartily supported books about controversial, but clinically important, topics. More recently, Julia Pastore expertly facilitated the writing of this book at all stages and provided outstanding editorial input.

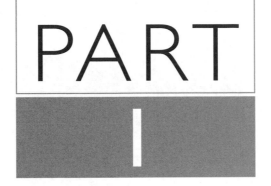

PART

I

Introduction

Alternative Medicine and Lifestyle Medicine

Multiple sclerosis (MS) is a common disease of the nervous system. Most people with MS use some form of conventional medical therapy, and there are well-established approaches for using these therapies to treat those with MS. In addition to conventional medicine, many people with MS also use some form of complementary and alternative medicine (CAM) and there is growing evidence and interest in the effects of lifestyle factors, such as diet and exercise, on MS. In fact, there is now evidence that various CAM therapies and lifestyle factors have beneficial—as well as harmful—effects on MS. Unfortunately, although CAM and lifestyle factors may have a significant impact on MS, they are often *not* included in the formal treatment plans that are developed by MS health professionals. It may even be difficult for people with MS—as well as health professionals—to obtain unbiased and practical information about the MS-relevant aspects of these nonmedication approaches. To improve this situation, this book provides evidence-based, MS-relevant information about CAM and lifestyle medicine and also provides guidance on how to safely and thoughtfully develop an MS treatment approach that utilizes CAM and lifestyle medicine alongside conventional medicine.

Before considering the relevance of CAM and lifestyle medicine to MS, it is important to understand the approach of conventional medicine to this disease. Dramatic advances have occurred recently in the field of MS research. Through scientific studies, we now have a significantly increased understanding of the disease process itself. Also, clinical studies using experimental medications have yielded a remarkable array of therapies that slow the disease process and alleviate MS-related symptoms.

Who Develops MS?

MS is a common neurologic disease that affects 350,000 to 400,000 people in the United States. Women are diagnosed with the disease about twice as frequently as are men. Although MS may affect people in all age groups, it is typically diagnosed between the ages of 20 and 40 years. A striking relationship exists between the prevalence of MS and the geographic area in which an individual lived during childhood. In general, an individual has a higher risk of developing MS if he or she grew up in an area that is far from the equator and a lower risk if the childhood years were spent near the equator.

How Does MS Affect the Nervous System?

In contrast to many diseases that affect a single part of the human body, MS affects two different body systems: the immune system and the nervous system. The immune system is not a distinct organ like the brain or liver. Instead, it is composed of many different types of molecules and cells (known as white blood cells) that travel through the bloodstream. The immune cells use chemical messages to protect the body from attack by bacteria, viruses, and cancers. MS is believed to be an *autoimmune condition* in which the immune system is excessively active and actually attacks the nervous system.

The *central nervous system* (CNS) is the part of the nervous system involved in MS. The CNS includes the brain, spinal cord, and optic nerves. The nerves in the CNS communicate with each other through long, wire-like processes that have a central fiber (*axon*) surrounded by an insulating material (*myelin*). In MS, the immune system cells produce inflammation that injures the myelin. In addition, damage occurs to the axon and the nerve cell itself. This damage is known as *degeneration,* which is the process that occurs in aging-related neurological diseases such as Alzheimer's disease and Parkinson's disease. The injury to the myelin and axons results in a slowing or blocking of nerve impulses that prevents the affected parts of the nervous system from functioning normally.

The cause of MS is not entirely clear. It is believed that two important factors are involved in developing the disease, one of which is environmental and the other genetic. The characteristic geographic distribution of MS indicates that an environmental factor is present. Many recent studies indicate that an important environmental factor is vitamin D, which mildly suppresses the immune system and thus could be protective against MS. Because vitamin D becomes active with sunlight exposure, those who live farther from the equator (with less-direct sunlight exposure) may have lower levels of vitamin D and higher risks of developing MS. Other environmental factors that appear to increase the risk of MS include infectious mononucleosis ("mono") as a teenager and cigarette smoking.

The presence of a genetic factor is indicated by family studies that demonstrate a hereditary predisposition to MS. Some genetic diseases are "dominant" and are clearly passed down through generations. MS is not passed on in such a well-defined pattern. Rather, there may exist an inherited predisposition to the disease that must be present in addition to an environmental agent to cause disease. Recent genetic studies indicate that multiple genes, many of which are related to immune system function, play a role in increasing the risk of developing MS. Ongoing, intensive research efforts are aimed at identifying specific genes that increase the risk of developing MS or affect the severity of the disease.

What Symptoms Do People With MS Experience?

The symptoms of MS depend on which areas of the brain and spinal cord develop MS *lesions*. For example, if the nerve that is involved in vision (the optic nerve) develops a lesion, blurring of vision occurs. This is referred to as *optic neuritis*. If a lesion develops in the part of the brain that produces movement on the left side of the body, left-sided weakness develops. In addition to visual blurring and weakness, other common MS symptoms include fatigue, depression, urinary difficulties, walking unsteadiness, stiffness in the arms or legs, tingling, and numbness.

The time course over which MS lesions develop and the number and location of lesions is different for each individual. Consequently, the time frame in which symptoms occur and the specific types of symptoms experienced are unique for each person. Also, as a result of the large variability of lesions between individuals, MS varies greatly in severity. Some people may have rare, mild attacks over their lifetime and may not experience any permanent symptoms, whereas others may develop severe, permanent symptoms over a relatively short period.

MS symptoms may occur episodically or may progress continuously. Episodes of symptoms are known as *relapses, attacks*, or *exacerbations*. Usually, some improvement in symptoms occurs after an attack. This improvement is referred to as a *remission*. In contrast to these relapsing-remitting symptoms, some people have symptoms that develop slowly and then progressively worsen over time with no clear remissions. These symptoms are referred to as *progressive*.

Specific combinations of relapsing-remitting and progressive symptoms are the basis for classifying MS. People who experience attacks and then improve have *relapsing-remitting MS*. This is the most common type of MS. At the time of diagnosis, about 85% of people with MS are classified as having relapsing-remitting MS. Some people who initially have relapsing-remitting disease may subsequently develop progressive symptoms. This is known as *secondary-progressive MS*. Those who have exclusively progressive symptoms from the onset of the disease, which constitutes only about 10% of people at the time of diagnosis, have *primary-progressive MS*, whereas those with *progressive-relapsing MS, which make up about 5% of those with MS,* have progressive symptoms from the onset (as occurs with *primary-progressive MS*), but also experience intermittent relapses. Some people who have experienced only one relapse may be diagnosed with *clinically isolated syndrome (CIS)* instead of MS. CIS is a condition that has a high risk of developing into MS.

Conventional Medical Therapy for MS

Dramatic breakthroughs have been made recently in the treatment of MS. In the past, no particularly effective therapies were available to change the course of disease. Since 1993, remarkable advances have led to Food and Drug Administration (FDA) approval of 10 medications for slowing down the disease course of MS. These drugs are referred to as *disease-modifying therapies*. In addition to these therapies, there is a long and diverse *pipeline* of MS drugs in development.

The currently available disease-modifying medications may be given by pill, injection, or intravenous administration:

- Pills
  - Fingolimod (Gilenya)
  - Teriflunomide (Aubagio)
  - Dimethyl fumarate (Tecfidera)
- Injections:
  - Interferons: interferon beta-1b (Betaseron and Extavia), interferon beta-1a once-weekly (Avonex), and interferon beta-1a three-times-weekly (Rebif)
  - Glatiramer acetate (Copaxone)
- Intravenous
  - Natalizumab (Tysabri)
  - Mitoxantrone (Novantrone)

These drugs decrease the number and severity of relapses, slow the progression of the disease, and decrease the development of new brain lesions. All of these medications have side effects, some of which are serious. Thus, it has become increasingly important in MS treatment to monitor closely for side effects and carefully balance the risks and benefits of therapies.

Because of the therapeutic effects of the FDA-approved medications, all people with MS should be strongly considered for treatment with one of these drugs. A 2008 statement by the National Multiple Sclerosis Society emphasizes the importance of treatment. The statement recommends treatment with these medications should be considered in all people with relapsing forms of MS and also in those with a CIS, the condition that has a high risk of developing into MS.

In addition to these medications, several other medications are used to treat MS. Steroid-based approaches are used for exacerbations. Steroids may be taken orally (prednisone, dexamethasone) or intravenously (methylprednisolone or Solu-Medrol). Also, a drug that increases the body's own production of steroids may be taken by injection (corticoptropin injection or Acthar) at the time of an attack. Some chemotherapy medications that are not FDA-approved for MS, including methotrexate, azathioprine (Imuran), and cyclophosphamide (Cytoxan), are used occasionally in an attempt to slow disease progression.

Given the wide range of symptoms caused by MS, multiple treatment approaches are possible. Therapies for symptoms include medications and non-medication-based approaches, such as physical therapy, occupational therapy, speech therapy, and psychotherapy. Common MS symptoms that are treated using these therapies include fatigue, depression, weakness, incoordination, walking difficulties, stiffness, bowel and bladder disorders, and sexual difficulties. Recent FDA-approved symptomatic therapies for MS include dalfampridine (Ampyra), which may improve walking, and dextromethorphan/quinidine (Nuedexta), which may alleviate uncontrollable laughing or crying.

(For more information on conventional approaches to MS, see the other, more extensive texts in this area in the "Additional Readings" section at the end of this chapter.)

Complementary, Alternative, Lifestyle, and Integrative Medicine

Beyond conventional medicine, there are many, many other approaches that may provide benefit—as well as harm—to those living with MS. These other approaches may be broadly categorized as CAM and lifestyle medicine. A term that is inclusive of all of these diverse healing methods is *integrative medicine*.

Complementary and Alternative Medicine

There are many different terms that are used in this area. The most general term is *unconventional medicine*, which refers to therapies that are not widely taught in medical schools or generally available in hospitals. The term *complementary medicine* refers to unconventional therapies that are used *in addition* to conventional medicine, while the term *alternative medicine* is used to describe unconventional treatments that are used *instead* of conventional medicine. The more inclusive term for both of these approaches is *CAM*. An even more inclusive term is *integrative medicine*, which refers generally to the combined use of unconventional medicine and conventional medicine.

CAM includes a vast array of therapies. To categorize these diverse and often unrelated therapies, multiple schemes have been proposed, several of which have been developed by the National Institutes of Health (NIH). This is one NIH scheme, with representative examples of therapies:

- Biologically based therapies—Dietary supplements, diets, bee venom therapy, hyperbaric oxygen
- Mind-body therapies—Guided imagery, hypnosis, meditation
- Alternative medical systems—Traditional Chinese medicine, Ayurveda, homeopathy
- Manipulative and body-based therapies—Chiropractic, reflexology, massage
- Energy therapies—Therapeutic touch, magnets

Lifestyle Medicine

As with CAM, there are many different definitions of lifestyle medicine. Generally, lifestyle medicine refers to daily habits and practices, such as diet and exercise, that are incorporated into conventional medical care in order to lower the risk for disease or, if disease is already present, to assist in the treatment of disease. Thus, lifestyle medicine aims to prevent and treat disease and also, more generally, to promote good health. Importantly, lifestyle factors are often two-edged swords—adhering to healthy lifestyle approaches, such as proper nutrition, exerts positive health effects, but leading an unhealthy lifestyle, such as poor nutrition, causes and worsens diseases.

Many different lifestyle approaches may be used. Commonly used strategies include:

- Nutrition
- Exercise
- Stress management
- Smoking cessation

While medications are often thought to be the best approach to treating a disease, it has been increasingly recognized that healthy lifestyle approaches are also very important—and perhaps the most important—strategy in treating, as well as preventing, multiple diseases. Hundreds of studies demonstrate that lifestyle practices play an important role in many diseases, including diabetes, obesity, high blood pressure, and heart disease.

Evidence is growing that a long list of other diseases, including MS, are also significantly impacted by daily habits and practices. For example, lack of physical activity, smoking, and some dietary factors, such as high salt intake and low vitamin D levels, may increase the risk of developing MS or increase the severity of the disease. Furthermore, in those with MS, the presence of other lifestyle-associated diseases, such as diabetes, high blood pressure, and heart disease, maylead to more rapid progression of neurological disability and lower quality of life.

Which Approach Belongs in Which Category?

In spite of these formal definitions, the distinction between CAM, lifestyle medicine, and conventional medicine is not always clear. For example, physical activity is often a component of conventional medicine, yet may also be categorized as lifestyle medicine and CAM. Similarly, some dietary interventions, such as vitamin D supplementation, may be classified as CAM, lifestyle medicine, or conventional medicine. An excessive focus on classifying and compartmentalizing therapies is not helpful—putting specific therapies in different treatment"turfs"with different practitioners and specialists may"disintegrate"care and ultimately detract from bringing all of the many potentially beneficial MS therapies together into an integrated, broad-based approach that is readily accessible to people with MS.

Integrative Medicine

The term *integrative medicine* refers to an approach that aims to optimize health and healing by decompartmentalizing all of the various therapeutic approaches. Integrative medicine is sometimes defined as the combination of CAM and conventional medicine. Actually, integrative medicine is much broader. It emphasizes health and wellness of the whole person through the use of conventional medicine, CAM, and lifestyle strategies within a supportive clinician-patient relationship.

CAM Is Popular in the General Population and in MS

Many studies have documented that CAM is used frequently in the general population in the United States. One well-known large study was conducted in 1997 and was reported in the medical literature in 1998 by Dr. David Eisenberg (1). In this landmark study of more than 2,000 people, approximately 42% used some form of CAM. It was estimated that 629 million visits were made to practitioners of alternative medicine; this was greater than the number of visits to all primary care physicians in that year. Nearly half of the people were using CAM without the advice of a physician or a CAM practitioner, which demonstrates the need for increased communication in this area between patients and health care providers.

More recent U.S. studies indicate that the use of CAM continues at a similar level and will continue in the future. In several large studies, approximately 40% of Americans were found to use some form of CAM (2–5). Another U.S. study found that CAM use is not a short-lived fad (6). In this report, CAM use by the age of 33 was evaluated relative to birth date. For those born before 1945, about 30% of respondents used CAM. The percentage of CAM users rose to about 50% for those born between 1945 and 1964, and was even higher, about 70%, for those born between 1965 and 1979. This study also found that nearly one-half of people who tried a specific form of CAM continued to use that CAM therapy more than 20 years later. Overall, this study indicates that CAM is not a short-lived phenomenon because some CAM therapies are used long-term and CAM use in general is higher among younger people.

Many studies have evaluated CAM use specifically in those with MS. One of the earliest studies in this area was conducted in Massachusetts and California in the 1990s (7). Approximately 60% of people had used CAM, and, on average, people used two to three different types of CAM. Subsequent studies have investigated CAM use in people with MS in the United States and have produced extremely variable results. CAM use among people with MS has ranged from 30% to 100%. As a whole, these studies indicate that at least 50% of people with MS use some form of CAM (8–16).

The use of CAM among people with MS is not simply an American phenomenon. Studies in other countries indicate similar results for the percentage of people with MS who use CAM: 65% to 80% in Australia, 70% in Canada, 27% to 55% in Denmark, 45% to 60% in Nordic countries, 41% in Spain, and 70% in Germany (17–24).

In surveys of people with MS and of the general population, a consistent finding is that CAM usually is used in conjunction with conventional medical therapy. Approximately 80% to 90% of people who use CAM also use conventional medicine. This leaves a relatively small fraction of people who use CAM in a truly alternative manner. These findings indicate that CAM usually is used in a complementary way.

People with MS use a wide range of CAM therapies. Those that appear to be especially popular include massage, dietary supplements, diets, chiropractic medicine, acupuncture, meditation and guided imagery, and yoga.

The reasons why people with MS pursue CAM are as varied as the different CAM modalities used. "Curing MS" is not a frequently cited reason for using CAM. Common reasons include decreasing the severity of MS-associated symptoms, increasing control, improving health, and using a method that accounts for the interrelation of mind, body, and spirit. Some people are drawn to CAM because of the lack of effectiveness of conventional medications and anecdotal reports of benefits or recommendations from friends, relatives, or physicians. One study of CAM use in people with MS and other chronic diseases concluded that CAM was an important component for self-care and was not generally embraced as a rejection of conventional medicine or an unrealistic search for a cure (25).

Underutilized Tools in the Toolbox

CAM and lifestyle approaches are often underutilized tools in the "MS toolbox." It is recognized that they are important factors to address in treating the disease. CAM is of high interest, and is used widely, in those with MS. In addition, both CAM and lifestyle approaches have beneficial as well as harmful effects on the disease. Despite the recognized importance of these "nonmedication" strategies, multiple barriers significantly limit their use.

Books and Other Written Material

For CAM in particular, the information available to the general public in books, magazines, and the Internet is vast but of variable quality. For CAM that is relevant to MS, the amount of information is limited and the quality also is variable. To attempt to understand the type of information that is available on CAM and MS, we conducted an informal survey of the popular literature on CAM several years ago. At two local bookstores, we found 50 CAM books written for a lay audience. In some books, MS was incorrectly defined as a form of muscular dystrophy. Other books made the erroneous—and potentially dangerous—statement that, because MS is an immune disorder, it is important to take supplements that stimulate the immune system. In fact, MS is an immune disorder, but it is characterized by an excessively active immune system; thus, immune-stimulating supplements actually may be harmful. On average, the CAM books recommended five or six therapies for MS. In 20% of them, 10 or more therapies were recommended. It was rare for books to discourage the use of any CAM treatment. Interestingly, none had the same recommended therapies.

Products and CAM/Lifestyle Practitioners

In addition to books, information about CAM and lifestyle strategies may be obtained from vendors of products, CAM practitioners, and others such as nutritionists and physical trainers. Unfortunately, product vendors, such as people who sell supplements, often exaggerate claims about their products. Practitioners of CAM and lifestyle approaches (as well as product vendors) sometimes have limited experience with MS and are not certain how their therapy relates to a complex disease process such as MS.

Physicians and Other Mainstream Health Care Providers

Physicians and other conventional medicine providers are potential sources of information and could play a valuable role in developing a treatment plan that utilizes CAM and lifestyle medicine in combination with conventional medicine. However, there are multiple barriers and challenges in this area. First, in the area of CAM, most conventional health providers have little or no training or experience. As a result, they may have little or no MS-relevant CAM information. In addition, for various reasons, some conventional health providers may find CAM unappealing or even repulsive. With lifestyle medicine, conventional health providers may also feel challenged. Many may find lifestyle medicine more palatable than CAM but, as with CAM, they may have little or no formal training, experience, or information. Further, they may feel that they lack the skills, time, or appropriate clinician–patient relationship to produce long-lasting changes in lifestyle, such as diet or physical activity. Indeed, producing changes in lifestyle may be extremely difficult and time-consuming, and it requires skills that are very different from those used to prescribe or administer medications and other conventional therapies. Paradoxically, the remarkable advances in conventional medical therapy for MS may actually prevent well-intentioned conventional health providers from using or discussing CAM and lifestyle medicine. The intensive safety and effectiveness monitoring and complex decision making that are required for using these drugs may consume all of the time that is available for a standard medical appointment. In addition, staying up-to-date and well-informed about all of the various conventional MS therapies may be an enormous challenge on its own for health care providers—to then also stay well-informed about the vast number of MS-relevant CAM and lifestyle approaches may simply not be possible for many.

Evidence for Safety and Effectiveness: Differences in Perspective

An additional challenge in this area is that conventional health providers and people with MS may have very different views about information on conventional therapies, CAM therapies, and lifestyle strategies. Physicians view the use of basic science and rigorous clinical trial methods as a powerful tool to develop new disease understanding and new therapies. In contrast, people with MS may agree that this process is powerful, but that it is also slow and thus may yield limited advances during their lifetimes. Also, they may believe the complexity of these studies is excessively rigorous, especially for many CAM and lifestyle strategies that have little or no risk and are known to provide general health benefits.

The "gold standard" for developing new therapies is a randomized, controlled clinical trial. This clinical testing employs specific and rigorous methods, including the use of a placebo-treated group, "blinding" of patients and investigators (so that neither patients nor investigators know who has received placebo and who has received active medication), and randomly selecting those who will receive placebo or active medication. Physicians and other mainstream health care providers generally use therapies only after they have been found to be effective in these well-designed clinical trials. FDA approval generally requires two randomized, controlled trials that are of the highest quality ("Class I") and show that the benefit outweighs the risk. Through the rigorous clinical trial methods, a black-and-white distinction exists between those therapies that have been proven effective and those that have not.

For CAM therapies and many lifestyle approaches, there may not be such a black-and-white distinction, but rather shades of gray. For example, some CAM and lifestyle approaches have not undergone definitive and rigorous large-scale clinical testing, but scientific studies in animals or limited clinical studies in people have produced promising results. These types of therapies generally are not incorporated into mainstream medicine and are not thought to be the "standard of care." However, people with a disease may have significant interest in such promising therapies, especially if they are relatively safe and inexpensive. In addition, some of these promising CAM and lifestyle approaches may provide other health benefits, which may make them even more appealing to people with a disease. An example of this situation in MS is vitamin D supplementation and other dietary strategies—these approaches have possible, but not definite, effectiveness in MS but they do have definite general health benefits.

Another difference in patient–physician perspective occurs with proven mainstream therapies. Conventional medications that are 30% to 60% effective at slowing down the disease process may represent a major advance for physicians and other health care providers but, for people with MS, these therapies may be seen as 40% to 70% away from a cure (which would be 100% effective).

In some areas of CAM, the same set of facts is viewed negatively by conventional medicine and positively by some people with MS. This emphasizes the importance of first establishing the facts about a therapy and then realizing that these facts may be interpreted differently by mainstream health care providers and people with MS. Under some circumstances, it is as if two different cultures exist: that of the health care provider and that of the person who has the disease. These two cultures may have strikingly different belief systems.

The difference in perspective becomes especially apparent when a physician develops a disease. In this situation, a dramatic shift may occur in an individual's attitudes about what constitutes an appropriate medical therapy. In MS, there have been several published examples of this shift in perspective.

Dr. George Jelinek is an Australian physician who has MS. Although he was not trained as a neurologist, he has devoted some of his career to MS-related writing and research. Much of his MS work actually highlights the differences between patient and physician perspectives and aims to study, and increase the use of, appropriate lifestyle and CAM approaches in MS treatment.

He writes: "Although a specialist emergency physician with typically conservative medical background, I have also experienced MS from a patient's perspective… Studies which have not 'proven' the treatment to be beneficial but which suggest a major benefit look much more interesting when you actually have the disease, especially when the treatment has other health benefits as well…Despite [its] effectiveness, lifestyle change is often not promoted" (26).

Two English physicians with MS have also written on this topic. With reference to evening primrose oil, a fatty acid dietary supplement, Dr. Alexander Burnfield states: "I started taking it before the research was published and, being only human, take it just in case I get worse if I stop. This is, I know, an unscientific and emotional response, and the logical-doctor part of me is quite shocked" (27). Dr. Elizabeth Forsythe writes whimsically about diet and MS: "It is what you feel in your own body and mind that is the most important thing, and it is very easy for doctors and patients to forget that. I believe that a little of what you fancy does do you good!" (28).

Transforming Challenge into Opportunity

There are challenges with incorporating CAM and lifestyle medicine into MS care. However, addressing these challenges and overcoming them provides a great opportunity to improve the quality of care for those with MS.

An encouraging aspect of the current situation is that a plethora of MS-relevant CAM and lifestyle information already exists but is underutilized or inappropriately utilized. Thus, one of the greatest challenges now is *not* to "start from scratch" and develop new therapies—that can be a long, expensive, and uncertain path. Rather, the challenge is to take currently available information about existing approaches and thoughtfully incorporate this information into MS therapy. This book aims to do this by providing MS-relevant, objective information about the safety and effectiveness of CAM and lifestyle approaches (Part 3) and also by providing guidelines on integrating these approaches with conventional medicine (Part 2). Having all of this information in one resource that is objective and easily accessible to people with MS as well as health professionals creates common ground upon which people with MS and their health care providers may communicate openly and work together to develop broad-based, safe, and effective treatment plans.

Additional Readings
Websites

www.neurologycare.net—CAM website that is maintained by Dr. Allen Bowling

www.nationalmssociety.org—website of the National MS Society of the United States

Books

Bauer B, ed. *Mayo Clinic Book of Alternative Medicine and Home Remedies.* New York, NY: Time Home Entertainment; 2013.

Bourdette D, Yadav V, Shinto L. Multiple sclerosis. In: Oken BS, ed. *Complementary Therapies in Neurology: An Evidence-Based Approach.* New York, NY: Parthenon Publishing Group; 2004:291–302.

Bowling AC. Complementary and alternative medicine in multiple sclerosis. In: Geisser B, ed. *Primer on Multiple Sclerosis.* New York, NY: Oxford University Press; 2011:369–381.

Bowling AC. Complementary and alternative medicine: practical considerations. In: Rae-Grant A, Fox R, Bethoux F, eds. *Multiple Sclerosis and Related Disorders: Diagnosis, Medical Management, and Rehabilitation.* New York, NY: Demos; 2013:243–249.

Burnfield A. *Multiple Sclerosis: A Personal Exploration.* London, UK: Souvenir Press; 1997.

Cassileth BR. *The Alternative Medicine Handbook.* New York, NY: W.W. Norton; 1998.

Ernst E, Pittler MH, Wider B. *The Desktop Guide to Complementary and Alternative Medicine: An Evidence-Based Approach.* Edinburgh, UK: Mosby; 2006.

Forsythe E. *Multiple Sclerosis: Exploring Sickness and Health.* London, UK: Faber and Faber; 1988.

Freeman L. *Mosby's Complementary and Alternative Medicine: A Research-Based Approach.* St. Louis, MO: Mosby; 2004.

Institute of Medicine. Committee on the Use of Complementary and Alternative Medicine by the American Public. *Complementary and Alternative Medicine in the United States.* Washington, DC: National Academies Press; 2005.

Jelinek G. *Overcoming Multiple Sclerosis.* Crows Nest, Australia: Allen & Unwin; 2009.

Kalb RC. *Multiple Sclerosis: The Questions You Have—The Answers You Need.* New York, NY: Demos Medical Publishing; 2011.

Kalb RC, Giesser B, Costello K. *Multiple Sclerosis for Dummies.* Hoboken, NJ: John Wiley & Sons; 2012.

Kennedy P, ed. *The Can Do Multiple Sclerosis Guide to Lifestyle Empowerment.* New York, NY: Demos; 2013.

Micozzi MS, ed. *Fundamentals of Complementary and Alternative Medicine.* Philadelphia, PA: Saunders Elsevier; 2011.

Navarra T. *The Encyclopedia of Complementary and Alternative Medicine.* New York, NY: Checkmark Books; 2005.

Polman CH, Thompson AJ, Murray TJ, McDonald WI. *Multiple Sclerosis: The Guide to Treatment and Management*. New York, NY: Demos Medical Publishing; 2006.

Rakel D. *Integrative Medicine*. Philadelphia, PA: Elsevier; 2012.

Rippe JM, ed. *Lifestyle Medicine*. Boca Raton, FL: CRC Press; 2013.

Russell M, Bowling AC. *The Everything Health Guide to Multiple Sclerosis*. Avon, MA: Adams Media; 2009.

Schapiro RT. *Managing the Symptoms of Multiple Sclerosis*. New York, NY: Demos Medical Publishing; 2007.

Spencer JW, Jacobs JJ. *Complementary/Alternative Medicine: An Evidence-Based Approach*. St. Louis, MO: Mosby; 2003.

Synovitz LB, Larson KL. *Complementary and Alternative Medicine for Health Professionals: A Holistic Approach to Consumer Health*. Burlington, MA: Jones and Bartlett Learning; 2013.

Journal Articles

Bell IR, Caspi O, Schwartz GE, et al. Integrative medicine and systemic outcomes research: issues in the emergence of a new model for primary health care. *Arch Int Med*. 2002;162:133–140.

Berkman CS, Pignotti MG, Cavallo PF, et al. Use of alternative treatments by people with multiple sclerosis. *Neurorehab Neural Repair*. 1999;13:243–254.

Bowling AC. Complementary and alternative medicine and multiple sclerosis. *Neurol Clin North Am*. 2011;29:465–480.

Bowling AC. Complementary and alternative medicine in multiple sclerosis: dispelling common myths about CAM. *Int J MS Care*. 2005;7:42–44.

D'hooghe MB, Nagels G, DeKeyser J, Haentjens P. Self-reported health promotion and disability progression in multiple sclerosis. *J Neurol Scis*. 2013;325: 120–126.

Eisenberg D, Davis R, Ettner S, et al. Trends in alternative medicine use in the United States, 1990-1997: results of a follow-up national survey. *JAMA*. 1998;280:1569–1575.

International Multiple Sclerosis Genetics Consortium. Analysis of immune-related loci identifies 48 new susceptibility variants for multiple sclerosis. *Nat Genet*. 2013;45:1353–1360.

Jelinek GA, Hassed CS. Managing multiple sclerosis in primary care: are we forgetting something? *Qual Prim Care*. 2009;17:55–61.

Marrie RA, Horwitz RI. Emerging effects of comorbidities on multiple sclerosis. *Lancet Neurol*. 2010;9:820–828.

Okoro CA, Zhao G, Li C, Balluz LS. Has the use of complementary and alternative medicine therapies by US adults with chronic disease-related functional limitations changed from 2002-2007? *J Altern Complement Med*. 2013;19:217–223.

Shinto L, Yadav V, Morris C, Lapidus JA, Senders A, Bourdette D. Demographic and health-related factors associated with complementary and alternative medicine (CAM) use in multiple sclerosis. *Mult Scler*. 2006;12:94–100.

Stoll SS, Nieves C, Tabby DS, Schwartzman R. Use of therapies other than disease-modifying agents, including complementary and alternative medicine, by patients with multiple sclerosis: a survey study. *J Am Osteopath Assoc*. 2012;112:22–28.

Yadav V, Bever C, Bowen J, et al. Summary of evidence-based guideline: complementary and alternative medicine in multiple sclerosis: report of the guideline development subcommittee of the American Academy of Neurology. *Neurology*. 2014;82:1–10.

Yadav V, Shinto L, Bourdette D. Complementary and alternative medicine for the treatment of multiple sclerosis. *Expert Rev Clin Immunol*. 2010;6:381–395.

Placebos and Nocebos

Placebos and the "placebo effect" provide valuable insights into treating disease and evaluating medical therapies, whether conventional or unconventional. Discussions of medical therapies usually focus on the effectiveness of the therapy and not on the placebo response. However, placebos produce beneficial effects and, though not fully understood, both the placebo effect and its lesser known opposite, the "nocebo effect," have important implications in the treatment of many medical conditions, including multiple sclerosis (MS).

Placebos and the Placebo Effect

A placebo is generally thought of as a "dummy pill" or "sugar pill." More formally, a placebo is a therapy that is not believed to have a specific effect on the disease or the condition for which it is given. *Placebo* is derived from Latin and means, "I will please." A placebo may be given in the form of a substance or a procedure. The *placebo effect* is the response of a person's condition to the placebo.

Many dramatic examples of the placebo effect exist. One of the early examples in medical literature involved a woman with excessive nausea and vomiting during pregnancy. She was told she was being given a medication for nausea but was actually given syrup of ipecac, which is known to induce vomiting and is sometimes given to children who have swallowed a possibly toxic substance. The woman in this study actually had improvement in her nausea.

A well-known study of the placebo effect was reported in 1955 by Dr. Harry Beecher (1). He described the placebo effect in a variety of conditions, including the common cold, pain after surgery, headache, and seasickness. Overall, symptoms were improved in 35% of the people who were given the placebo. Subsequent studies of a variety of medical conditions found placebo effects that were frequently in the range of 30% to 40%. In some studies, placebos have been 70% effective.

As would be expected, a placebo effect occurs in studies of people with MS. A notable response to placebos has been observed in studies of therapy for MS itself, as well as for MS-related symptoms. In older MS studies, from 1935 to 1950, a variety of ineffective therapies produced 60% to 70% improvement. In research studies using interferon beta-1b (Betaseron), the first U.S. Food and Drug Administration (FDA)-approved immune therapy for MS, the number of MS attacks was determined for people taking Betaseron and for another group taking placebo. The placebo-treated group had a 28% decrease in the rate of MS attacks. Similarly, the placebo group showed decreased attack rates of 33% in trials with intramuscular interferon beta-1a (Avonex), 13% with subcutaneous interferon beta-1a (Rebif), and 43% with glatiramer acetate (Copaxone). Importantly, in all these trials, the study drug was significantly more effective than the placebo, and this finding is the basis for the FDA approval of these and other medications.

Several explanations can be given for the decrease in MS attack rates observed with placebos. This may represent the natural course of the disease, or it may be an artifact of statistics (referred to as *regression to the mean*), but it also may represent a genuine placebo effect.

Placebo responses also have occurred in studies that use biological tests to monitor disease activity. Magnetic resonance imaging (MRI) is frequently used in MS clinical trials. An MRI study of a small number of people with MS found that the placebo-treated group had an approximately 20% reduction in the development of new brain lesions (2). This finding was not statistically significant, but this may have been due to the small number of people in the study. A particularly interesting finding occurred in a study of an experimental medication, alpha-interferon (3). People with MS were given alpha-interferon or placebo and monitored. A component of the monitoring included measurement of the activity of an immune cell known as a *natural killer cell*. As expected, the group treated with alpha-interferon showed a 52% increase in natural killer cell activity. However, the placebo group also showed an increase in natural killer cell activity that was nearly identical to that of the alpha-interferon group.

Placebo effects have been observed in other MS clinical studies, including those of medications for MS symptoms. For MS-associated fatigue, the placebo effect in clinical trials has been as high as 50%. In one clinical trial of MS fatigue, the therapeutic effect of the placebo was actually larger than that of the active medication (4).

These studies suggest that the mind may have a powerful influence over the symptoms of a disease and perhaps even on the underlying disease process.

The Nocebo Effect

Many people are not familiar with the nocebo response. With this response, which is essentially the opposite of the placebo effect, people expect that a specific "therapy" will produce a negative health outcome and then that negative outcome does indeed occur.

In one well-known nocebo study, participants were told that a liquid would make them vomit and then were asked to swallow the liquid. The liquid was actually a mixture of water and sugar. Nevertheless, approximately 80% of those in the study vomited.

Nocebo effects are common in clinical trials. Approximately 25% of those in trials experience some type of nocebo response—the most common nocebo responses are headaches, drowsiness, and weakness. They occur even in those who are in the placebo group, receiving some type of dummy pill or other inactive therapy. A prominent nocebo response was reported in a review of 100 MS clinical trials over a 20-year time period (5). In participants in trials for MS symptoms, such as muscle stiffness or fatigue, 25% had a nocebo response. An even higher nocebo response of 74% was seen in those in trials of disease-modifying therapies. As might be expected, higher nocebo responses occur in the earlier phases of drug testing, when drug safety is less certain.

Mechanisms of Placebo and Nocebo Responses

The ways in which placebos and nocebos produce their responses has been extensively studied but is still not fully understood. Several important factors have been identified. These include the setting in which the therapy is provided as well as the attitudes and mindsets of the clinicians and the people being treated. The expectation of the person being treated is thought to be particularly important. Specifically, positive expectations are a major factor in producing placebo responses. Placebos create optimism and hope that there will be improvement in one's health. In contrast, negative health expectations underlie nocebo responses. Depression and anxiety increase the possibility of nocebo responses.

At the molecular level, several potential mechanisms have been identified. Endorphins, the pain-relieving molecules synthesized by the human body, have been implicated in the placebo-induced alleviation of pain. Placebo responses in some neurological conditions, especially Parkinson's disease, have been associated with a specific neurochemical known as dopamine.

Placebo effects on the immune system in conditions such as MS may occur through complex immune system–nervous system interactions. The nervous system and the immune system do not appear to function independently but rather are components of a network in which they communicate and alter each other's activities. For example, the brain alters the production of hormones that then affect the immune system. Also, nerve fibers have connections with the immune system and the chemical messengers of the immune system and nervous system *cross-communicate*.

Placebos and Unconventional Medicine

Placebos and the placebo effect are important when considering conventional medicine and complementary and alternative medicine (CAM). In conventional medicine, the placebo effect often is disregarded or minimized. In clinical trials of experimental drugs, the placebo response is simply subtracted from the effect of the drug. Also, a certain level of discomfort exists for placebos within conventional medicine. Dr. Jay Katz states:"... if placebos were to be acknowledged as effective in their own right, it would expose large gaps in medicine's and in doctors' knowledge about underlying mechanisms of care and relief from suffering" (6).

For studies of MS, which is an extremely individualized, variable, and unpredictable disease, it is clear that any evaluated therapy must be compared with a placebo. Sometimes CAM therapies are touted on the basis of the experience of individuals—these are known as *anecdotes*. Because of the placebo effect and the fact that MS may remain stable with no therapy or that full recovery may occur after an MS attack, it is important not to rely heavily on treatment benefits based only on anecdotes. Whether a therapy is conventional or unconventional, definitive claims of effectiveness must be based on studies of large numbers of people, some of whom are treated with placebos.

Finally, an important difference between conventional medicine and CAM may relate to the placebo effect. It has been stated that much of the history of conventional medicine is actually the history of the placebo effect because medicine has not, until recently, had particularly effective therapies. Physicians in the past may have relied very heavily on establishing relationships with patients and may have become skilled at administering ineffective therapies in a way that maximized the placebo response.

Modern mainstream medicine has undergone significant changes. It has become more technological. Much of medicine is now focused on the body alone, instead of on the body and the mind. Decreased insurance reimbursement has generally led to briefer physician visits. With all these changes, many physicians lack the resources and time to nurture strong patient relationships and to develop optimal methods for administering therapies. In contrast to the past history of medicine, some of the recent history of American medicine may be the history of *removing* the placebo effect from clinical practice.

In contrast to physicians, many practitioners of CAM spend more time with patients and rely more on positive interpersonal skills to interact with and treat them. This may be true for practitioners in areas such as acupuncture, homeopathy, and massage. A single session with these practitioners may last 60 minutes or longer and involve a detailed discussion of many topics, whereas physician visits are often 10 to 20 minutes or shorter and often focus exclusively on diseases, symptoms, diagnostic tests, and drug therapies. Regardless of the effectiveness of their therapies, some practitioners of CAM may be more skilled and more comfortable than are physicians with using the power of the placebo effect.

Incorporating Placebo and Nocebo Concepts Into Treatment

Placebos and nocebos are sometimes viewed as annoying aberrations. They are unpredictable, and, in spite of extensive clinical and scientific research, they are not fully understood. However, they impact health positively as well as negatively and thus offer valuable insights into healing that should be used to guide treatment approaches for chronic conditions such as MS.

Specific strategies may be used to maximize placebo responses and minimize nocebo effects. Generally, these strategies involve cultivating the hope, optimism, and empowerment that occurs with placebos and simultaneously identifying and addressing negative feelings and expectations. Ideally, these placebo–nocebo strategies are thoughtfully incorporated into the ways in which the various therapies for a medical condition are provided. Attention to the ways in which therapies are provided—and also making use of a wide range of conventional, CAM, and lifestyle approaches—are critical components of *integrative medicine*.

Within conventional medicine, CAM, and lifestyle medicine, there are practical approaches that may be taken to address placebo and nocebo issues:

- Conventional Medicine

  At some level, it is tempting to consider using placebos in clinical practice. However, that is generally considered unethical because it could significantly interfere with the trust between patients and clinicians. However, other approaches may be used. It is important for people to feel confident and positive about the care that they receive. Generally, this may be achieved within mainstream medicine by seeking out health professionals who provide personal encouragement, respect the individual values of patients, and are thought to be trustworthy, reassuring, and straightforward. One specific conventional therapy that may be particularly beneficial in this area—but underutilized—is psychotherapy. This approach may improve conditions, such as anxiety and depression, which interfere with maximizing placebo effects and minimizing nocebo responses.

■ CAM and Lifestyle Medicine

As with conventional medicine, it is important to work with CAM and lifestyle practitioners who provide positive support and instill confidence and trust. Many specific CAM and lifestyle approaches are relevant to placebos and nocebos. For example, relaxation strategies, such as meditation and guided imagery, may, like placebo responses, tap into powerful mind–body connections. Exercise programs may provide relaxation and empowerment. Spirituality and prayer may provide hope, optimism, and other beneficial effects, especially for those who are already spiritual. A blend of spirituality and exercise may be found with some unconventional exercise approaches such as tai chi and yoga. Alternative medical systems, such as traditional Chinese medicine or Ayurveda, may be helpful for those who use conventional medicine but also have skepticism about it and want clinicians with entirely different approaches to disease and treatment. Finally, one's social network may be optimized by surrounding oneself with friends and family who provide positive support and avoiding those who are negative and discouraging.

It may be challenging to determine which CAM and lifestyle strategies are appropriate for a specific person with MS and then how to blend those strategies into a broad-based treatment plan that is supportive and encouraging.

Additional Readings

Books

Brody H. *The Placebo Response: How You Can Release the Body's Inner Pharmacy for Better Health*. New York, NY: HarperCollins; 2011.

Evans D. *Placebo: The Belief Effect*. London, UK: HarperCollins; 2003.

Harrington A, ed. *The Placebo Effect: An Interdisciplinary Exploration*. Cambridge, UK: Harvard University Press; 1997.

Kennedy P. *The Can Do Multiple Sclerosis Guide to Lifestyle Empowerment*. New York, NY: Demos Medical Publishing; 2012.

Moerman D. *Meaning, Medicine, and the Placebo Effect*. Cambridge, UK: Cambridge University Press, 2002.

Oken B. Placebo effect: clinical perspectives and potential mechanisms. In: Oken BS, ed. *Complementary Therapies in Neurology: An Evidence-Based Approach*. New York, NY: Parthenon Publishing Group; 2004:209–230.

Seligman MEP. *Authentic Happiness*. New York, NY: Free Press; 2002.

Shapiro AK, Shapiro E. *The Powerful Placebo: From Ancient Priest to Modern Physician*. Baltimore, MD: Johns Hopkins University Press; 2000.

Tindle H. *Up: How Positive Outlook Can Transform Our Health and Aging.* New York, NY: Hudson Street Press; 2013.

Journal Articles

Artemiadis AK, Anagnostouli MC, Alexopoulos EC. Stress as a risk factor for multiple sclerosis onset or relapse: a systematic review. *Neuroepidemiology.* 2011;36:109–120.

Barrett B, Muller D, Rakel D, Rabago D, Marchand L, Scheder JC. Placebo, meaning, and health. *Persp Biol Med.* 2006;49:178–198.

Barsky AJ, Saintfort R, Rogers MP, Borus JF. Nonspecific medication side effects and the nocebo phenomenon. *JAMA.* 2002;287:622–627.

Benedetti F. Recent advances in placebo research. *Int J Pain Med Pall Care.* 2005;4:2–7.

Benedetti F, Lanotte M, Lopiano L, Colloca L. When words are painful: unraveling the mechanisms of the nocebo effect. *Neuroscience.* 2007;147:260–271.

Bowling AC. Placebos and nocebos—techniques to optimize MS management? *Momentum.* Spring 2011;4(2):45–47.

Brown RF, Tennant CC, Dunn SM, Pollard JD. A review of stress-relapse interactions in multiple sclerosis: important features and stress-mediating and -moderating variables. *Mult Scler.* 2005;11:477–484.

Deckx N, Lee WP, Berneman ZN, Cools N. Neuroendocrine immunoregulation in multiple sclerosis. *Clin Dev Immunol.* 2013;2013:705232. (epub).

Enck P, Benedetti F, Schedlowski M. New insights into the placebo and nocebo responses. *Neuron.* 2008;59:195–206.

Fassler M, Meissner K, Schneider A, Linde K. Frequency and circumstances of placebo use in clinical practice-a systematic review of empirical studies. *BMC Med.* 2010;8:15.

Finniss DG, Kaptchuk TJ, Miller F, Benedetti F. Biological, clinical, and ethical advances of placebo effects. *Lancet.* 2010;375:686–695.

Hirsch RL, Johnson KP, Camenga DL. The placebo effect during a double blind trial of recombinant alpha2 interferon in multiple sclerosis patients: immunological and clinical findings. *Neuroscience.* 1988;39:189–196.

Hroibjartsson A, Gotzsche PC. Placebo interventions for all clinical conditions. *Cochrane Database Syst Rev.* 2010;(1):CD003974. doi:10.1002/14651858. CD003974.pub3.

La Mantia L, Eoli M, Salmaggi A, Milanese C. Does a placebo-effect exist in clinical trials on multiple sclerosis? Review of the literature. *Ital J Neurol Sci.* 1996;17:135–139.

Papadopoulos D, Mitskiostas DD. Nocebo effects in multiple sclerosis trials: a meta-analysis. *Mult Scler*. 2010;16:816–828.

Pollo A, Benedetti F. The placebo response: neurobiological and clinical issues of neurological relevance. *Progr Brain Res*. 2009;175;283–294.

Torem MS. Mind-body hypnotic imagery in the treatment of auto-immune disorders. *Am J Clin Hypn*. 2007;50:157–170.

Welsh CJ, Steelman AJ, Mi W, et al. Neuroimmune interactions in a model of multiple sclerosis. *Ann N Y Acad Sci*. 2009;1153:209–219.

Important Precautions About Complementary and Alternative Medicine, Lifestyle Medicine, and Multiple Sclerosis

This book provides much detailed information about specific types of complementary and alternative medicine (CAM) and lifestyle medicine. This information is intended to assist people in assessing these approaches within the unique context of multiple sclerosis (MS). In addition to this specific information, some general ideas are important to understand and may be helpful in the decision-making process about CAM and lifestyle medicine:

- *When making decisions about CAM and lifestyle medicine, recognize that this is an individual decision.* Conclusive evidence about the effectiveness and safety of most forms of CAM and lifestyle medicine is not available. This book provides a review of the information that is available. The way in which this information is used and the decision about whether to pursue CAM and lifestyle approaches rests with the individual. Ultimately, individuals must decide for themselves about using these strategies, and they must assume the risks and responsibilities of pursuing a specific therapy.

- *Be aware of when it is reasonable to pursue CAM and lifestyle approaches.* It is reasonable to consider therapies outside of conventional medicine for some situations. For example, it is reasonable to consider CAM or lifestyle approaches for symptoms that are of low intensity, such as mild muscle stiffness or mild pain. These approaches also may be worth pursuing for conditions in which conventional medical therapy is ineffective or only partially effective. Forms of CAM and lifestyle medicine to consider are those that are possibly effective, are probably safe, are of low or moderate cost, and require a reasonable amount of effort. On the other hand, severe symptoms, such as prominent muscle stiffness or excruciating pain, or a serious disease process—such as MS—should not be treated *solely* with CAM or lifestyle medicine. In these situations, it may be reasonable to utilize these approaches *in addition to* conventional therapy. CAM therapies should not be pursued if little or no reliable information is available about effectiveness, safety, or cost. Therapies to avoid are those that are probably ineffective or unsafe or involve high expense or great effort.

■ *Have a plan for using CAM and lifestyle medicine.* Several steps must be taken when using any form of CAM and lifestyle medicine:

- Evaluate and address the reason(s) for wanting to use CAM and lifestyle medicine.

- Obtain accurate information about effectiveness, safety, cost, and effort involved.

- If the therapy or strategy is chosen, discuss it with your physician, monitor your response, and discontinue the treatment when appropriate.

- It is important to include a physician or other conventional health provider in this process because many practitioners and vendors of CAM and lifestyle products and services do not have a conventional medical provider's broad knowledge base about the diagnosis and treatment of medical conditions.

■ *Realize that information about most forms of CAM and lifestyle medicine is incomplete.* Many forms of conventional medical therapy have undergone rigorous testing for effectiveness and safety. In contrast, data are limited for many CAM and lifestyle therapies, especially in terms of specialized studies of people with MS or studies of the effects of therapies on immune system activity. As a result, often it is only possible to make a "best guess" about the effectiveness and safety of these approaches. As more studies are done in this area, some of these "best guesses" may be found to be incorrect. For example, a therapy that is currently thought to be "possibly effective" or "probably safe" may conceivably be found, after further studies, to be definitely ineffective or definitely unsafe. Thus, a certain amount of risk is involved in pursuing these approaches. In terms of slowing down the MS disease process, no "magic cure" exists. No forms of CAM or lifestyle medicine have undergone sophisticated clinical testing similar to that used to prove the efficacy of the Food and Drug Administration (FDA)-approved "disease-modifying drugs" for MS. As a result, these conventional therapies should be considered by all people with MS.

- *Be aware of the "telltale signs" of unreliable forms of CAM and lifestyle medicine.* Several features often indicate that a therapy has not been well studied, is provided by an unreliable source, or is being promoted with exaggerated claims. Some of these "telltale signs" are:

  - Heavy reliance on testimonials: The benefits of a therapy sometimes are reported in accounts known as *testimonials*, which may not be entirely accurate and which describe the treatment response of a single person, as opposed to that of a large, well-studied group of people.

  - Strong claims about effectiveness: Terms such as *amazing* and *miraculous* should raise suspicions. If it sounds too good to be true, it probably is.

  - A single therapy is claimed to be effective for many different medical conditions.

  - The composition of a therapy is "secret."

  - Little or no objective information is available on effectiveness, safety, or cost.

  - Therapy involves inpatient treatment, injections, or intravenous medication.

  - An antiscience or anticonventional medicine attitude prevails: This may be conveyed through claims of "conspiracies" or through the unwillingness of a CAM/lifestyle practitioner to work cooperatively with a physician.

- *Recognize that MS is a disease that involves excessive immune system activity.* In some lay books on CAM, MS is described as an immune disorder, and it is then assumed that therapies that stimulate the immune system should be beneficial for MS. Some books may even recommend 5 to 10 supplements that activate the immune system. Using this faulty reasoning, therapies recommended for MS are sometimes the same as those recommended for acquired immunodeficiency syndrome (AIDS) and cancer. Also, the vague term *immunomodulator* sometimes is used to describe supplements that appear to stimulate the immune system. This approach and these recommendations are inaccurate and potentially dangerous. Although MS is, indeed, an immune disorder, it generally involves too much, not too little, immune-system activity. Consequently, CAM therapies that increase the activity of the immune system could worsen the disease process. In contrast to MS, AIDS and cancer may benefit from treatment that activates the immune system. Thus, in general, immune-stimulating therapies that may be helpful for AIDS and cancer may actually be harmful for MS.

■ *Do not confuse scientific evidence with clinical evidence.* Potential MS thera-pies may be evaluated scientifically through "test tube" experiments or by using an animal model of MS known as experimental allergic encephalo-myelitis (EAE). The most important (and most expensive and laborious) test of a therapy, however, is to give it to people with MS and to carefully monitor their response. It is essential to realize that scientific studies are imperfect and that therapies that are promising in scientific experiments are not necessarily clinically effective therapies for people with MS. A long list of experimental compounds are effective in suppressing the immune system or treating EAE but are ineffective for treating people with MS. Some therapies (e.g., interferon-gamma, lenercept, and antibodies to tumor necrosis factor [TNF]) are effective in treating animal models of MS but actually worsen disease in people with MS.

■ *For dietary supplements, use a "single bullet" rather than "shotgun" approach.* In the past, some believed that dietary supplements had ben-eficial effects or no effects at all. This led some to advocate for "shotgun" approaches that utilized a large number of supplements and assumed that the many supplements would be therapeutic or "neutral." In fact, many studies over the past 20 years have shown that modest doses of commonly used vitamins and minerals may actually have adverse effects, including increasing the risk for heart disease, various forms of cancers, and overall mortality. Thus, supplements, like drugs, may have negative health effects. Given this situation, it is important to use more of a "single bullet" approach with supplements. In other words, if supplements are used, the number of supplements should be limited and specific sup-plements should be used only after careful consideration of safety and effectiveness information.

■ *Avoid misconceptions about supplements.* Many misconceptions are some-times promoted by the vendors of supplements. These misconceptions include:

- Compounds are sometimes claimed to be safe and beneficial if they are "natural." Although some natural compounds are safe and beneficial, some are toxic (e.g., the deadly chemicals that are present in poisonous mushrooms and many other plants), and many are not effective ther-apies for any disorder.

- *More is not necessarily better.* It is sometimes believed that the use of high doses of a single supplement or a large number of different supplements is more beneficial than the use of low doses or a single supplement; however, in most cases, supplements in high doses or large numbers are probably not more effective and may, in fact, be more likely to produce side effects.

- *Combinations of supplements with conventional medications have not been fully investigated.* Supplements are sometimes taken in addition to conventional medications. In general, the effectiveness and safety of these "combination therapies" have not been investigated. Notably, some situations exist in which combination therapy is less effective or more likely to produce side effects than single-treatment therapy.

The precautions discussed in this introduction have been incorporated into the discussions in this book. These guidelines should be helpful for evaluating CAM and lifestyle therapies not mentioned here or for assessing CAM and lifestyle therapies for conditions other than MS.

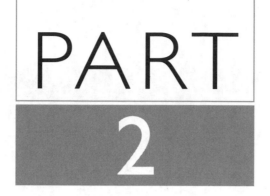

PART

2

Optimal Health With Multiple
Sclerosis: A Seven-Step Guide to
Integrating Lifestyle, Alternative,
and Conventional Medicine

Introduction

Multiple sclerosis (MS) may have widespread effects on physical, cognitive, and emotional function. Conventional medicine as well as lifestyle approaches and unconventional medicine have beneficial effects on MS. Given this situation, there is great opportunity to wisely make use of these diverse treatment approaches to optimize health in those with MS. However, this opportunity is often *not* taken advantage of in MS. Instead, MS treatment is often focused primarily on administering and monitoring the safety and effectiveness of immunological drugs that slow the course of the disease. While these medications are extremely important in treating MS, an excessive focus on them may actually detract from optimizing health. Specifically, a narrow focus on MS medications may limit the use of other approaches that have therapeutic effects on MS, maintain physical and psychological wellness, and prevent and manage many other medical conditions that may adversely affect MS or general health and well-being.

This part of the book describes an integrative approach to MS that includes the use of conventional, lifestyle, and unconventional medicine. The approach has seven steps that incorporate a wide range of lifestyle approaches in combination with conventional and unconventional therapies. This approach was developed on the basis of scientific and clinical evidence—the evidence regarding the lifestyle and unconventional medicine approaches is reviewed in detail in Part 3 of this book. This seven-step approach is designed to be individualized. For each step, multiple treatment options are provided—options should be chosen to meet individual needs and orientations. Overall, this integrative approach aims to wisely and thoughtfully use all available methods to slow down the disease course of MS, decrease the severity of MS symptoms, optimize general health, and, ultimately, allow people with MS to live full and meaningful lives.

The seven steps of this approach are summarized below:

- Step 1—Disease-Modifying Medications

- Step 2—Diet, Dietary Supplements, and Weight Management

- Step 3—Tobacco and Alcohol Use

- Step 4—Physical Activity

- Step 5—Personal and Social Well-Being

- Step 6—Prevention and Management of Other Medical Conditions

- Step 7—Symptom Management

General Concepts

There are multiple concepts that are fundamental to this seven-step approach. First, *the typical lifestyle of Westernized countries has adverse effects on multiple sclerosis (MS) and general health*. It has been known for decades that the risk for many common Western medical problems, such as diabetes, obesity, and heart disease, is increased by components of the Western lifestyle, such as physical inactivity and diets that are high in salt, fat, and calories. More recent evidence indicates that some of these lifestyle factors also increase the risk for MS and, in those with MS, may increase the severity of the disease. These observations indicate that MS and general health may be improved by changing some core features of the typical Western lifestyle. Minimizing or eliminating these unhealthy lifestyle factors is central to several of the steps in this integrative approach to MS.

Another important concept in this seven-step strategy is that *other medical conditions have adverse effects on MS*. There is growing recognition that other medical problems have negative effects on those with MS. While this may seem obvious, it has not, until recently, been a focus of attention in the medical community. Multiple studies indicate that the presence of other medical conditions may lead to more rapid progression of disability in those with MS. This effect has been observed with many common diseases, including asthma, arthritis, high blood pressure, high cholesterol, heart disease, and diabetes. Also, quality of life in those with MS is worsened by the presence of other medical conditions. Studies indicate that as the number of other diseases increases in those with MS, the quality of life decreases. Another way of viewing these findings is that preventing and managing other medical conditions is important for optimal neurological function and quality of life in those with MS—this concept underlies several of the steps in this seven-step strategy.

A final idea that is central to this seven-step approach is that *some of the most beneficial treatment approaches may be those that use the "built-in resources" of the human body and do not require any medications, supplements, devices, or technology*. In the past few decades, there have been remarkable advances in the diagnosis and treatment of many medical conditions, including MS. During this time period, many people may have developed an unrealistic and ultimately unhealthy reliance on therapeutic approaches that are external to the human body, such as medications, dietary supplements, and medical devices. The human body has remarkable internal resources, such as the ability to change physical, cognitive, and emotional functions. However, optimizing the use of these internal resources requires understanding of, and experience with, one's body, which may be a skill that is lacking in our current culture that is focused on externally administered therapies. In this way, our generation may be an aberration of human history—relative to our ancestors, we may be much more technologically advanced but may also be much less skilled at tapping into our body's own internal resources. Some of the approaches that are outlined in this seven-step method may provide education and skills to optimize body function without the use of medications or devices. For example, yoga, tai chi, and Pilates may allow one to learn about the physicality of the body and then use that understanding to improve physical function. Importantly, in contrast to the "quick fix" that may occur with therapies such as medications and surgery, it may take several months to acquire the education and beneficial skills associated with methods that use one's internal resources.

Helpful Strategies

Specific strategies may allow one to use this approach more successfully. Some of these strategies are common to any broad-based, integrative approach to health—others are unique to multiple sclerosis (MS):

- **The most effective and long-lasting changes in lifestyle are usually those that are small and consistent**

  When making lifestyle changes, it is tempting to make large changes at once. However, these grand, New-Year's-resolution types of approaches are usually not successful. Rather, success usually comes with small changes that are instituted methodically over an extended period of time. An example of this approach would be an exercise program that begins with just 2 minutes per session for 3 days per week— if 2 minutes are added to the session every 2 weeks, then, after about 6 months, one is exercising for 30 minutes three times weekly.

- **An MS diagnosis may be a powerful source of motivation for lifestyle change**

  Some people with MS comment that their MS diagnosis was one of the best "gifts" they received in life. In making this surprising observation, which often occurs 5 to 20 years after the diagnosis, people explain that the MS was the force that motivated them to live a healthy and meaningful life. Indeed, one of the most important factors for successfully changing one's lifestyle, such as diet or exercise, is motivation. Finding this motivation in an MS diagnosis is a way to transform the challenge of the diagnosis into an opportunity. Stated differently, the disease of MS may, paradoxically, lead one to live a healthier life.

■ *Excessive focus on one therapy may detract from, or be used to avoid, other valuable approaches*

There are several ways in which excessive focus on a single therapy is unhealthy in MS. For example, within the conventional medical care of MS, excessive focus on administering and monitoring the safety and effectiveness of MS medications may detract from using other therapies that provide important therapeutic effects. Likewise, focusing on one specific unconventional therapy may limit the use of other approaches, such as healthy lifestyle changes. In some cases, excessive focus on one treatment may actually be used to avoid the challenge of making a difficult lifestyle change or addressing an aspect of one's medical condition. For example, it may be "easier" (but less healthy) to focus on taking one specific dietary supplement than to address challenging emotional issues or make important, fundamental lifestyle changes, such as losing weight or quitting smoking. With regard to the seven-step approach to MS, it is important to make ongoing efforts to follow all of the steps and to be thoughtful and balanced in one's approach to each of these steps.

■ *One must be responsible and accountable and advocate for oneself*

Successful use of this seven-step approach requires self-advocacy, responsibility, and personal accountability. For conventional medical approaches, the health care system has many services and resources but *does not* have personal advocates. As a result, one must advocate for oneself and seek out appropriate and high-quality medical care. In this seven-step approach, different steps require consulting with different health professionals— identifying and working with professionals who are appropriate for one's situation is largely dependent on the individual. For unconventional and lifestyle approaches, one must be aware of precautions in these areas and proceed responsibly. For many approaches, especially lifestyle strategies such as nutrition, exercise, and tobacco and alcohol use, the ultimate accountability for adhering to these approaches is with the individual, not a health provider, friend, or family member.

■ *Find joy and meaning!*

This integrative, seven-step model is aimed at optimizing health in MS. Some of the steps, such as taking medications, are tasks that are not particularly enjoyable but must be done. However, several of the steps, such as exercise, diet, and personal and social well-being, have components that extend beyond one's health. They are important components of a full and rich life. Thus, thoughtful and personalized pursuit of this "medical treatment approach" may actually add joy and meaning to one's life.

Step 1: Disease-Modifying Medications

At this time, the best available evidence for modifying the course of disease in MS is with one of the Food and Drug Administration (FDA)-approved disease-modifying medications. These medications are approved for use in those with relapsing, not progressive, forms of MS. There are a total of 10 FDA-approved medications. In the United States, nine of these are commonly used—one of the approved medications, mitoxantrone (Novantrone), is not generally used because of concerns that the risks outweigh the benefits. Some of these drugs are given in pill form, while others are given intravenously or injected under the skin or into the muscle. The nine commonly used medications may be categorized by the ways in which they are administered:

- Pills
  - Fingolimod (Gilenya)
  - Teriflunomide (Aubagio)
  - Dimethyl fumarate (Tecfidera)

- Injections:
  - Interferons: interferon beta-1b (Betaseron and Extavia), interferon beta-1a once-weekly (Avonex), and interferon beta-1a three-times-weekly (Rebif)
  - Glatiramer acetate (Copaxone)

■ Intravenous

   • Natalizumab (Tysabri)

It is important to note that in the above classification scheme, there are six medication classes: three are pills, two are injections, and one is intravenous. Each class produces its therapeutic effects through distinct biochemical actions, known technically as *mechanisms of action*. These different mechanisms of action for different classes of drugs are a "good news-bad news" situation for MS treatment. The good news is that if one takes a drug in one class and it is not effective, then drugs in any of the other five classes have the potential to work better because they work through different mechanisms. The bad news is that if one takes a drug in one class and it is effective, then it is possible that there may be less effectiveness with drugs in other classes.

Although the MS medications have different mechanisms of action, they have several features in common:

■ For people with relapsing forms of MS, *all* of these medications:

   • Decrease the risk of attacks

   • Probably slow disability progression

   • Decrease MRI activity

■ Likewise, *none* of these medications:

   • Cure MS

   • Treat MS symptoms

   • Are approved for use, or have definite therapeutic effects, in progressive MS

All of these medications have potential side effects, some of which are serious. Thus, it is very important to weigh the risks and benefits of these medications and to do appropriate testing, such as blood tests and MRIs, before and during treatment. Also, these medications may interact with other drugs as well as dietary supplements and herbs (see *Appendix 2* and Part 3 chapters on *Ayurveda; Herbs, Acupuncture and Traditional Chinese Medicine;* and *Vitamins, Minerals, and Other Nonherbal Supplements*).

Additional Information and Guidance

Decisions about using MS medications should be made by consulting with one's neurologist. Other resources that may be helpful include:

■ Website

   • www.nationalmssociety.org—website of the National MS Society of the United States

- Books
  - *Multiple Sclerosis for Dummies*, by RC Kalb, B Giesser, and K Costello. Hoboken, NJ: John Wiley & Sons, 2012.
  - *Multiple Sclerosis: The Questions You Have—The Answers You Need*, by RC Kalb. New York: Demos Medical Publishing, 2011.
  - *The Everything Health Guide to Multiple Sclerosis*, by M Russell and AC Bowling. Avon, MA: Adams Media, 2009.

Step 2: Diet, Dietary Supplements, and Weight Management

The topic of diet and MS generates much confusion and controversy. The possible role of diet in MS was first proposed more than 50 years ago. Over the past several decades, many studies of diet and MS have been conducted. However, in spite of these studies, there are many unanswered questions. *Contrary to what is sometimes stated in books and websites, there is not definite evidence that a specific diet slows down the course of MS.* However, as outlined in several chapters of Part 3 of this book, multiple dietary approaches may be beneficial for MS and also are known to prevent and manage many other medical conditions, such as diabetes and heart disease, which may have negative effects on MS.

Weight Management

Weight management is an extremely important aspect of diet in MS. In those who have MS, obesity may worsen MS symptoms. Also, obesity may increase the risk for other diseases, such as diabetes, heart disease, and arthritis, which may worsen quality of life and neurological disability in MS. Weight management may be a valuable yet underutilized strategy to prevent or manage symptoms and also to optimize neurological function and quality of life in those with MS. See *Obesity and Weight Management* chapter for additional details.

Dietary Components

The relative intake of specific components of the diet may be beneficial for MS as well as general health. Those that are discussed in detail in other chapters include:

■ Fats

- A diet that, relative to the average American, is *lower* in saturated fat and *higher* in polyunsaturated fat may have beneficial effects on MS and also help prevent and manage many other medical conditions, including heart disease, stroke, diabetes, and obesity.

- See *Fats* chapter for additional details.

■ Fiber

- Consumption of the recommended amount of fiber, which is significantly *higher* than the average U.S. intake, helps manage and prevent constipation (a common MS symptom) as well as many other serious medical conditions, including heart disease, diabetes, cancer, and obesity.

- See *Fiber* chapter for additional details.

■ Salt

- Dietary intake of the recommended amount of salt, which is significantly *lower* than the intake of the average American, may have beneficial effects on MS and lower the risk of many other conditions, including heart disease, high blood pressure, stroke, congestive heart failure, and kidney disease.

- See *Salt* chapter for additional details.

■ Vitamin D

- Vitamin D intake (with foods and supplements) and sunlight exposure that produces normal blood levels of vitamin D may have therapeutic effects on MS as well as osteoporosis, which is relatively common in MS, and multiple other medical conditions.

- See *Vitamins, Minerals, and Other Nonherbal Supplements* chapter for additional details.

■ Vitamin B_{12}

- High intake of vitamin B_{12} through food and supplements is not needed for most people with MS. However, those with MS who have low blood levels of vitamin B_{12} should be supplemented with vitamin B_{12} in the form of pills or injections.

- See *Vitamins, Minerals, and Other Nonherbal Supplements* chapter for additional details.

There are other major dietary components that have not been studied specifically in MS but are known to be important in preventing and managing other serious medical problems:

- Fruits and vegetables
  - Servings of fruits and vegetables, which should take up *most* of the plate, should be *higher* than those of the average American. A diet that is rich in fruits and vegetables may prevent heart disease, high blood pressure, diabetes, and cancer.

- Protein
  - The daily intake of appropriate amounts of healthy, protein-rich foods, which is not typical of the average American, decreases the intake of saturated fat—a strategy which, as previously noted, may have beneficial effects on MS and help prevent and manage other serious diseases, including heart disease, stroke, diabetes, and obesity.
  - Protein intake should be primarily in the form of foods that are low in saturated fats, such as lean meat, seafood, low-fat or fat-free dairy products, legumes (beans and peas), and tofu and other soy products.

- Grains (breads, cereals, pastas, rice)
  - Whole grains contain more fiber and other healthful nutrients than refined grains. Higher intake of whole grains has been associated with decreased risk of heart disease, stroke, diabetes, and obesity.
  - At least half of grain intake should be in the form of whole-grain products, such as brown rice and whole-grain breads, pastas, and cereals.

- Potassium
  - Intake of the daily recommended amount (4,700 mg), which is significantly *higher* than the U.S. average intake, decreases the risk of osteoporosis, which is relatively common in those with MS, and also counters the blood pressure-raising effect of sodium and reduces the chance of developing kidney stones.

- Calcium
  - Calcium plays an important role in maintaining bone density and preventing osteoporosis. The recommended daily intake of calcium is 1,000 to 1,200 mg, which is somewhat *lower* than that of the average American.

Overview

All of these dietary findings about MS and general health may be combined to develop a diet and dietary supplement approach that is appropriate for those with MS. To summarize such an approach:

- Diet

  - Follow the general approach of the "Healthful Diet Strategies" or specific eating plans of the "Dietary Approaches to Stop Hypertension (DASH) Diet" or similar diets.

  - Consume an appropriate number of calories.

- Supplements: Consider vitamin D, fish oil, and multivitamins. If vitamin B_{12} deficiency is present, use vitamin B_{12} supplements. Cautiously use other supplements.

The remainder of this section describes these diet and dietary supplement approaches in detail.

Diets

General Approach: "Healthful Diet Strategies"

This general approach meets the 2010 recommendations of the U.S. Dietary Guidelines that were developed by the U.S. Department of Agriculture (USDA) and the U.S. Department of Health and Human Services. Similar strategies may be found in the "My Plate" nutrition guide developed by the USDA (www.choosemyplate.gov). These dietary strategies result in a diet that is quite different from that of the average American:

- Decrease total fat in diet to 20% to 35% of calories

  - Mainly use plant oils, such as sunflower, safflower, canola, olive, and soybean

- Limit saturated fat intake to 10% or less of calories

  - Decrease animal-based food, such as full fat cheese, processed meats, and dairy desserts like ice cream

  - Decrease highly processed snack food, such as cakes and cookies

- Decrease *trans fats*, which are also known as "partially hydrogenated oils"

  - Limit intake of fried food and baked goods that contain these fats

- Fill most of plate with fruits and vegetables

- Eat fish at least two times per week

- Eat lean meats and poultry

- Eat whole-grain, high-fiber foods

- Limit salt intake

- Consume appropriate number of daily calories

Specific Diets: "DASH Diet" and Similar Diets

There are several well-studied diets that, like the general strategies just described, incorporate approaches that may be helpful for MS and are definitely beneficial for general health. These include the "DASH Diet" as well as the Therapeutic Lifestyle Changes (TLC) Diet, Mayo Clinic Diet, and Mediterranean Diet.

The DASH Diet and related diets are generally highly regarded by nutrition authorities. In 2014, *U.S. News and World Report* surveyed 22 nationally recognized nutrition experts about "Best Diets." These experts were asked to independently rate 32 different diets on the basis of seven criteria, including nutritional completeness, ease of use, ability to produce short- and long-term weight loss, and safety and effectiveness in managing and preventing heart disease and diabetes. The diet that received the highest overall score was the DASH Diet. Other diets that ranked in the "top 5" included the TLC Diet, Mayo Clinic Diet, and Mediterranean Diet.

The DASH Diet is relatively simple because it does not require special foods or recipes. Instead, it calls for a certain number of daily servings from specific food groups. The amount of food that is eaten daily is dependent on one's gender, age, and level of physical activity.

The DASH Diet is rich in vegetables, fruits, whole grains, fish, poultry, low-fat or fat-free dairy products, beans, seeds, and nuts. It is relatively low in salt, sugars, fats, and red meats. Also, it is low in saturated fat and high in fiber, calcium, potassium, and protein.

Additional user-friendly information about the DASH Diet, TLC Diet, Mayo Clinic Diet, and Mediterranean Diet may be found through the website of *US News and World Report* (http://health.usnews.com/best-diet).

Dietary Supplements
Vitamin D

Many people with MS may have low vitamin D levels. For those with low levels, modest doses of vitamin D supplements (4,000 IU or less daily) that raise the vitamin D level to 30–55 ng/mL may have beneficial effects on MS, osteoporosis, and other medical conditions (see the *Vitamins, Minerals, and Other Nonherbal Supplements* chapter).

Vitamin B$_{12}$

A small subgroup of people with MS may have vitamin B$_{12}$ deficiency, which produces neurological injury and may mimic MS. People with MS who have vitamin B$_{12}$ deficiency should be treated with vitamin B$_{12}$ pills or injections (see the *Vitamins, Minerals, and Other Nonherbal Supplements* chapter).

Fish Oil and Other Polyunsaturated Fatty Acids

There is limited and conflicting evidence about the potential benefits of fish oil and other fatty acid supplements in MS. If supplements are taken, a modest approach is to take fish oil at a dose that provides 1 to 2 g of EPA (eicosapentanoic acid) and DHA (docosahexanoic acid) daily and, to avoid possible vitamin E deficiency, to take modest doses of vitamin E, such as 100 IU daily (see *Fats* chapter).

Multivitamins

The use of multivitamins in MS has not been well studied. The clearest indication for the use of multivitamins in MS is for those who have unhealthy diets that do not provide adequate intake of vitamins and minerals (see *Vitamins, Minerals, and Other Nonherbal Supplements* chapter).

Other Supplements

Other dietary supplements and herbs should be used with caution in MS. Many of these products have significant toxicity, have never been studied for safety in MS, may produce MS-relevant side effects, or may interact with medications that are commonly used to treat MS (see *Appendix 2*).

Step 3: Tobacco and Alcohol Use

Tobacco

In one large North American study, it was reported that about 20% of those with MS smoke. Smoking has multiple adverse effects in MS. It has been associated with an increased risk of developing progressive MS and more severe neurological disability. Also, smoking increases the risk for many other diseases. Some of these other diseases, such as heart disease, asthma, and stroke, may increase the disability and lower the quality of life in those with MS. For those with MS who smoke, stopping smoking is absolutely essential for optimizing health. See the *Tobacco and Smoking Cessation* chapter for additional information.

Alcohol

Alcohol should be used appropriately with those that have MS. Alcohol does not have clear adverse effects on the course of MS. However, alcohol, even in moderation, may interact with multiple MS medications and could provoke some MS symptoms. Excessive alcohol use, which has been reported in 15% to 40% of people with MS, has many serious health effects. If alcohol is used, it should be consumed in moderation:

- Nonpregnant women and everyone over age 65: one drink per day
- Men under age 65: two or fewer drinks per day
- Pregnant women: avoid alcohol use

Additional information about alcohol and MS may be found in the *Alcohol* chapter.

Step 4: Physical Activity

Physical activity is an inexpensive, simple, and generally safe approach that may produce remarkable health benefits for those with MS. Exercise studies in MS indicate that the most consistent improvement is in walking, weakness, and fatigue. Also, exercise may improve many other MS symptoms, including anxiety, anger, depression, bowel and bladder difficulties, pain, sleeping difficulties, muscle stiffness (spasticity), and cognitive problems.

Beyond its direct effects on MS, exercise has general health benefits. Exercise reduces the risk of stroke and heart disease, lowers blood pressure, improves blood lipids (cholesterol), decreases weight, prevents and aids in the management of diabetes and osteoporosis, decreases the risk of multiple cancers, and decreases the overall risk of death. Using exercise to prevent or manage these various medical conditions may secondarily have positive effects on MS since some of these conditions may worsen neurological function and quality of life when they occur in combination with MS.

There are conventional and unconventional approaches to physical activity. Conventional approaches involve standard exercise programs, which may be developed by working with a physical therapist. Hydrotherapy, or water exercise, may be especially well-suited for people with MS who have leg weakness or walking difficulties. Unconventional exercise programs that may provide beneficial effects for those with MS include tai chi, yoga, and Pilates, all of which are discussed in separate chapters of this book. Importantly, many conventional and unconventional exercise programs may be modified for those with disabilities.

More details about physical activity and MS are available in the *Exercise* chapter.

Step 5: Personal and Social Well-Being

For people with MS and also the general population, optimal health means physical as well as mental health. However, in the American culture and health care system, there is often much more focus on physical health than mental health. Lay people and health professionals may not be attentive, comfortable, or skilled at maintaining optimal mental health. Also, when mental health problems arise, lay people and clinicians may be challenged with identifying and appropriately treating the issues.

Important mind–body processes are involved in the complex interplay between mental and physical health. Placebo as well as nocebo responses are examples of mind–body processes that are important in MS and also in general health (see *Placebos and Nocebos* chapter).

Many factors are involved in maintaining mental health. These include finding meaning and enjoyment in one's life; having healthy, supportive relationships; and, for many, pursuing religious or spiritual activities.

Mental health issues often present in the form of depression and anxiety. Both of these conditions are common in the general population and in those with MS.

This book provides information in many areas relevant to personal and social well-being. For treating anxiety and depression, many different conventional, unconventional, and lifestyle medicine approaches are available and are discussed in *Step 7: Symptom Management*.

Many lifestyle and unconventional medicine strategies may be beneficial for optimizing mental health, and, in appropriate situations, for treating mental health conditions. Some of these approaches, as well as psychotherapy, may be valuable ways to gain insight into one's emotional self and acquire skills to improve one's mental health. Lifestyle and unconventional medicine approaches that may be beneficial in this area are listed below. All of these approaches are discussed in detail in specific chapters in Part 3:

- Exercise (see *Exercise* chapter)

- Unconventional exercise, such as tai chi, yoga, Pilates, Feldenkrais, and Tragerwork (see chapters on each of these therapies)

- Mind–body methods, such as meditation, guided imagery, and mindfulness (see chapters on each of these therapies)

- Alternative medical systems, such as traditional Chinese medicine and Ayurveda (see *Acupuncture and Traditional Chinese Medicine* and *Ayurveda* chapters)

- Spirituality and prayer (see *Prayer and Spirituality* chapter)

Step 6: Prevention and Management of Other Medical Conditions

Among health professionals and people with MS, there is sometimes an "MS-centric" approach in which MS is evaluated and treated in isolation. In fact, other medical conditions are common in those with MS and these conditions may have significant adverse effects on MS. As noted earlier, a wide array of medical conditions, including asthma, heart disease, diabetes, and arthritis, has been associated with worsening disability and quality of life in people with MS. Also, unhealthy lifestyle factors, such as smoking, unhealthy eating, and physical inactivity, may have direct negative effects on MS but may also increase the risk for many of these other medical conditions that may secondarily have negative effects on MS. Due to this situation, optimal health in MS depends not only on treating MS itself but also on preventing and managing other diseases through conventional medical care and also appropriate lifestyle strategies.

The rich and complex interplay of MS, other medical problems, and lifestyle factors creates a potent situation. For example, high quality general medical care and healthy lifestyle factors may work together to create positive synergies that improve overall health and quality of life. On the other hand, low quality general medical care and unhealthy lifestyle factors may negatively synergize and lead to high disability, poor general health, and low quality of life.

Several strategies may be used to prevent and manage other medical conditions. First, for general medical care, it is important to have a primary care provider who is not entirely dependent on specialists. The primary care provider should be devoted to, and competent in, broad-based medical and lifestyle approaches.

For other medical care, clinicians, including neurologists, should also be skilled in medical and lifestyle approaches and should be willing, if needed, to work with the primary care provider. Finally, the person who is receiving care should be aware, informed, responsible, and accountable for adhering to diagnostic and treatment plans.

There are multiple lifestyle and unconventional medical approaches that have beneficial effects on general health. The most important of these approaches are actually included in the previous four steps of this seven-step approach:

- Step 2—Diet, Dietary Supplements, and Weight Management
- Step 3—Tobacco and Alcohol Use
- Step 4—Physical Activity
- Step 5—Personal and Social Well-Being

Step 7: Symptom Management

MS may produce more than 20 different symptoms. There are standard approaches for the diagnosis and conventional medical treatment of these symptoms. This is a very large topic that is well described in other publications:

- ■ Website
  - • www.nationalmssociety.org—website of the National MS Society of the United States
- ■ Books
  - • *Multiple Sclerosis for Dummies*, by RC Kalb, B Giesser, and K Costello. Hoboken: John Wiley & Sons; 2012.
  - • *Multiple Sclerosis: The Questions You Have—The Answers You Need*, by RC Kalb. New York: Demos Medical Publishing; 2011.
  - • *Managing the Symptoms of Multiple Sclerosis*, by RT Schapiro. New York: Demos Medical Publishing; 2007.
  - • *The Everything Health Guide to Multiple Sclerosis*, by M Russell and AC Bowling. Avon, Massachusetts: Adams Media; 2009.

An exhaustive review of MS symptom management is not the focus of the remainder of this chapter. Rather, this section describes lifestyle and unconventional medicine therapies that may be effective for specific symptoms. The quality of the evidence supporting the use of some of these therapies in MS is variable and, in many cases, not as substantial as that for conventional medical therapies—detailed descriptions of these lifestyle and unconventional approaches, including the evidence supporting their use in MS, may be found in the relevant chapters of Part 3 of this book. In spite of the limited evidence for some of these therapies, they may be valuable, nonmedication approaches that are preferred by some people with MS. Also, since this approach to symptom management is generally not considered in detail in conventional medical care, the potential benefits of some of these therapies may be relatively untapped.

Lifestyle and Unconventional Therapies That May Improve Many Different Symptoms

People with MS may experience a wide range of symptoms. These symptoms may be physical, such as muscle stiffness, weakness, or walking difficulties. Also, symptoms may be emotional, such as depression or anxiety, or "invisible," such as fatigue.

In conventional medicine, one therapy is usually prescribed for one specific symptom. As a result, there are not many conventional therapies that are effective for multiple symptoms. However, among unconventional and lifestyle approaches, some may actually be effective for multiple MS symptoms and also beneficial for general health. In addition, these approaches may be inexpensive and generally safe. Therefore, these approaches may be low-cost, low-risk methods to relieve multiple MS symptoms and provide general health benefits.

The approach with the greatest number of potential health benefits is exercise:

■ Exercise

- May improve multiple MS symptoms, including anxiety, anger, cognitive problems, depression, bowel and bladder difficulties, fatigue, pain, sleeping difficulties, spasticity, walking problems, weakness.

- Also, may provide general health benefits, including decreased risk of heart disease and stroke, lowering of blood pressure, improved blood lipids (cholesterol), weight reduction, prevention and treatment of diabetes and osteoporosis, decreased risk of multiple cancers, and overall decreased risk of death.

The following is a listing of the multiple MS symptoms and general health conditions that may be treated with other lifestyle and unconventional approaches:

■ Acupuncture

- Anxiety, bladder and bowel difficulties, depression, dizziness, fatigue, pain, sleeping difficulties, and weakness.

■ Cooling

- Bladder problems, cognitive difficulties, fatigue, incoordination, sexual difficulties, spasticity, speech problems, tremor, visual difficulties, walking problems, and weakness.

■ Guided Imagery

- Anxiety, depression, fatigue, pain, and sleeping difficulties.

- Hippotherapy
  - Bladder and bowel problems, depression, pain, spasticity, walking difficulties, weakness.

- Massage
  - Anxiety, depression, constipation, muscle stiffness (spasticity), pain, and walking.

- Meditation
  - Anxiety, depression, fatigue, insomnia, pain, cognitive problems, and self-esteem.
  - Also, possible general health benefits, including reduction of blood pressure and improved blood glucose control.

- Mindfulness
  - Anxiety, depression, fatigue, pain, and sleeping difficulties.

- Music Therapy
  - Anxiety, depression, self-esteem, coping, cognitive problems, incoordination, pain, sleeping problems, and walking difficulties.

- Tai chi
  - Anxiety, depression, fatigue, coordination, sleeping problems, weakness, and walking difficulties.

- Yoga
  - Anxiety, depression, fatigue, bladder function, pain, spasticity, weakness, and walking difficulties.
  - Also, possible general health benefits, including reduction of blood pressure and weight loss.

Symptoms That May Be Relieved With Specific Lifestyle and Unconventional Therapies

Note: For each symptom, see the text entries for an overview and for specific therapies see the charts that follow these overviews. Detailed information about the specific therapies may be found in the relevant chapters in *Part 3*.

Anxiety and Stress

Anxiety and stress occur frequently among those with MS. Approximately one-third of people with MS experience anxiety. Anxiety may be underdiagnosed and undertreated in MS.

Conventional Medical Therapy

Conventional medical therapy in this area is often very effective. It typically involves the use of antianxiety medications. In addition, anxiety may be treated with psychotherapy, which may be underutilized for this condition. Anxiety and stress may be due to multiple causes, some of which may be the result of medical conditions. As a result, a physician should be consulted about the possible causes of anxiety before considering complementary and alternative medicine (CAM) therapies.

Possibly Effective Lifestyle and Unconventional Therapies

In general, CAM therapies for anxiety have not been studied extensively. The evidence supporting the use of conventional medical therapy, especially antianxiety medications, is much stronger than that for CAM therapy.

Other Unconventional Therapies

Homeopathy generally is safe but is of uncertain effectiveness for anxiety. Kava kava should be avoided because of possible liver toxicity. Valerian is sometimes recommended for anxiety, but most studies of this herb have been for its use in insomnia.

ANXIETY AND STRESS	
CONVENTIONAL TREATMENTS	**UNCONVENTIONAL AND LIFESTYLE TREATMENTS**
■ Anti-Anxiety Medications ■ Psychotherapy	Possibly Effective ■ Acupuncture ■ Biofeedback ■ Exercise ■ Feldenkrais ■ Guided Imagery ■ Hypnosis ■ Massage ■ Meditation ■ Mindfulness ■ Music Therapy ■ Prayer and Spirituality ■ Tai Chi ■ Therapeutic Touch ■ Yoga
	Uncertain ■ Homeopathy ■ Valerian
	CAUTION ■ Kava kava

Bladder Problems

MS may affect bladder function in several ways, including causing problems with storing urine, emptying urine, incontinence, and urinary tract infections (UTIs).

Conventional Therapy

It is important to undergo a medical evaluation for impaired urinary function, such as frequency and incontinence. Conventional therapy for bladder difficulties usually involves medications and lifestyle changes. Catheterization and surgical therapies may be indicated for more severe difficulties. People with recurrent UTIs should undergo a medical evaluation because it is important to determine the underlying cause of the UTIs.

Possibly Effective Lifestyle and Unconventional Therapies

Lifestyle and unconventional medicine approaches may be reasonable in some situations and should be discussed with a physician.

For UTI prevention, cranberry juice may be effective and is of low risk. Its effectiveness relative to the conventional approach with prescription antibiotics has not been investigated.

For UTI treatment, conventional treatment with antibiotics should be used because the effectiveness of unconventional approaches for treating UTIs, including cranberry juice, is not established. Also, people with MS and UTIs should attempt to eliminate the infection as quickly as possible because the infection may worsen neurological symptoms.

BLADDER PROBLEMS	
CONVENTIONAL TREATMENTS	**UNCONVENTIONAL AND LIFESTYLE TREATMENTS**
■ Medications ■ Lifestyle Changes ■ Catheterization (for severe difficulties) ■ Surgical Therapy (for severe difficulties) ■ Antibiotics (for UTI)	Possibly Effective for UTI ■ Cranberry Juice
	Possibly Effective for Bladder Function ■ Acupuncture ■ Biofeedback ■ Cooling ■ Exercise (Kegel) ■ Hippotherapy ■ Yoga
	Uncertain ■ Bearberry (Uva ursi) ■ Marijuana Extracts
	CAUTION ■ Vitamin C

Multiple unconventional therapies have produced promising results for urinary function.

Other Unconventional Therapies

Vitamin C is sometimes recommended for preventing and treating UTIs. However, studies do not indicate that vitamin C is effective in these situations. Also, it carries a theoretical risk in MS because of its immune-stimulating activity. Bearberry, or uva ursi, is also sometimes recommended for UTIs. The effectiveness and safety of this herb have not been established. Specific extracts of marijuana, which are not available in the United States, have shown benefit for urinary frequency.

Bowel Problems

Several MS-associated bowel problems occur, the most common of which is constipation. Rarely, diarrhea or incontinence may occur.

Conventional Therapy

The conventional therapy of bowel problems usually involves developing a *bowel program,* with changes in fluid and food intake, including increased fiber consumption. Medication approaches, such as stool softeners and laxatives, are also sometimes used.

Possibly Effective Unconventional Therapies

A low-risk therapy for constipation is psyllium, which is FDA-approved for this use. Some additional unconventional and lifestyle therapies have produced promising results.

BOWEL PROBLEMS	
CONVENTIONAL TREATMENTS	UNCONVENTIONAL AND LIFESTYLE TREATMENTS
■ Bowel Program ■ Stool Softeners ■ Laxatives	Definitely Effective ■ Psyllium
	Possibly Effective ■ Acupuncture ■ Biofeedback ■ Exercise ■ Hippotherapy ■ Massage

Colds and Flu—Prevention or Decreasing Duration

Colds and flu are of interest to people with MS because these viral infections may trigger MS attacks. Thus, any measure that prevents or decreases the duration of colds and flu may be helpful.

Conventional Therapy

Conventional medical approaches in this area include flu vaccination and flu medications (Relenza, Tamiflu, and amantadine). Also, infection with cold or flu viruses may be prevented by simple measures such as avoiding exposure to infected people, frequent hand washing, and avoiding touching the face with the hands.

Possibly Effective Lifestyle and Unconventional Therapies

Despite some claims, no highly effective alternative cure is available for colds and flu. For the flu, there is not any unconventional therapy that has been shown to be as effective as the flu medications. As a result, people with MS who have flu symptoms should strongly consider these medications.

Homeopathy is low risk but of unproven benefit in this area. A variety of supplements have produced positive results in some, but not all, studies. However, these therapies are theoretically risky for people with MS because they may stimulate the immune system and thus may potentially worsen MS. These therapies include echinacea, garlic, vitamin C, and zinc.

| COLDS AND FLU – PREVENTION OR DECREASING DURATION ||
CONVENTIONAL TREATMENTS	UNCONVENTIONAL AND LIFESTYLE TREATMENTS
■ Flu vaccination ■ Flu medications ■ Preventive measures	Uncertain ■ Homeopathy
	CAUTION ■ Echinacea ■ Garlic ■ Vitamin C ■ Zinc

Coordination Problems

In MS, coordination may be impaired in the arms and legs. Several factors may contribute to incoordination, including tremor, weakness, muscle stiffness, and numbness.

Conventional Therapy

Mainstream approaches to incoordination usually involve occupational therapy measures, such as the use of special devices and compensatory techniques.

Possibly Effective Lifestyle and Unconventional Therapies

Small studies in people with MS and in people with other conditions suggest that some unconventional therapies may improve or compensate for incoordination.

COORDINATION PROBLEMS	
CONVENTIONAL TREATMENTS	**UNCONVENTIONAL AND LIFESTYLE TREATMENTS**
■ Occupational Therapy	Possibly Effective ■ Cooling ■ Music Therapy ■ Pets ■ Tai Chi

Depression

Approximately 50% of people with MS experience depression. This condition may be serious and, consequently, should be evaluated and treated by a physician.

Conventional Therapy

Conventional therapy for depression is definitely effective and includes antidepressant medication and psychotherapy. Psychotherapy may be quite effective yet be underutilized in the treatment of depression.

Possibly Effective Lifestyle and Unconventional Therapies

As mentioned, complaints of depression warrant evaluation by a conventional medical approach. For mild to moderate depression, some unconventional and lifestyle therapies may be considered with the supervision of a physician. Two low-risk and low-cost therapies that are probably effective are exercise and St. John's Wort.

Many other unconventional and lifestyle approaches are possibly effective and of low risk. Further studies are needed to determine whether these therapies are definitely effective.

Other Unconventional Therapies

Homeopathy is safe but of uncertain effectiveness for depression. One dietary supplement, 5-HTP, is possibly beneficial but also may be unsafe. DHEA (dehydroepiandrosterone) is of unproven benefit and may be harmful.

DEPRESSION	
CONVENTIONAL TREATMENTS	**UNCONVENTIONAL AND LIFESTYLE TREATMENTS**
■ Antidepressants ■ Psychotherapy	Probably Effective ■ Exercise ■ St. John's Wort

(*continued*)

DEPRESSION (*continued*)	
CONVENTIONAL TREATMENTS	**UNCONVENTIONAL AND LIFESTYLE TREATMENTS**
	Possibly Effective ■ Acupuncture ■ Feldenkrais ■ Guided Imagery ■ Hippotherapy ■ Massage ■ Meditation ■ Mindfulness ■ Music Therapy ■ Prayer and Spirituality ■ SAMe (S-adenosylmethionine) ■ Tai Chi ■ Yoga
	Uncertain ■ Homeopathy
	CAUTION ■ 5-HTP ■ DHEA

Fatigue

MS-associated fatigue is the most common disabling symptom in MS. Fatigue has multiple causes, including the MS disease process itself, depression, medication side effects, and other medical conditions.

Conventional Therapy

Because of the multiple factors involved in fatigue, a physician or other health care provider should evaluate this symptom and determine the underlying cause. For fatigue due to MS, multiple treatment options are available, including several medications such as amantadine (Symmetrel), modafinil (Provigil), and armodafinil (Nuvigil).

Unconventional Therapies

After a medical evaluation, unconventional and lifestyle therapies may be considered for mild fatigue or for fatigue that does not respond to conventional treatment. Several unconventional and lifestyle options are possibly effective for fatigue, but many have not undergone rigorous evaluation in MS.

Limited research indicates that ginkgo biloba may be effective for MS-associated fatigue. Asian ginseng may be effective for MS fatigue, but it may also activate the immune system. Acetyl-L-carnitine is of uncertain benefit for fatigue in MS.

Several supplements have unclear effects on fatigue and may be unsafe. These include androstenedione, DHEA, Siberian ginseng, and spirulina.

FATIGUE	
CONVENTIONAL TREATMENTS	**UNCONVENTIONAL AND LIFESTYLE TREATMENTS**
■ Amantadine (Symmetrel) ■ Modafinil (Provigil) ■ Armodafinil (Nuvigil)	Possibly Effective ■ Acupuncture ■ Caffeine, including caffeine tablets, coffee, and other caffeine-containing herbs ■ Cooling ■ Exercise ■ Feldenkrais ■ Guided Imagery ■ Hypnosis ■ Magnets and Electromagnetic Therapy ■ Meditation ■ Mindfulness ■ Tai Chi ■ Yoga
	Uncertain ■ Ginkgo Biloba ■ Acetyl-L-Carnitine
	CAUTION ■ Asian Ginseng ■ Androstenedione ■ DHEA ■ Siberian Ginseng ■ Spirulina

Pain

Pain occurs at some point in about 50% of those with MS. There are many different types of MS-associated pain and many different underlying causes, including MS lesions and joint or muscle pain due to weakness or spasticity.

Conventional Therapy

The mainstream treatment of pain depends on its type and severity. Therapies include anti-inflammatory medications, specific medications that are effective for nerve-related pain, and physical therapy.

Unconventional Therapies

Unconventional and lifestyle approaches may be worth considering if pain is mild or not completely alleviated by conventional approaches. Feldenkrais and homeopathy are generally safe but are of uncertain effectiveness for MS-related pain. In MS studies, pain has been relieved by specific marijuana extracts that are not available in the United States.

PAIN	
CONVENTIONAL TREATMENTS	**UNCONVENTIONAL AND LIFESTYLE TREATMENTS**
■ Anti-inflammatory medication ■ Medication for nerve-related pain ■ Physical Therapy	Possibly Effective ■ Acupuncture ■ Biofeedback ■ Exercise ■ Guided Imagery ■ Hippotherpy ■ Hypnosis ■ Massage ■ Meditation ■ Mindfulness ■ Music Therapy ■ Pilates ■ Tai Chi ■ Therapeutic Touch ■ Yoga
	Uncertain ■ Feldenkrais ■ Homeopathy ■ Marijuana Extracts

Sexual Problems

MS may cause sexual difficulties, including decreased libido, erection difficulties, and reduced genital sensation. Physical or psychological causes for these sexual problems also may be present.

Conventional Therapy

Because of the complexities in this area, conventional medical evaluation aims to first identify the underlying problem and then provide appropriate treatment. Conventional measures include medications, lubricants, sexual techniques, and counseling.

Possibly Effective Lifestyle and Unconventional Therapies

For sexual difficulties in MS, it is best to be evaluated by a physician or other health care provider who can determine the underlying cause. Few unconventional therapies have been examined in this area. Cooling has produced possibly beneficial results, but further studies are needed to determine whether it is definitely effective. Also, there are claims that yoga and Pilates improve sexual function. It is possible that these therapies could indeed be beneficial for sexual function, but this possibility has not undergone rigorous clinical investigation.

Other Unconventional Therapies

Yohimbe, an herbal supplement, may be beneficial for erectile difficulties, but it also may produce significant side effects. DHEA, another supplement, is claimed to be helpful for sexual difficulties. However, it is of unclear benefit and may cause adverse effects.

SEXUAL PROBLEMS	
CONVENTIONAL TREATMENTS	UNCONVENTIONAL AND LIFESTYLE TREATMENTS
■ Counseling ■ Lubricants ■ Medications ■ Sexual techniques	Uncertain ■ Cooling ■ Pilates ■ Yoga
	CAUTION ■ DHEA ■ Yohimbe

Sleep Problems

Sleep disorders are more likely to occur in people with MS than in the general population. Also, stiffness and spasms may contribute to sleeping difficulties.

Conventional Therapy

Conventional medical evaluation for a sleep problem initially involves determining the underlying cause. People with MS are at risk for many different sleep disorders, including sleep apnea, periodic limb movements of sleep, and restless legs syndrome. Treatment of sleep disorders includes medications, devices, and surgery.

Possibly Effective Lifestyle and Unconventional Therapies

A mainstream medical evaluation should be obtained for sleeping problems. Lifestyle and unconventional therapies may be considered for mild sleeping difficulties or those that are not fully responsive to conventional measures.

Other Unconventional Therapies

Homeopathy is a low-risk approach of uncertain effectiveness for sleep problems. Several supplements are promoted for insomnia. As discussed elsewhere in this book, melatonin may be beneficial. However, in people with MS, melatonin carries a theoretical risk because of its possible immune-stimulating activity. 5-HTP, another supplement, has unclear effectiveness for insomnia and may be harmful. Marijuana has produced positive results in some studies. Kava kava sometimes is recommended for insomnia, but most studies of this herb have actually only evaluated its effectiveness for anxiety. In any case, kava kava should be avoided because of possible liver toxicity.

SLEEP PROBLEMS	
CONVENTIONAL TREATMENTS	**UNCONVENTIONAL AND LIFESTYLE TREATMENTS**
■ Medications ■ Devices ■ Surgery	Possibly Effective ■ Acupuncture ■ Biofeedback ■ Exercise ■ Feldenkrais ■ Guided Imagery ■ Hypnosis ■ Meditation ■ Mindfulness ■ Music Therapy ■ Pilates ■ Tai Chi ■ Valerian
	Uncertain ■ Homeopathy ■ Marijuana

(continued)

SLEEP PROBLEMS (*continued*)	
CONVENTIONAL TREATMENTS	UNCONVENTIONAL AND LIFESTYLE TREATMENTS
	CAUTION ■ 5-HTP ■ Kava Kava ■ Melatonin

Spasticity (Muscle Stiffness)

MS may cause spasticity, or muscle stiffness. This usually is due to MS-associated nervous-system injury. MS may also produce spasms, a related symptom characterized by brief, strong muscle contractions.

Conventional Therapy

The mainstream approach to spasticity frequently begins with simple exercise techniques developed with a physical therapist. Oral medications such as lioresal (Baclofen) and tizanidine (Zanaflex) are often used. For spasticity that does not respond to these medications, injections of medications or other specialized therapeutic techniques may be beneficial.

Possibly Effective Lifestyle and Unconventional Therapies

Unconventional and lifestyle approaches may be worth considering for spasticity that is mild or spasticity that is not fully controlled with conventional therapy.

Other Unconventional Therapies

"Subjective spasticity" may be improved with tetrahydrocannabinol (THC) and standardized marijuana extracts, which are not available in the United States. Pilates is a low-risk therapy claimed to be effective in this area, but it has not been formally studied.

SPASTICITY (MUSCLE STIFFNESS)	
CONVENTIONAL TREATMENTS	UNCONVENTIONAL AND LIFESTYLE TREATMENTS
■ Physical Therapy ■ Lioresal (Baclofen) ■ Tizanidine (Zanaflex)	Possibly Effective ■ Cooling ■ Exercise ■ Hippotherapy ■ Magnets and Electromagnetic Therapy

(continued)

SPASTICITY (MUSCLE STIFFNESS) (*continued*)	
CONVENTIONAL TREATMENTS	UNCONVENTIONAL AND LIFESTYLE TREATMENTS
	Possibly Effective ■ Massage ■ Tai Chi ■ Yoga
	Uncertain ■ Marijuana Extracts ■ Pilates

Thinking (Cognitive) Problems

MS may impair cognitive function. As with the physical effects of MS, the cognitive effects may be quite variable from one person to another.

Conventional Therapy

A conventional approach to cognitive problems includes evaluation of cognitive function and assessment for depression or anxiety, both of which may affect thinking processes. Treatment may involve rehabilitation in identified areas of weakness and appropriate therapy for significant depression or anxiety.

Possibly Effective Lifestyle and Unconventional Therapies

Limited studies in people with MS have indicated beneficial effects with cooling, exercise, meditation, and music therapy, but further studies are needed to evaluate whether these therapies are definitely effective.

THINKING (COGNITIVE) PROBLEMS	
CONVENTIONAL TREATMENTS	UNCONVENTIONAL AND LIFESTYLE TREATMENTS
■ Rehabilitation ■ Therapy for Depression or Anxiety	Possibly Effective ■ Cooling ■ Exercise ■ Meditation ■ Music Therapy

Walking Problems

MS often causes walking difficulties. This may be the result of impaired leg function caused by weakness, stiffness, clumsiness, or numbness.

Conventional Therapy

The evaluation and treatment of walking difficulties generally is done by physical therapists. Treatment usually involves an individualized physical therapy program. Also, dalfampridine (Ampyra) is a medication that is FDA approved specifically to improve walking in those with MS. Other therapies include medications for spasticity and assistive devices, such as braces, canes, and walkers.

Possibly Effective Lifestyle and Unconventional Therapies

It may be reasonable to consider unconventional and lifestyle strategies for walking difficulties that are mild or do not respond well to conventional approaches. In limited studies, multiple low-risk CAM therapies have produced promising beneficial effects for people with walking difficulties.

WALKING PROBLEMS	
CONVENTIONAL TREATMENTS	**UNCONVENTIONAL AND LIFESTYLE TREATMENTS**
■ Physical Therapy ■ Dalfampridine (Amprya) ■ Medications for Spasticity ■ Assistive Devices (braces, canes, walkers)	Possibly Effective ■ Cooling ■ Exercise ■ Feldenkrais ■ Hippotherapy ■ Massage ■ Music Therapy ■ Pets ■ Pilates ■ Tai Chi ■ Yoga

Weakness

The nervous system injury in MS frequently produces weakness of the arms and legs. A lack of physical activity also may produce weakness through a process of physical deconditioning.

Conventional Therapy

Conventional medicine relies on physical and occupational therapists to determine which muscles are weak and to develop an individualized exercise program to strengthen these muscles.

Possibly Effective Lifestyle and Unconventional Therapies

It may be reasonable to use unconventional and lifestyle strategies for mild weakness or for weakness that does not respond significantly to conventional therapy. Limited studies in MS and other conditions indicate that several therapies may improve or compensate for weakness.

Other Unconventional Therapies

Creatine does not appear to be effective for MS-associated weakness. Androstenedione, a supplement that has been claimed to increase strength, has not been shown to be effective and may actually be harmful.

WEAKNESS	
CONVENTIONAL TREATMENTS	**UNCONVENTIONAL AND LIFESTYLE TREATMENTS**
■ Physical Therapy ■ Occupational Therapy	Possibly Effective ■ Acupuncture ■ Cooling ■ Exercise ■ Hippotherapy ■ Pets ■ Pilates ■ Tai Chi ■ Yoga
	Ineffective ■ Creatine
	CAUTION ■ Androstenedione

Additional Readings

Websites

www.neurologycare.net—CAM website that is maintained by Dr. Allen Bowling

www.nationalmssociety.org—website of the National MS Society of the United States

Books

Bauer B, ed. *Mayo Clinic Book of Alternative Medicine and Home Remedies*. New York, NY: Time Home Entertainment; 2013.

Duyff RL. *American Dietetic Association Complete Food and Nutrition Guide*. Boston, MA: Houghton Mifflin Harcourt; 2012.

Geisser B, ed. *Primer on Multiple Sclerosis*. New York, NY: Oxford University Press; 2011.

Kalb RC. *Multiple Sclerosis: The Questions You Have—The Answers You Need*. New York, NY: Demos Medical Publishing; 2011.

Kalb RC, Giesser B, Costello K. *Multiple Sclerosis for Dummies*. Hoboken, NJ: John Wiley & Sons; 2012.

Katz DL. *Nutrition in Clinical Practice*. Philadelphia, PA: Lippincott Williams & Wilkins; 2008.

Kennedy P, ed. *The Can Do Multiple Sclerosis Guide to Lifestyle Empowerment*. New York, NY: Demos; 2013.

Rae-Grant A, Fox R, Bethoux F, eds. *Multiple Sclerosis and Related Disorders: Diagnosis, Medical Management, and Rehabilitation*. New York, NY: Demos; 2013.

Ratey JJ. *Spark: The Revolutionary New Science of Exercise and the Brain*. New York, NY: Little, Brown and Company; 2008.

Rippe JM, ed. *Lifestyle Medicine*. Boca Raton, FL: CRC Press; 2013.

Russell M, Bowling AC. *The Everything Health Guide to Multiple Sclerosis*. Avon, MA: Adams Media; 2009.

Salem Y, Csiza L, Harrison M, See J. *Aquatic Exercise and Multiple Sclerosis: A Healthcare Professional's Guide*. Cherry Hill, NJ: MS Association of America; 2013. [available from the MS Association of America].

Schapiro RT. *Managing the Symptoms of Multiple Sclerosis*. New York, NY: Demos Medical Publishing; 2007.

U.S. Dept. of Agriculture and U.S. Dept. of Health and Human Services. *Dietary Guidelines for Americans, 2010*. Washington, DC: U.S. Govt. Printing Office; 2010.

Journal Articles

Anon. Best diets 2014. *U.S. News and World Report* 2014; http://health.usnews.com/best-diet.

Bowling AC. Complementary and alternative medicine and multiple sclerosis. *Neurol Clin North America*. 2011;29:465–480.

D'hooghe MB, Nagels G, DeKeyser J, Haentjens P. Self-reported health promotion and disability progression in multiple sclerosis. *J Neurol Scis*. 2013;325:120–126.

Goodman S, Gulick EE. Dietary practices of people with multiple sclerosis. *Int J MS Care*. 2008;10:47–57.

Hadgkiss EJ, Jelinek GA, Weiland TJ, et al. Health-related quality of life outcomes at 1 and 5 years after a residential retreat promoting lifestyle modification for people with multiple sclerosis. *Neurol Sci.* 2013;34:187–195.

Jelinek GA, Hassed CS. Managing multiple sclerosis in primary care: are we forgetting something? *Qual Prim Care.* 2009;17:55–61.

Manzel A, Muller DN, Hafler D, Erdman SE, Linker RA, Kleinewietfeld M. Role of "Western diet" in inflammatory autoimmune diseases. *Curr Allergy Asthma Rep.* 2014;14:404.

Marrie RA, Hanwell H. General health issues in multiple sclerosis: comorbidities, secondary health conditions, and health behaviors. *Continuum.* 2013;19:1046–1057.

Marrie RA, Horwitz RI. Emerging effects of comorbidities on multiple sclerosis. *Lancet Neurol.* 2010;9:820–828.

Marrie RA, Horwitz, RI, Cutter G, Tyry T, Vollmer T. Association between comorbidity and clinical characteristics of MS. *Acta Neurol Scand.* 2011;124:135–141.

Marrie RA, Horwitz, RI, Cutter G, Tyry T. Cumulative impact of comorbidity on quality of life in MS. *Acta Neurol Scand.* 2012;125:180–186.

Ramsaransing GS, Mellema SA, De Keyser J. Dietary patterns in clinical subtypes of multiple sclerosis: an exploratory study. *Nutr J.* 2009;8:36.

Schwartz S, Leweling H. Multiple sclerosis and nutrition. *Mult Scler.* 2005;11:24–32.

Timmerman GM, Stuifbergen AK. Eating patterns in women with multiple sclerosis. *J Neurosci Nurs.* 1999;31:152–158.

Von Geldern G, Mowry EM. The influence of nutritional factors on the prognosis of multiple sclerosis. *Nat Rev Neurol.* 2012;8:678–689.

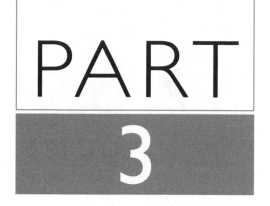

PART
3

Types of Lifestyle and Unconventional Medicine

Acupuncture and
Traditional Chinese Medicine

✓ **Acupuncture**

⚠ **Asian Proprietary Medicine**

⚠ **Chinese Herbal Medicine**

Acupuncture is one of many components of what is known as traditional Chinese medicine (TCM), a multimodal healing method that has been in use for more than 2,000 years. TCM is used by approximately one-fourth of the world's population. In Western countries, the use of TCM, especially acupuncture, has grown over the past two decades. Between 2002 and 2007 in the United States, acupuncture use increased by about 1 million people. It is now estimated that a few million Americans are treated with acupuncture yearly.

The recognition of acupuncture by Western medicine is not entirely new. In the late 1800s, Sir William Osler, one of the most honored and respected physicians and medical educators, wrote a textbook of medicine in which he recommended acupuncture for low back pain and sciatica. In 1901, *Gray's Anatomy*, a classic medical text, also referred to acupuncture as a treatment for sciatica.

There are multiple components of TCM. In addition to acupuncture, they include herbal medicine, diet/nutrition, exercise, meditation, and massage. Tai chi, which is discussed elsewhere in this book, is also a component of TCM. This chapter discusses acupuncture as well as two types of herbal medicine: Asian herbal medicine and Asian proprietary (or patent) medicine.

✅ Acupuncture

Acupuncture is based on a complex theory of body functioning that is very different from the Western biologic approach. Briefly, it is believed that a free flow of energy or qi passes through 12 major pathways or meridians on the body. There is also a balance of opposites, known as yin and yang. Disease is believed to result from a disruption in the normal flow of this energy.

Treatment Method

Acupuncture involves the insertion of thin, solid, metallic needles into specific points on the meridians. It is believed that this alters the flow of energy and thereby produces improvement. Approximately 400 acupuncture points exist. Fortunately, not all these are used in a single session! Four to 12 points are typically used in a session.

For those wary of needles, methods other than needle insertion may be used to stimulate acupuncture points. The application of finger pressure to these points is known as acupressure or, in Japan, shiatsu. Small hot cups are placed on points with *cupping*, and electrically stimulated needles are used with electroacupuncture. Transcutaneous electrical nerve stimulation (TENS), a variant of electroacupuncture, sometimes is used. In moxibustion, smoldering fibers of an herb, Asian mugwort or "moxa," are placed on acupuncture points or are used to heat needles that are then placed in acupuncture points.

How could a needle stuck into the skin possibly provide pain relief and other medical benefits? Many answers to this question have been proposed. As noted, from a TCM perspective, the insertion of needles is believed to alter the flow of energy in such a way that it produces therapeutic effects. From a Western scientific viewpoint, various possible mechanisms have been explored. One explanation for the pain-relieving effects of acupuncture is that it releases *opioids,* chemicals produced by the body that decrease pain. Other studies indicate that levels of another chemical, *serotonin,* are altered by acupuncture. It has been hypothesized that the changes in blood flow induced by needle insertion may have therapeutic effects. Studies on the brain using MRI indicate that acupuncture may change the activity in specific pain-related brain regions. Acupuncture also may decrease stress or, in some situations, act as a placebo. In the end, it may be found that multiple processes are involved.

Studies in Multiple Sclerosis and Other Conditions

A large number of studies have evaluated the effectiveness of acupuncture. Unfortunately, many of these studies have been small and not well conducted.

In an early attempt to provide an objective review of acupuncture, a 12-member panel was convened by the National Institutes of Health (NIH) in 1997 (1). This landmark study concluded that there existed "clear evidence" for acupuncture's effectiveness in relieving nausea and vomiting associated with surgery, chemotherapy, and possibly pregnancy. Evidence for effectiveness also was found for pain after dental procedures and several other types of pain. The report concluded that "the data in support of acupuncture are as strong as those for many accepted Western medical therapies" and that acupuncture was a "reasonable option" for some conditions.

In the specific area of multiple sclerosis (MS), it is surprising how few studies of acupuncture have actually been done. In an early Canadian study in 1974, acupuncture treatment in eight people with MS was associated with mild and brief benefits (2). In 1986, a very small study of two people with MS showed that multiple symptoms improved (3).

Interesting and contrary results have been obtained in small studies of the effects of acupuncture on MS-associated muscle stiffness, which is also known as spasticity. One study evaluated four people with MS—two of these people were wheelchair-bound and the other two were able to walk (4). Improvement in spasticity was seen in the two people who were able to walk but not in those who were wheelchair-bound. A 1986 study of 28 people with MS evaluated responses to stimulation at acupuncture sites (5). Interestingly, acupuncture sites were more sensitive in people with MS, and needle insertion actually provoked stiffness and muscle spasms. These findings may simply reflect a generalized MS-associated skin hypersensitivity or vulnerability to muscle stiffness.

Several small symptom-related studies have been conducted in MS. One small study of 14 people with secondary progressive MS reported improvement in a psychological measure of anxiety, depression, and irritability (the psychological component of a test known as the MS Impact Scale 29) (6). Another study of electroacupuncture in 31 people with MS found improvement in overall quality of life, including improvement in pain and depression (7). An investigation of 40 people with MS evaluated the effects of using acupuncture in addition to a fatigue medication, amantadine, in people whose fatigue was not adequately relieved by the amantadine alone. The study found that acupuncture improved fatigue in 25% of these people (8). Finally, a study of 35 people with MS-associated bladder difficulties found significant reduction in how often people needed to urinate and also improvement in people's ability to hold their urine (9).

Some studies have evaluated the effectiveness of acupuncture for symptoms and conditions that may occur with MS. In these studies, however, the underlying disease was not MS. Limited studies suggest beneficial effects of acupuncture for weakness in people with strokes. In studies of variable quality in other conditions, it has been found that acupuncture may be effective for other symptoms that may occur with MS, including anxiety, bladder dysfunction, bowel difficulties (constipation), depression, dizziness, fatigue, pain (including headache, facial pain, low back pain, and neck pain), sleeping difficulties, and tremor. In the area of general health, some studies indicate that acupuncture may mildly reduce blood pressure.

An important issue for MS is whether acupuncture has an effect on the immune system. At this time, the impact of acupuncture on immune-system activity is not well understood. Although no studies have been done specifically in people with MS, two studies in experimental allergic encephalomyelitis (EAE), the animal model of MS, indicate that electroacupuncture is associated with less severe disease and potentially beneficial immune system effects (10,11). In studies of immune-system activity in people with various forms of cancer and rheumatoid arthritis, acupuncture has been associated with stimulating, inhibiting, and having no effect on the immune system. Further studies are needed to clarify this area.

Side Effects

In general, acupuncture is a well-tolerated procedure. The most common side effects are mild and include soreness, bruising, and bleeding at needle sites and dizziness. There are very rare reports of more serious side effects, including breaking of needles and collapsing of a lung (pneumothorax). Infections may occur (including AIDS and hepatitis), especially if needles are reused. One recent large review of acupuncture safety studies reported a total of five acupuncture-related fatalities in the medical literature. Serious complications of acupuncture are often caused by poorly trained or negligent acupuncturists.

For people with MS, it is important to realize that acupuncture may produce drowsiness in up to one-third of people in the general population. As noted, limited studies in MS indicate that fatigue may actually be improved. If acupuncture does produce sedation in someone with MS, this could conceivably be worse in people who already have MS-associated fatigue or in those who take potentially sedating medication such as baclofen (Lioresal), tizanidine (Zanaflex), or diazepam (Valium).

Other rare risks are associated with acupuncture. People with damaged or prosthetic heart valves should probably not be treated with acupuncture because of the risk of infection. People who take blood-thinning medication (warfarin or Coumadin) or who have bleeding disorders may occasionally experience bruising or, more rarely, bleeding complications. Electroacupuncture may produce heart-rhythm abnormalities in people with a pacemaker, and the fumes from moxibustion may worsen breathing in people with asthma. Acupuncture to the chest should be done with caution or avoided to prevent lung or heart injury. These and other precautions of acupuncture are shown in Table 3.1.

TABLE 3.1 PRECAUTIONS WITH ACUPUNCTURE USE

Avoid with:	Blood-thinning medication (warfarin or Coumadin) or bleeding disorder Damaged or prosthetic heart valves Pacemaker (electroacupuncture)
Use caution with:	Immune-suppressing drugs or conditions Pregnancy Metal allergy Acupuncture sites in thorax (risk of lung or heart injury)

Practical Information

Acupuncture usually is done once or twice weekly. Sessions are typically 30 to 60 minutes and cost $60 to $150. The length of time required for a course of treatment varies. If a beneficial response occurs, it should usually be noted after six to ten sessions. The length of a complete course of treatment depends on the specific symptoms and the underlying disease process. A longer treatment course may be necessary for MS and other chronic diseases.

There are approximately 20,000 licensed acupuncturists in the United States. Organizations that can be helpful in obtaining information about acupuncture and locating an acupuncturist include:

- American Association of Acupuncture and Oriental Medicine, P.O. Box 96503, #44114, Washington, DC 20090 (866-455-7999) (www.aaaomonline.org)

- National Certification Commission for Acupuncture and Oriental Medicine 76 South Laura St., Suite 1290, Jacksonville, FL 32202 (904-598-1005) (www.nccaom.org)

- A listing of physicians or osteopaths who have acupuncture training is available from the American Academy of Medical Acupuncture, 1970 E. Grand Ave., Suite 330, El Segundo, CA 90245 (310-364-0193) (www.medicalacupuncture.org)

Conclusion

Acupuncture usually is well tolerated, but rare adverse effects do occur. Studies of MS and acupuncture are limited. In studies of variable quality, MS-associated symptoms that have responded to acupuncture include anxiety, bladder difficulties, bowel difficulties (constipation), depression, dizziness, fatigue, pain (including headache, facial pain, low back pain, and neck pain), sleeping difficulties, and weakness. Acupuncture may mildly reduce blood pressure.

⚠ Asian Proprietary Medicine (or Asian Patent Medicine)

Asian proprietary medicine, also known as Asian patent medicine, is a form of Asian herbal medicine. Preparations of this type of medicine usually contain mixtures of herbs as well as animal parts and minerals.

Several studies of the chemical composition of these preparations have found that they frequently contain potentially toxic ingredients. Some studies indicate that approximately one-third of these products contain drugs or dangerous metals. Drugs that have been found include diazepam (Valium), steroids, and prescription asthma medications. Toxic metals sometimes found in these products are arsenic, mercury, lead, and cadmium.

Because of the possible presence of these toxic ingredients, Asian proprietary medicine should be avoided or used with extreme caution.

⚠ Asian Herbal Medicine

Asian herbal medicine, which includes Chinese and Japanese herbal therapy, involves the use of herbal preparations that are often complex mixtures of many different herbs. Chinese herbal medicine frequently is used in combination with acupuncture, but it also may be used on its own. Asian herbal medicine may be administered in several different ways, including as tablets, pills, powders, capsules, or tinctures. Raw herbs or extracts of herbs also may be used.

When considering the use of Asian herbal medicine, it is essential to know which specific herbs are being used and to recognize that the full range of effectiveness and toxicity has not been fully established for any of these herbal preparations. These issues and other important factors related to herbal medicine in general are discussed in more detail in the section on herbs. In addition, the chapter of this book on herbs has information on some Asian herbs, including *Asian ginseng, astragalus,* dong-quai, ephedra (ma huang), *Ginkgo biloba,* and licorice (see *Herbs*).

Transforming Chinese Herbal Medicine Into Conventional MS Medication

Interestingly, fingolimod (Gilenya)—the first Food and Drug Administration (FDA)-approved oral MS drug—actually has its origins in Chinese herbal medicine. In the 1990s, scientists in Japan conducted studies to determine if any Chinese herbal medicines had unique effects on the immune system. In their studies of a fungus that is used to promote longevity in TCM (*Isaria sinclairii*), they did indeed identify a molecule with novel immune effects. This molecule was slightly altered chemically, subjected to years of rigorous animal and human testing, and was ultimately approved for use in MS by the FDA in 2010.

Studies of Chinese Herbal Medicine in MS and Other Conditions

There are multiple studies of Chinese herbal medicine in MS. Unfortunately, these studies are not rigorous or well-designed. Thus, the safety and effectiveness of Chinese herbal medicine in MS is not known. Of note, the reports of most of these studies are published in Chinese and are in the Chinese medical literature, but limited English translations are available for some (12).

One study evaluated the effects of Ping Fu Tang, a mixture of 17 different herbs (13). In this study, 45 people with MS were monitored for nearly 3 years. Two groups were followed: a treatment group that received the herbal therapy, and a control group that was treated with conventional Western medicine or a combination of Western and Chinese medicine. The group that received the herbal therapy had a significant decrease in attack rate compared to the control group. Unfortunately, the results of this study are difficult to interpret because of limited reporting about the characteristics of the people in the study, the way in which the study was conducted, and the type of monitoring that was performed.

Several other studies of the use of Chinese herbal medicine in MS have been reported (14). In 1990, one Chinese study reported beneficial effects with herbal treatment in 35 people with MS. In 1995, another study reported by the same research group found that Ping Fu Tang decreased the rate of MS attacks. Several other MS studies of Chinese herbal medicine (as well as Japanese herbal medicine) have been conducted. Paradoxically, in one of these studies, an herb that appears to stimulate the immune system, *Ganoderma lucidum*, was reported to slow the disease course in five people with MS. Overall, because these studies are not available in English, it is impossible to rigorously evaluate them or to make any clear conclusions about the research results.

Several specific Chinese herbs modulate or suppress the activity of the immune system and therefore could be therapeutic for MS. These herbs include *Ginkgo biloba* (see *Herbs* chapter), Re Du Qing, *Berberis*, *Stephania tetrandra*, and *Tripterygium wilfordii*.

A compound from *Stephania tetrandra*, tetrandrine, has produced promising results in scientific studies. This chemical suppresses the immune system through mechanisms that are different from several conventional medications. In addition, tetrandrine appears to produce additional immune-suppressing effects when it is given in combination with conventional medications. One study showed that tetrandrine decreased the severity of EAE, the animal model of MS. Further research is needed in this area.

One of the more extensively studied immune-suppressing Chinese herbs is *Tripterygium wilfordii*, also known as Thunder God Vine, *threewingnut*, or lei-gong-teng. Scientific studies indicate that this herb decreases the activity of T cells and other specific components of the immune system. In addition, it lessens the severity of EAE. One study conducted in China following 10 people with MS found that *T. wilfordii* produced "significant" improvement in eight people and mild improvement in two people. *T. wilfordii* has been studied primarily in autoimmune disorders other than MS. Beneficial effects have been noted in animals with an experimental form of lupus. Some clinical improvement has been noted in people with rheumatoid arthritis and lupus.

At this time, studies are too limited for this herb to be recommended specifically for MS or other autoimmune conditions. In addition, use of this herb has been associated with serious side effects (see the following section).

There are interesting recent parallels between *T. wilfordii* and fingolimod (Gilenya). As in the early stages of fingolimod development, rigorous biochemical studies of *T. wilfordii* have led to the identification of a molecule with novel immune system effects. It is possible that this molecule from *T. wilfordii*, triptolide, could ultimately be developed into a treatment for MS (and other immunological and neurological conditions).

Side Effects

If considering Asian herbal medicine, people with MS should be aware of individual herbs or herbal mixtures that may stimulate the immune system (Table 3.2). The immune-stimulating effects of these herbs have been shown in scientific tests or in laboratory animals. Their effects on humans in general or on people with MS have not been specifically investigated. Thus, the immune-stimulating activity of the herbs represents a theoretical risk for people with MS.

Fu-zheng therapy, a type of Chinese herbal medicine, is believed to improve the ability of the body to defend itself. Two herbs used in Fu-zheng therapy, *astragalus* and *Ligustrum lucidum*, have been shown to activate immune cells. *Asian ginseng*, which is present in many different types of Chinese herbal medicine, has diverse effects on the immune system, including stimulating effects. Green tea contains potent antioxidant compounds, which also may produce immune-stimulating activity; this is discussed elsewhere in this book (see "Coffee and Other Caffeine-Containing Herbs" in the *Herbs* chapter).

Some types of Japanese herbal medicine have immune-stimulating properties (see Table 3.2). Some of these mixtures also are used in Chinese medicine; for example, the Japanese herbs kakkan-to and shosaiko-to are the same as the Chinese herbs ge-gen-tang and xiao-chai-hu-tang, respectively.

TABLE 3.2 ASIAN HERBAL MEDICINE THAT MAY STIMULATE THE IMMUNE SYSTEM

Chinese	Japanese
Asian ginseng (Panax ginseng)	*Bupleurum*
Acanthopanax obovatus	*Cordyceps*
Angelica sinensis (dong quai)	Kakkan-to
Artemisia myriantha	Kanzo-bushi-to
Artemisia annua	Shosaiko-to
Astragalus (Astragalus membranaceus)	
Bupleurum	
Cordyceps	
Coix	
Dendrobium	
Epimedium sagittatum	
Ge-gen-tang	
Green tea	
jiaogulan	
Ligustrum lucidum	
Maitake mushroom	
Reishi mushroom (*Ganoderma lucidum*)	
Salvia miltiorrhiza	
Shiitake mushroom (*Lentinus edodes*)	
Sophora flavescens	
Xiao-chai-hu-tang	

TABLE 3.3 POTENTIALLY TOXIC ASIAN HERBS

Aristolochia fangchi	Guiji
Baijiaolia	Jin bu yuan
Bushi	Licorice
Caowu	Ma huang (ephedra)
Chuanwa	Naoyanghua
Datura preparations	*Tripterygium wilfordii* (thunder
Fuzi	god vine)
Guangfangji	Yangjinhua

Toxic effects have been associated with the use of some types of Asian herbal medicine (Table 3.3). These effects are not specific to MS. These herbs should be used with caution. Serious toxic effects on multiple body organs have been associated with some of these herbs. *T. wilfordii* has caused stomach upset, infertility, and, on one occasion, death. Less significant toxicity has been observed with the regular use of licorice, which may produce high blood pressure and low blood levels of potassium. The use of *ma huang* (ephedra) has been associated with increased blood pressure, other dangerous cardiac and neurologic side effects, and, rarely, death. Due to safety concerns, the FDA banned the sale of ephedra products in the United States on December 30, 2003.

There are multiple other safety concerns with Asian herbal medicine. For example, there are cases in which herbs have been misidentified or mislabeled. Some preparations may be contaminated with microorganisms, pesticides, and heavy metals. Also, the ways in which these herbs interact with prescription medications have not been well studied. Finally, the long-term safety of Asian herbal medicine is generally not known.

Practical Information

Chinese herbal medicine should be obtained from a trained herbalist. Monthly costs are approximately $20 to $60.

Conclusion

Acupuncture and Asian herbal medicine, both of which are components of TCM, should be approached very differently by people with MS.

Acupuncture is of low risk and possibly beneficial for a variety of MS-associated symptoms. Studies of variable quality indicate that acupuncture may improve anxiety, bladder difficulties, bowel difficulties (constipation), depression, dizziness, fatigue, pain (including headache, facial pain, low back pain, and neck pain), sleeping difficulties, and weakness. Thus, acupuncture may be a reasonable treatment option for some with MS. Also, acupuncture may mildly reduce blood pressure.

In contrast, Asian herbal medicine should be approached with caution. There is no convincing evidence that Asian herbal medicine has any therapeutic effects in MS. The herbs may stimulate the immune system and may be toxic or contaminated. Also, the interaction of the herbs with drugs and the safety of long-term use of the herbs has not been well studied.

Additional Readings

Books

Bauer B, ed. *Mayo Clinic Book of Alternative Medicine and Home Remedies.* New York, NY: Time Home Entertainment; 2013:120–123.

Bowling AC. Complementary and alternative medicine in multiple sclerosis. In: Geisser B, ed. *Primer on Multiple Sclerosis.* New York, NY: Oxford University Press; 2011:369–381.

Bowling AC. Complementary and alternative medicine: practical considerations. In: Rae-Grant A, Fox R, Bethoux F, eds. *Multiple Sclerosis and Related Disorders: Diagnosis, Medical Management, and Rehabilitation.* New York, NY: Demos; 2013:243–249.

Filshie J, White A. *Medical Acupuncture A Western Scientific Approach.* Edinburgh, UK: Churchill Livingstone; 1998.

Jellin JM, Gregory PJ, Batz F, et al. *Pharmacist's Letter/ Prescriber's Letter Natural Medicines Comprehensive Database.* Stockton, CA: Therapeutic Research Faculty; 2014.

Lin Y-C. Acupuncture and traditional Chinese medicine. In: Oken BS, ed. *Complementary Therapies in Neurology.* London, UK: Parthenon Publishing; 2004: 113–125.

Micozzi MS, ed. *Fundamentals of Complementary and Alternative Medicine.* Philadelphia, PA: Saunders Elsevier; 2011:403–437.

Navarra T. *The Encyclopedia of Complementary and Alternative Medicine.* New York, NY: Checkmark Books; 2005:2–5.

Rakel D. *Integrative Medicine.* Philadelphia, PA: Elsevier; 2012.

Synovitz LB, Larson KL. *Complementary and Alternative Medicine for Health Professionals.* Burlington, MA: Jones & Bartlett Learning; 2013: 97–120.

Journal Articles

Borchers AT, Hackman RM, Keen CL, Stern JS, Gershwin ME. Complementary medicine: a review of immunomodulatory effects of Chinese herbal medicines. *Am J Clin Nutr.* 1997;66:1303–1312.

Bowling AC. Complementary and alternative medicine and multiple sclerosis. *Neurol Clin North Am.* 2011;29:465–480.

Bowling AC. Complementary and alternative medicine in multiple sclerosis: dispelling common myths about CAM. *Int J MS Care.* 2005;7:42–44.

Bowling AC. Learning from traditional Chinese medicine and Ayurveda. *Momentum.* Summer 2010:48–50.

Bunchorntavakul C, Reddy KR. Review article: herbal and dietary supplement hepatotoxicity. *Aliment Pharmacol Ther.* 2013;37:3–17.

Chan TYK, Critchley JAJH. Usage and adverse effects of Chinese herbal medicines. *Human Exp Toxicol.* 1996;15:5–12.

Chon TY, Lee MC. Acupuncture. *Mayo Clin Proc.* 2013;88:1141–1146.

Donnellan CP, Shanley J. Comparison of the effect of two types of acupuncture on quality of life in secondary progressive multiple sclerosis: a preliminary single-blind randomized controlled trial. *Clin Rehabil.* 2008;22:195–205.

Efferth T, Kaina B. Toxicities by herbal medicines with emphasis to traditional Chinese medicine. *Curr Drug Metab.* 2011;12:989–996.

Ernst E, Lee MS, Choi TY. Acupuncture: does it alleviate pain and are there serious risks? A review of reviews. *Pain.* 2011;152:755–764.

Finnegan-John J, Molassiotis A, Richardson A, et al. A systematic review of complementary and alternative medicine interventions for the management of cancer-related fatigue. *Integr Cancer Ther.* 2013;12:276–290.

Foroughipour M, Bahrami Taghanaki HR, Saeidi M, et al. Amantadine and the place of acupuncture in the treatment of fatigue in patients with multiple sclerosis: an observational study. *Acupunct Med.* 2013;31:27–30.

Genuis SJ, Schwalfenberg G, Siy A-K, Rodushkin I. Toxic element contamination of natural health products and pharmaceutical preparations. *PLoS One.* 2012;7:e49676.

Ho LJ, Lai JH. Chinese herbs as immunomodulators and potential disease-modifying antirheumatic drugs in autoimmune disorders. *Curr Drug Metab.* 2004;5:181–192.

Lai JH. Immunomodulatory effects and mechanisms of plant alkaloid tetrandrine in autoimmune diseases. *Acta Pharmacol Sin.* 2002;23:2093–1101.

Liu J, Gao Y, Kan BH, Zhou L. Systematic review and meta-analysis of randomized controlled trials of Chinese herbal medicine in treatment of multiple sclerosis. *Zhong Xi Yi He Xue Bao.* 2012;10:141–153. [in Chinese].

Miller RE. An investigation into the management of the spasticity experienced by some patients with multiple sclerosis using acupuncture based on traditional Chinese medicine. *Compl Ther Med.* 1996;4:58–62.

NIH Consensus Development Panel on Acupuncture. *JAMA.* 1998;280: 1518–1524.

Quispe-Cabanillas JG, Damasceno A, von Glehn F, et al. Impact of electroacupuncture on quality of life for patients with relapsing-remitting multiple sclerosis under treatment with immunomodulators: a randomized study. *BMC Complement Altern Med.* 2012;12:209.

Rabinstein AA, Shulman LM. Acupuncture in clinical neurology. *Neurologist.* 2003;9:137–148.

Tjon Eng Soe SH, Kopsky DJ, Jongen PJH, de Vet HC, Oei-Tan CL. Multiple sclerosis patients with bladder dysfunction have decreased symptoms after electro-acupuncture. *Mult Scler.* 2009;15:1376–1377.

Wang J, Xiong X, Liu W. Acupuncture for essential hypertension. *Int J Cardiol.* 2013;169:317–326.

Wang Y, Mei Y, Feng D, Xu L. Triptolide modulates T-cell inflammatory responses and ameliorates experimental autoimmune encephalomyelitis. *J Neurosci Res.* 2008;86:2441–2449.

Wheway J, Agbabiaka TB, Ernst E. Patient safety incidents from acupuncture treatments: a review of reports to the National Patient Safety Agency. *Int J Risk Saf Med.* 2012;24:163–169.

Wu J-J, Ai C-Z, Liu Y, et al. Interactions between phytochemicals from traditional Chinese medicines and human cytochrome P450 enzymes. *Curr Drug Metabol.* 2012;13:599–614.

Xi L, Zhiwen L, Huayan W, et al. Preventing relapse in multiple sclerosis with Chinese medicine. *J Chin Med.* 2001;66:39–40.

Zhang L-H, Huang Y, Wang L-W, et al. Several compounds from Chinese traditional and herbal medicine as immunomodulators. *Phytother Res.* 1995;9: 315–322.

Zheng Y, Zhang WJ, Wang XM. Triptolide with potential medicinal value for diseases of the central nervous system. *CNS Neurosci Ther.* 2013;19:76–82.

Alcohol

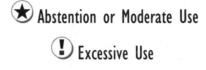

★ Abstention or Moderate Use

! Excessive Use

Consuming alcohol has benefits as well as risks. For some medical conditions, moderate amounts of alcohol may actually be beneficial. However, when taken in excess, alcohol causes significant health problems. A growing number of studies are evaluating the relevance of alcohol use to those with multiple sclerosis (MS).

Approaches to Alcohol Use

If alcohol is used, it should be used in moderation. Definitions of moderation are based on the number of "drinks"—one drink equals five ounces of wine, 12 ounces of beer, or 1 ¼ ounces of 80-proof liquor. Moderation is defined as:

- Nonpregnant women and everyone over age 65: one drink per day
- Men under age 65: two or fewer drinks per day
- Pregnant women: avoid alcohol use

Studies in MS and Other Conditions

Limited studies in MS have evaluated alcohol abuse and also the effects of alcohol on the risk of developing MS and on the progression of the disease. Misuse or excessive intake of alcohol has been reported in 15%–40% of those with MS. Excessive use has been associated with men and also those who are younger and more educated. Of note, in one study, only about one-quarter of those who were misusing alcohol were actually given advice about decreasing or abstaining from alcohol from health providers. Research on alcohol's effects on the risk of developing MS have produced mixed results—some studies indicate that alcohol has no effect while others indicate it may decrease the risk of developing MS. Similarly, variable results have been obtained in studies of alcohol's effects on disease activity—some indicate a mildly beneficial effect but others do not. Additional research is needed to understand more clearly the effects of alcohol on the risk of MS and on the course of the disease.

In other medical conditions, moderate alcohol use has been associated with beneficial effects. Alcohol may increase levels of "good cholesterol" ("HDL" or high-density lipoprotein) and decrease the risk of heart disease.

Side Effects

Mild to moderate amounts of alcohol may produce multiple side effects, including decreased alertness, reduced cognitive function, impaired coordination, walking difficulties, fatigue, and increased reaction time. The side effects of alcohol may be more pronounced in those with MS. Indeed, some people with MS observe that the negatives of alcohol outweigh the positives after being diagnosed, and, perhaps related to this observation, one study found that people with MS were more likely to abstain from alcohol after being diagnosed than prior to the diagnosis. There is no evidence that moderate alcohol use, relative to abstaining, exerts negative effects on the disease course of MS.

Alcohol, especially in excess, may have significant health effects. It may increase triglycerides in the blood, raise blood pressure, and interfere with the effectiveness of blood pressure medications. Also, alcohol use has been associated with increased risk of various forms of cancer, including cancers of the breast, liver, throat, mouth, and esophagus. Alcohol use should be avoided in women who are pregnant and also in those who plan to drive or do work that requires high levels of attention and skill.

Alcoholism, which is addiction to alcohol, can be life-threatening. It may lead to death from accidents, suicide, toxic effects of alcohol on the liver and other organs, and malnutrition.

Alcohol may interact with many different medications, some of which are commonly used in MS. Some MS disease-modifying medications have possible liver toxicity, including interferons (Avonex, Betaseron, Extavia, and Rebif), fingolimod (Gilenya), teriflunomide (Aubagio), and natalizumab (Tysabri). Alcohol use with these medications could increase the risk of liver toxicity. Other common MS medications that may interact with alcohol include sleeping medications and antidepressant medications—alcohol in combination with these drugs may produce excessive sedation. Also, over-the-counter pain medications, which are frequently used by those with MS, may interact with alcohol. Acetaminophen (Tylenol) may increase the risk of alcohol-associated liver toxicity, while aspirin and nonsteroidal inflammatory drugs (NSAIDs) such as ibuprofen (Motrin), may increase the risk of alcohol-related stomach bleeding.

Conclusion

If alcohol is consumed, it should be used in moderation. Moderate alcohol use does not have any known adverse effects on the disease course of MS. Alcohol may interact with multiple MS medications. Excessive alcohol use should be avoided.

Additional Readings

Books

Bauer B, ed. *Mayo Clinic Book of Alternative Medicine and Home Remedies.* New York, NY: Time Home Entertainment; 2013:188–194.

Duyff RL. *American Dietetic Association Complete Food and Nutrition Guide.* Boston, MA: Houghton Mifflin Harcourt; 2012.

Jellin JM, Batz F, Hitchens K. *Natural Medicines Comprehensive Database.* Stockton, CA: Therapeutic Research Faculty; 2014.

Journal Articles

Beier M, D'Orio V, Spat J, Shuman M, Foley FW. Alcohol and substance use in multiple sclerosis. *J Neurol Sci.* 2014;338:122–127.

D'hooghe MB, Haentjens P, Nagels G, De Keyser J. Alcohol, coffee, fish, smoking and disease progression in multiple sclerosis. *Eur J Neurol.* 2012;19:616–624.

D'hooghe MB, Nagels G, Bissay V, De Keyser J. Modifiable risk factors influencing relapses and disability in multiple sclerosis. *Mult Scler.* 2010;16:773–785.

Foster M, Zivadinov R, Weinstock-Guttman B, et al. Associations of moderate alcohol consumption with clinical and MRI measures in multiple sclerosis. *J Neuroimmunol.* 2012;243:61–68.

Hedstrom AK, Hillert J, Olsson T, Alfredsson L. Alcohol as a modifiable lifestyle factor affecting multiple sclerosis risk. *JAMA Neurol.* 2014;71:300–305.

Massa J, O'Reilly EJ, Munger KL, Ascherio A. Caffeine and alcohol intakes have no association with risk of multiple sclerosis. *Mult Scler.* 2013;19:53–58.

Overs S, Hughes CM, Haselkorn JK, Turner AP. Modifiable comorbidities and disability in multiple sclerosis. *Curr Neurol Neurosci Rep.* 2012;12:610–617.

Ponsonby AL, Lucas RM, Dear K, et al. The physical anthropometry, lifestyle habits and blood pressure of people presenting with a first clinical demyelinating event compared to controls: the Ausimmune study. *Mult Scler.* 2013;19: 1717–1725.

Turner AP, Hawkins EJ, Haselkorn JK, Kivlahan DR. Alcohol misuse and multiple sclerosis. *Arch Phys Med Rehab.* 2009;90:842–848.

Weiland TJ, Hadgkiss EJ, Jelinek GA, Pereira NG, Marck CH, van der Meer DM. The association of alcohol consumption and smoking with quality of life, disability and disease activity in an international sample of people with multiple sclerosis. *J Neurol Sci.* 2014;336:211–219.

⑦ Aromatherapy

Aromatherapy is a type of healing that uses aromatic substances derived from plants. It was used in some form in ancient Egypt and ancient China. The type of aromatherapy currently used in the United States was originally developed in the early 20th century by Rene-Maurice Gattefosse, a French chemist.

Treatment Method

Aromatherapy is based primarily on the use of essential oils. These oils, which are of high quality and purity, are obtained from plants using a specialized distillation process or by cold pressing. More than 40 different essential oils are used. They may be used individually or as mixtures, and they are administered by direct application to the skin, mixing with bath water, or inhalation. Oils sometimes are applied to the skin by massage. In France, oils are sometimes taken internally by mouth or by the vagina or rectum. However, in general, oils should not be taken internally.

As with the other senses, the sense of smell serves an important role. Specific odors may trigger feelings and memories. Some studies have shown that certain odors may produce headaches or elicit relaxation. The nerve signals from the nose are transmitted to a part of the brain known as the *limbic system*, which is involved in emotion and motivation.

Although smell often is thought of as a "minor" sense in humans, it is actually the major sense for many animals. For these animals, chemicals known as *pheromones* are detected by the olfactory system and are important in mating and communication.

Although the sense of smell is important and olfactory signals are sent to a brain region involved in basic psychological processes, the mechanism by which administering specific odors may produce therapeutic effects is not clear.

Studies in Multiple Sclerosis and Other Conditions

Aromatherapy has not been systematically studied in people with multiple sclerosis (MS). A small preliminary study of two people with MS reported that a treatment program of aromatherapy and massage led to improvement in mobility, dressing ability, and personal hygiene (1). Studies of olfaction in MS indicate that 10% to 20% of people with the disease have an impaired sense of smell.

Only a limited number of studies detail the effects of aromatherapy on any medical condition, and those that do exist are generally of low quality. Many of the therapeutic claims about aromatherapy are based on tradition, not on actual clinical research.

Symptoms of MS that have been investigated in some aromatherapy research are anxiety, depression, pain, and insomnia. For anxiety, studies of variable quality indicate that beneficial effects may be obtained with the use of lavender oil, Roman chamomile oil, and neroli (orange) oil. However, no large, well-designed clinical studies have examined this antianxiety effect. Preliminary information suggests that a lower dose of antidepressant medication may be needed by depressed men when the medication is used in combination with aromatherapy using a citrus fragrance. Lavender has produced positive as well as negative results with childbirth-associated pain. Similarly, mixed results have been obtained in other studies of aromatherapy and pain. Several fragrances, especially lavender, have been evaluated in sleep studies in animals and humans. Some positive results have been reported, but these studies are of variable quality.

Aromatherapy has been studied in a few other unrelated conditions. Small studies on older people with dementia have produced mixed results. Inhalation of black pepper extract may decrease the craving for cigarettes. People with a form of baldness, alopecia areata, may benefit from scalp massage using a mixture of thyme, rosemary, lavender, and cedar-wood oils.

When aromatherapy is combined with massage, as is often the case, it may be difficult to distinguish the benefits of the oil from those of the massage. In limited studies, massage alone has been associated with several beneficial effects (see the *Massage* chapter).

Side Effects

Aromatherapy usually is well tolerated, but it is not risk-free. Side effects are most frequently reported with lavender, peppermint, tea oil, and ylang-ylang. The most common side effect is *contact dermatitis*, a rash that may occur when oil is applied to the skin. This type of allergic reaction may be detected by applying a small amount of oil to the skin and monitoring for a response for 24 hours. Cinnamon or clove oil should not be applied directly to the skin. Basil, fennel, lemon grass, rosemary, and verbena oils may cause skin irritation—the use of these oils should be discontinued if skin irritation occurs. Approximately 5% of people appear to be allergic to fragrances. Because of possible toxic effects, oil should not be taken internally by mouth or any other method (this is especially true for eucalyptus, hyssop, mugwort, thuja, pennyroyal, sage, and wormwood). Pregnant women probably should avoid aromatherapy because the use of some oils may lead to miscarriage. Odors may provoke headaches in people with migraines and cause breathing difficulties in those with asthma. Some oils (rosemary, fennel, hyssop, sage, wormwood) may cause seizures in people with epilepsy. Naphthalene-related compounds, such as menthol and camphor, should be avoided in those with a condition known as Glucose-6-phosphate dehydrogenase (G6PD) deficiency.

If aromatherapy is combined with massage, the possible side effects of massage should be kept in mind (see *Massage* chapter).

Practical Information

Aromatherapy may be obtained from a practitioner or may be self-administered. It is sometimes combined with herbal medicine or traditional Chinese medicine. Aromatherapy may be provided on an individual basis or as informational classes. Individual sessions typically cost $60 to $80 and last about 60 minutes. Classes cost about $30 for 60 to 120 minutes.

More information on aromatherapy and aromatherapists may be obtained from:

- Aromatherapy Registration Council (ARC) (www.aromatherapycouncil .org)

- National Association for Holistic Aromatherapy (NAHA) (www.naha .org), PO Box 27871, Raleigh, NC 27611 (919-894-0298)

Conclusion

Aromatherapy is of low risk and reasonable cost. The benefits of this therapy in people with MS have not been systematically studied. A small, preliminary study in MS found improvement in multiple symptoms using aromatherapy and massage. Some small clinical studies have found beneficial effects for anxiety, depression, pain, and insomnia, but these studies are of variable quality and some of the results have not been consistent. Further research is needed on the effects of aromatherapy on MS and other neurologic conditions.

Additional Readings

Books

Harris R. Aromatherapy. In: Micozzi MS, ed. *Fundamentals of Complementary and Alternative Medicine*. Philadelphia, PA: Saunders Elsevier; 2011:332–342.

Hirsh AR. Aromatherapy: art, science, or myth. In: Weintraub MI, Micozzi M, eds. *Alternative and Complementary Treatment in Neurologic Illness*. Philadelphia, PA: Churchill Livingstone; 2001:128–150.

Navarra T. *The Encyclopedia of Complementary and Alternative Medicine*. New York, NY: Checkmark Books; 2005:8–10.

Synovitz LB, Larson KL. *Complementary and Alternative Medicine for Health Professionals*. Burlington, MA: Jones & Bartlett Learning; 2013:159–177.

Vickers A. *Massage and Aromatherapy: A Guide for Health Professionals*. London, UK: Chapman & Hall; 1996.

Journal Articles

Cho MY, Min ES, Hur MH, Lee MS. Effects of aromatherapy on the anxiety, vital signs, and sleep quality of percutaneous intervention patients in intensive care units. *Evid Based Compl Alt Med*. 2013;2013:381381.

Howarth AL. Will aromatherapy be a useful treatment strategy for people with multiple sclerosis who experience pain. *Complement Ther Nurs Midwifery*. 2002;8:138–141.

Lee MS, Choi J, Posadzki P, Ernst E. Aromatherapy for health care: an overview of systematic reviews. *Maturitas*. 2012;71:257–260.

Lyttle J, Mwatha C, Davis KK. Effect of lavender aromatherapy on vital signs and perceived quality of sleep in the intermediate care unit: a pilot study. *Am J Crit Care*. 2014;23:24–29.

Ni CH, Hou WH, Kao CC, et al. The anxiolytic effect of aromatherapy on patients awaiting ambulatory surgery: a randomized controlled trial. *Evid Based Complement Alternat Med*. 2013;2013:927419.

Olapour A, Behaeen K, Akhondzadeh R, Soltani F, Al Sadat Razavi F, Bekhradi R. The effect of inhalation of aromatherapy blend containing lavender essential oil on cesarean postoperative pain. *Anesth Pain Med*. 2013;3:203–207.

Posadski P, Alotaibi A, Ernst E. Adverse effects of aromatherapy: a systematic review of case reports and case series. *Int J Risk Saf Med*. 2012;24:147–161.

Walsh E, Wilson C. Complementary therapies in long-stay neurology in-patient settings. *Nurs Stand.* 1999;13:32–35.

Wixted JT. Sleep aromatherapy curbs conditioned fear. *Nat Neurosci.* 2013; 16:1510–1512.

Yim VW, Ng AK, Tsang, HW, Leung AY. A review on the effects of aromatherapy for patients with depressive symptoms. *J Altern Complement Med.* 2009;15: 187–195.

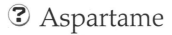# ? Aspartame

Some claims exist that aspartame, an artificial sweetener used in soft drinks, causes multiple sclerosis (MS) or worsens MS-associated symptoms. Much of the initial concern about aspartame and MS was raised through Internet postings in the late 1990s. Interest in the topic has waxed and waned since that time.

Treatment Method

It sometimes is recommended that people with MS avoid all drinks and foods that contain aspartame.

Studies in MS and Other Conditions

No well-conducted studies have shown that aspartame causes MS or worsens symptoms in most people with the disease. Of note, this area has not been subjected to rigorous clinical investigation. However, at this time, there are not any scientific or clinical studies that provide compelling evidence to warrant large-scale clinical studies.

Limited studies indicate that aspartame may provoke migraine headaches and worsen depression. Interestingly, one migraine medication that dissolves in the mouth, known as rizatriptan or Maxalt-MLT, actually contains aspartame and thus may worsen headache in those with aspartame-provoked migraines.

In terms of other neurologic disorders, clinical studies do not indicate that aspartame worsens Parkinson's disease or provokes seizures. In addition, there are not any studies that clearly demonstrate that aspartame is toxic to nerve cells or interferes with memory and learning.

Aspartame is of potential concern because the body may convert aspartame to methanol and then convert the methanol to formic acid, which may produce serious toxicity. However, consuming moderate or even large quantities of diet soft drinks does not significantly increase blood levels of methanol or formic acid.

In terms of other medical conditions, isolated reports raise concern that aspartame causes cancer. However, at this time, the vast majority of scientific and clinical studies do not indicate that aspartame causes cancer or increases the risk of any other serious medical condition.

For food additives such as aspartame, acceptable daily intake (ADI) values are determined through the use of safety information. In the United States, the daily ADI for aspartame is 50 mg/kg of body weight or approximately 25 mg/lb of body weight. For a 150-lb person, this translates to about 20 12-oz cans of diet soda daily.

Conclusion

Based on current information, no compelling reason exists for most people with MS to avoid aspartame. No evidence demonstrates that a reasonable intake of aspartame worsens MS or provokes MS-specific symptoms. Aspartame may provoke migraine headaches and depression.

Due to the limited information in this area, it is possible that a subgroup of people with MS could experience aspartame-related symptoms. To determine if one is in this subgroup, it would be reasonable and simple to discontinue aspartame use for a few days and note if any benefit occurs.

Additional Readings

Journal Articles

Aune D. Soft drinks, aspartame, and the risk of cancer and cardiovascular disease. *Am J Clin Nutr.* 2012;96:1249–1251.

Lipton RB, Newman LC, Cohen JS, Solomon S. Aspartame as a dietary trigger of headache. *Headache.* 1989;29:90–92.

Magnuson BA, Burdock GA, Doull J, et al. Aspartame: a safety evaluation based on current use levels, regulations, and toxicological and epidemiological studies. *Crit Rev Toxicol.* 2007;37:629–727.

Marinovich M, Galli CL, Bosetti C, Gallus S, LaVecchia C. Aspartame, low-calorie sweeteners and disease: regulatory safety and epidemiological issues. *Food Chem Toxicol*. 2013;60:109–115.

Newman LC, Lipton RB. Maxalt MLT-down: an unusual presentation of migraine in patients with aspartame-triggered headaches. *Headache*. 2001;41:899–901.

Schernhammer EA, Bertrand KA, Birmann BM, Sampson L, Willett WC, Feskanich D. Consumption of artificial sweetener- and sugar-containing soda and risk of lymphoma and leukemia in men and women. *Am J Clin Nutr*. 2012;96:1419–1428.

Soffritti M, Padovani M, Tibaldi E, Falcioni L, Manservisi F, Belpoggi F. The carcinogenic effects of aspartame: the urgent need for regulatory re-evaluation. *Am J Indust Med*. 2014;57:383–397.

Van dewn Eeden SK, Koepsell TD, Longstreth WT Jr, van Belle G, Daling JR, McKnight B. Aspartame ingestion and headaches: a randomized crossover trial. *Neurology*. 1994;44:1787–1793.

Walton RG, Hudak R, Green-Waite RJ. Adverse reactions to aspartame: double-blind challenge in patients from a vulnerable population. *Biol Psych*. 1993;34:13–17.

Whitehouse CR, Boullata J, McCauley LA. The potential toxicity of artificial sweeteners. *AAOHN J*. 2008;56:251–259.

Ayurveda

(!) **Ayurvedic Supplements**

(✓) **Yoga**

(✓) **Meditation**

(✓) **Massage**

Ayurveda was developed in India thousands of years ago and is the oldest known medical system still in use. Ayurveda means "knowledge (or science) of life" in Sanskrit, and its practice includes medicine and science as well as philosophy and religion. The form of Ayurvedic medicine now practiced is a modified version of the ancient form of this healing method. Ayurveda is still widely practiced in India. It has been popularized and promoted in the United States by Maharishi Mahesh Yogi and Dr. Deepak Chopra.

In Ayurveda, a harmonious relationship between mind, body, and spiritual awareness is believed to be important. The function of these entities is regulated by three physiologic principles known as doshas. Disease is claimed to be the result of an imbalance of the doshas, and treatment aims to restore dosha balance. As in traditional Chinese medicine (TCM), Ayurveda holds that an important life force, called prana, exists.

Treatment Method

Ayurveda consists of several components. As in TCM, pulse and tongue evaluation are important for diagnosis. Diet, exercise, lifestyle changes, and specific supplements are used therapeutically. Yoga, breathing exercises, massage, and meditation, discussed elsewhere in this book, are also components of Ayurveda. One type of Ayurvedic meditation, transcendental meditation (TM), was popularized by Maharishi Mahesh Yogi. Another important aspect of Ayurveda, panchakarma, is used for disease prevention. Panchakarma means "five processes" and includes massages, sweat baths, vomiting, enemas, and bloodletting (through the use of leeches).

One specific Ayurvedic supplement, known as ashwagandha, is sometimes specifically recommended for treating multiple sclerosis (MS). This supplement is derived from the roots of the *Withania somnifera* plant. This herb is one of several herbal components in a product known as *Protandim,* which is also sometimes recommended for MS.

Two primary types of Ayurveda are practiced outside India. Maharishi Ayur-Veda was started by Maharishi Mahesh Yogi and relies heavily on meditation. The other Ayurvedic school, advocated by Dr. Deepak Chopra, uses meditation in conjunction with other Ayurvedic methods.

Studies in MS and Other Conditions

No large published clinical studies have specifically investigated the effect of Ayurveda on MS or its symptoms. Some components of Ayurveda have been investigated individually. These include massage, meditation, and yoga, all of which are discussed elsewhere in this book. These therapies may be helpful for some symptoms that occur with MS, including fatigue, spasticity, pain, depression, and anxiety.

Ashwagandha, the Ayurvedic supplement sometimes recommended for MS, has been studied mainly in scientific and animal studies. In multiple studies, ashwagandha has been shown to stimulate the immune system. It also may produce sedating effects. Ashwagandha has not been studied in clinical trials in MS—as a result, it is not known if it has any therapeutic effects in MS.

Limited research has evaluated Ayurvedic supplements for other conditions. Preliminary studies indicate that Ayurvedic preparations may have effects on cardiovascular disease, cognitive function, diabetes, hepatitis, and arthritis. However, beneficial effects have not been reported in all studies in these conditions and many studies have significant limitations, including small numbers of participants, research design problems, and lack of placebo-treated groups. As with MS, further research is needed in these conditions.

Side Effects

Ayurveda should not be used in place of conventional medicine for treating MS. Some Ayurvedic preparations contain dangerous heavy metals, such as lead, arsenic, and mercury. These preparations have been associated with serious metal poisoning and should be avoided, even if they are claimed to be "deactivated" by heat. In the medical literature, there is a case report of a man with MS who developed anemia, vomiting, weight loss, and abdominal pain while taking Ayurvedic supplements. He was diagnosed with lead poisoning, and one of his Ayurvedic preparations had a very high lead level. One study of 70 different Ayurvedic herbal preparations found that 20% contained potentially harmful levels of certain metals.

Ashwagandha is sometimes recommended for MS. However, due to its immune-stimulating effects, this Ayurvedic supplement poses theoretical risks for people with MS. These effects also could interfere with the effectiveness of the Food and Drug Administration (FDA)-approved disease-modifying medications for MS. The sedating effects of ashwagandha could worsen MS fatigue or increase the sedating effects of some medications. Ashwagandha may interfere with thyroid medications.

Scientific studies indicate that other Ayurvedic supplements also influence the immune system. Immune-stimulating activity has been noted in isolated scientific studies of Kanakasava, Maharishi-4, Maharishi-5, *Boerhavia diffusa*, *Phyllanthus emblica*, *Nimba arishta*, and *Woodfordia fruticosa*. These preparations theoretically could be harmful to people with MS. Further studies are needed to determine if they are in fact dangerous.

Ayurvedic remedies have caused serious liver toxicity. There is a report of a woman with MS who experienced fatigue and gastrointestinal symptoms while using Ayurvedic medicine. Blood tests showed significant liver toxicity, which was attributed to two of her Ayurvedic supplements, *Azadirachta indica* and *Momordica charantia*. In other reports, Ayurvedic supplements containing *Heliotropium* species have been associated with liver toxicity, which in some cases has led to death. Chemicals that may produce liver or kidney toxicity have been found in several Ayurvedic herbs, including *Cassia auriculata*, *Crotalaria juncea*, *Crotalaria verrucosa*, and *Holarrhena antidysenterica*.

Practical Information

No program is in place for licensing Ayurvedic practitioners in the United States. Ayurveda is practiced by a variety of health care professionals, including physicians, chiropractors, and nutritionists. Initial visits with Ayurvedic practitioners last 1 to 3 hours; follow-up visits are 30 to 60 minutes. The initial evaluation costs between $90 and $225, and follow-up visits cost $60 to $90. Ayurveda usually is not covered by insurance. More information about Ayurveda and Ayurvedic medical practices may be obtained:

- National Ayurvedic Medical Association (www.ayurvedanama.org), 620 Cabrillo Ave., Santa Cruz, CA 95065 (800-669-8914)

- Ayurvedic Institute (www.ayurveda.com), 11311 Menaul Boulevard NE, Albuquerque, NM 87112 (505-291-9698)

Conclusion

Ayurveda is a multicomponent healing system with generally low risk and moderate cost. Some components of Ayurveda, including massage, meditation, and yoga, are of low risk and may provide beneficial effects for fatigue, anxiety, depression, pain, and spasticity (see *Massage*, *Meditation*, and *Yoga* chapters). However, another component of Ayurveda, the use of specific supplements, may produce serious side effects. This aspect of Ayurvedic treatment has not been fully studied in any medical condition, including MS. Ashwagandha, a specific Ayurvedic supplement sometimes recommended for MS, actually poses theoretical risks for people with MS because it could worsen the disease or decrease the therapeutic effects of some MS medications. Also, Ashwagandha could worsen MS fatigue and increase the sedating effects of some medications.

The overall assessment of Ayurveda is similar to that of TCM. Both of these multimodal healing methods may provide beneficial effects through some of their approaches, such as acupuncture and tai chi in TCM and massage, meditation, and yoga in Ayurveda. These approaches may be worth considering for some people with MS. However, the biologically based components of both of these healing systems, which are herbal medicine in TCM and supplements in Ayurveda, are generally of unknown safety and effectiveness, may pose theoretical risks in MS, and thus should be used with caution by people with MS.

Additional Readings

Books

Bauer B, ed. *Mayo Clinic Book of Alternative Medicine and Home Remedies.* New York, NY: Time Home Entertainment; 2013:142,143.

Jellin JM, Batz F, Hitchens K. *Natural Medicines Comprehensive Database.* Stockton, CA: Therapeutic Research Faculty; 2014.

Kaplan GP. Ayurvedic medicine. In: Oken BS, ed. *Complementary Therapies in Neurology.* London, UK: Parthenon Publishing; 2004:145–158.

Manyam BV. Ayurvedic approach to neurologic illness. In: Weintraub MI, Micozzi MS, eds. *Alternative and Complementary Treatment in Neurologic Illness.* New York, NY: Churchill Livingstone; 2001:68–74.

Pai S, Shanbhag V, Archarya S. Ayurvedic medicine. In: Kligler B, Lee R, eds. *Integrative Medicine: Principles for Practice.* New York, NY: McGraw-Hill; 2004:219–240.

Sharma HM. Contemporary Ayurveda. In: Micozzi MS, ed. *Fundamentals of Complementary and Alternative Medicine.* Philadelphia, PA: Saunders Elsevier; 2011:495–508.

Synovitz LB, Larson KL. *Complementary and Alternative Medicine for Health Professionals.* Burlington, MA: Jones & Bartlett Learning; 2013:79–96.

Journal Articles

Agarwal R, Diwanay S, Patki P, Patwardhan B. Studies on immunomodulatory activity of *Withania somnifera* (Ashwagandha) extracts in experimental immune inflammation. *J Ethnopharmacol*. 1999;67:27–35.

Bowling AC. Learning from traditional Chinese medicine and Ayurveda. *Momentum*. Summer 2010:48–50.

Bunchorntavakul C, Reddy KR. Review article: herbal and dietary supplement hepatotoxicity. *Aliment Pharmacol Ther*. 2013;37:3–17.

Genuis SJ, Schwalfenberg G, Siy A-K, Rodushkin I. Toxic element contamination of natural health products and pharmaceutical preparations. *PLOS One*. 2012;7:e49676.

Iuvone T, Esposito G, Capasso F, Izzo AA. Induction of nitric oxide synthase expression by *Withania somnifera* in macrophages. *Life Sci*. 2003;72:1617–1625.

Kanen BL, Perenboom RM. Chronic lead intoxication associated with Ayurvedic medication. *Ned Tijdschr Geneeskd*. 2005;149:2893–2896.

Khan S, Malik F, Suri KA, Singh J. Molecular insight into the immune up-regulatory properties of the leaf extract of Ashwagandha and identification of Th1 immunostimulatory chemical entity. *Vaccine*. 2009;27:6080–6087.

Mikolai J, Erlandsen A, Murison A, et al. In vivo effects of Ashwagandha (*Withania somnifera*) extract on the activation of lymphocytes. *J Alt Compl Med*. 2009;15:423–430.

Saper RB, Kales SN, Paquin J, et al. Heavy metal content of Ayurvedic herbal medicine products. *JAMA*. 2004;292:2868–2873.

Sarker MR, Nahar S, Shahriar M, Seraj S, Choudhuri MS. Preliminary study of the immunostimulating activity of an ayurvedic preparation, Kanakasave, on the splenic cells of BALB/c mice in vitro. *Pharmaceut Biol*. 2012;50:1467–1472.

Shah A, Juvekar AR. In vitro and in vivo immunostimulatory activity of Woodfordia fruticosa flowers on non-specific immunity. *Pharm Biol*. 2010;48:1066–1072.

Tremlett H, Fu P, Yoshida E, Hashimoto S. Symptomatic liver injury (hepatotoxicity) associated with administration of complementary and alternative products (Ayurveda-AP-Mag Capsules) in a beta-interferon-treated multiple sclerosis patient. *Eur J Neurol*. 2011;18:e78,e79.

Yamada K, Hung P, Park TK, Park PJ, Lim BO. A comparison of the immunostimulatory effects of the medicinal herbs Echinacea, ashwagandha, and Brahmi. *J Ethnopharmacol*. 2011;137:231–235.

Ziauddin M, Phansalkar N, Patki P, Diwanay S, Patwardhan B. Studies on the immunomodulatory effects of Ashwagandha. *J Ethnopharmacol*. 1996;50:69–76.

Bee Venom Therapy and Other Forms of Apitherapy

! **Bee Venom Therapy**

? **Bee Pollen, Propolis, Raw Honey, and Royal Jelly**

Bee venom therapy, used by some people with multiple sclerosis (MS), is one type of *apitherapy*. This term refers to the use of bees or bee products to treat medical conditions. It is estimated that 5,000 to 10,000 people with MS in the United States use bee venom therapy.

Apitherapy has been used for thousands of years. It was used in ancient Egypt. In ancient Greece, Hippocrates used bee venom to treat arthritis. Bee venom therapy has been used by famous leaders, including Charlemagne, Ivan the Terrible, and Charles the Great.

In more recent times, apitherapy, especially bee venom therapy, has been recommended by some people for MS and other autoimmune conditions, such as rheumatoid arthritis, lupus, and scleroderma. In the United States, Charles Mraz, also known as "The Bee Man," first advocated bee venom therapy during the 1930s. He initially obtained beneficial effects on his own arthritis with bee venom therapy and subsequently recommended the treatment to people with arthritis and other inflammatory conditions, including MS. He claimed that the bee sting produces inflammation at the site of the sting and that the body then mounts an anti-inflammatory response. This anti-inflammatory response is believed to act not only against the sting but also against other inflammatory processes in the body.

A more recent advocate of bee venom therapy is Pat Wagner, known as "The Bee Lady." She has MS and claims to have used bee venom therapy effectively to treat herself.

⚠ Bee Venom Therapy

A variety of insects, collectively referred to as"bees,"may inject venom through a burning sting. Honeybees generally are used in bee venom therapy. Along with wasps, yellow jackets, and hornets, honeybees are species in a family of insects known as Hymenoptera.

The venom of bees is produced by specialized cells. It has two purposes: to defend against attackers and to weaken or paralyze prey. Bee venom contains a mixture of substances. The pain and swelling that result from a bee sting are produced by chemicals, including histamine, dopamine, norepinephrine, and serotonin. Bee venom also contains several toxins that are known as apamin, melittin, mast-cell degranulating peptide, and monamine. Finally, bee venom contains proteins that are involved in allergic responses. These proteins (including phospholipase-A2 and hyaluronidase) activate some immune cells and stimulate the production of one specific type of antibody, immunoglobulin E (IgE).

Bee venom contains many different substances. At this time, it is not known exactly how each of these substances interacts with the body and what effect they might have on a disease process such as MS.

Treatment Method

In bee venom therapy, a bee usually is grasped with tweezers and put on a particular part of the body. Tweezers then are used to remove the stinger 10 to 15 minutes after the sting. Ice may be applied to the skin before and after the sting to decrease the pain. Bee venom therapy typically is done in three sessions each week, and 20 to 40 stings are done in each session.

Studies in MS and Other Conditions

Experimental studies indicate that the components of bee venom have biological actions that could affect an inflammatory disease such as MS. Various mixtures of venom proteins produced anti-inflammatory effects in several experimental studies. Other research has shown that two specific components of venom, melittin and adolapin, have anti-inflammatory properties. In contrast, other studies have shown that bee venom components actually cause an inflammatory response.

Interestingly, apamin, a chemical constituent of the venom, has some effects that could be beneficial for MS. Apamin inhibits the action of a component of the nerve cell known as the *potassium channel*. This is the same part of the nerve cell affected by the MS medication Ampyra (also known as dalfampridine and 4-aminopyridine), which improves walking. However, it is not clear that bee venom therapy produces high enough levels of apamin in the central nervous system to significantly inhibit potassium channels. Further studies are needed in this area.

To attempt to determine the effect of bee venom on MS, research has been conducted using experimental allergic encephalomyelitis (EAE), an animal form of MS. At this time, these studies are limited and have produced inconsistent results. One study found that the treatment had no effect or produced worsening (1), while another study reported beneficial effects (2).

Bee venom therapy has been evaluated on a limited basis in people with MS. Isolated accounts exist of individuals with MS who improved after this treatment (3). A small clinical study of bee venom therapy in nine people with progressive MS was conducted at Georgetown University (4). This study, which was designed primarily to assess safety, did not report any major adverse effects. Over the course of the study, four people experienced worsening, two had improvement, and the remainder did not have any significant change. The conclusion of this study states that more research is needed but also states that "there was little evidence to support the use of honeybee venom in the treatment of MS." A more recent study, conducted in 2004 in The Netherlands, is the largest and highest quality study to date (5). In this clinical trial, a *randomized crossover study*, 26 people with relapsing-remitting or secondary-progressive MS were randomly assigned to receive either no treatment or bee venom therapy for 24 weeks. After this initial phase, people "crossed over" to the other treatment method for another 24 weeks—that is, those who received no treatment were then treated with bee venom therapy and those who received bee venom therapy then received no treatment. Detailed clinical and MRI measures were used to monitor people during the study. No beneficial effects were found in terms of various MRI measures, numbers of attacks, neurologic disability, fatigue, and overall quality of life. Bee venom therapy was generally well tolerated. Although this is the largest study to date, it was still relatively small and thus did not have the "power" to detect small to moderate beneficial effects.

Side Effects

In general, bee venom therapy is well tolerated. The most common side effect is swelling and redness at the sting site. About 20% of people experience itching, hives, fatigue, or anxiety. Women appear to have more frequent and severe side effects than do men. In the clinical trial of bee venom therapy in The Netherlands, no severe side effects were noted (5). Mild side effects included itching, flulike symptoms, and tenderness, swelling, and redness near sting sites. In the Georgetown study, four of the nine participants dropped out of the study due to side effects, which included spasticity, walking difficulties, visual problems, and bowel and bladder dysfunction.

Death is a very rare, but obviously important, adverse effect. Approximately 40 cases of bee sting deaths occur annually in the United States. Bee sting deaths frequently are attributed entirely to severe allergic reactions (anaphylaxis), but many of these deaths actually may be due to heart attacks that occur as a result of the stress of a mild allergic reaction in combination with heat, dehydration, or underlying heart disease. Importantly, severe allergic reactions may occur in individuals who have no past history of reactions to bee stings. Because of the possibility of a severe allergic reaction, a bee sting kit (Epi-Pen Autoinjector) should be available if bee venom therapy is used.

People with MS should be aware of other rare side effects of bee venom therapy. One form of inflammation of the nervous system, known as *acute disseminated encephalomyelitis* (ADEM), has been associated with bee stings. This inflammation typically involves multiple areas in the brain and spinal cord.

There are rare reports of liver toxicity due to bee venom. These reports have typically been described in the general population, but there is one report of a 35-year-old woman with MS who developed liver toxicity with associated yellowing of the skin (*jaundice*) due to bee venom therapy.

For people with visual problems due to MS, it is sometimes recommended that bee stings be given to the temple or eyebrows. However, bee stings on or near the eye may actually produce MS side effects. One specific type of inflammation associated with bee stings in this area is *optic neuritis*. This condition involves inflammation of the nerve that connects the eye to the brain. Optic neuritis may produce mild or severe impairment of vision and is actually one of the more common conditions caused by MS. There have been reports of stings on or near the eye producing an MS-like form of optic neuritis in people who do not have MS. Bee stings on or near the eye have caused several other serious problems, including eye movement abnormalities, infections, and cataracts. Thus, contrary to some recommendations, it would be safest for people with MS (and people without MS) to *avoid bee stings in this area*.

Finally, it is important to note that no formal studies have evaluated the long-term safety of bee venom therapy. As a result, it is not known if chronic bee venom therapy use is associated with significant toxic effects that have yet to be identified.

⑦ Other Bee Products

A variety of bee products other than bee venom also are used in apitherapy. These products often are recommended for MS and those symptoms that may occur with the disease, such as fatigue, weakness, visual difficulties, and memory problems. No evidence suggests that these products are effective for MS or MS-associated symptoms.

Bee Pollen

Bee pollen, which is composed of plant pollens, plant nectars, and bee saliva, is sometimes recommended to lessen fatigue, increase strength, and improve many other ailments. It contains a variety of nutrients, but it also may be contaminated with rodent debris, bacteria, insects, and the eggs and feces of insects. Rarely, bee pollen may cause severe allergic reactions, especially in those with pollen allergies. Asthma may worsen after bee pollen use. Isolated reports suggest that liver toxicity may be associated with bee pollen. Pollen could increase the risk of liver toxicity associated with some MS medications, such as interferons and methotrexate. Bee pollen may interfere with blood-thinning medications. Studies of bee pollen use in college and high school athletes have not demonstrated improvement in physical performance. There are no clear reasons for consuming bee pollen because it has no clear therapeutic properties and may have adverse effects.

Propolis

Propolis, a waxlike material also known as "bee glue," is collected by bees from buds on poplar and conifer trees and is used to repair cracks in hives. It may be weakly effective in killing a variety of bacteria and viruses. Limited studies have shown both stimulation and suppression of immune system activity. Propolis may facilitate the healing of herpes lesions in the mouth ("cold sores") and genital area. One component of propolis, caffeic acid phenethyl ester (CAPE), has anti-inflammatory effects and, in one study, decreased the severity of disease in EAE, the animal model of MS. Whether propolis has an effect on MS is not known—no published clinical studies have been undertaken of propolis use in MS. No studies have systematically examined the safety of propolis use. Propolis may cause allergic reactions, especially in people with allergies to bees or bee products. One case of severe kidney toxicity has been associated with propolis.

Raw Honey

It is sometimes claimed that honey contains valuable minerals and vitamins. Actually, honey contains approximately 80% sugar and 20% water. The mineral and vitamin content of honey is very low. Honey applied to the skin may improve healing from burns. No clinical studies have been undertaken of honey use in MS. Honey consumption is generally safe.

Royal Jelly

Royal jelly is recommended for many conditions, including some MS-associated symptoms such as weakness, depression, cognitive difficulties, and sexual problems. Royal jelly is a white substance produced by worker bees and is important in the development of queen bees. It has many chemical constituents, including neopterin, which is a compound secreted by immune system cells, and royalisin, a protein that has antibiotic activity. As with propolis, a small number of studies suggest that royal jelly may activate or suppress the immune system. No clinical studies exist of royal jelly use in MS. In people with asthma or a hyper-allergic condition known as *atopy*, royal jelly may provoke allergic symptoms, including itching, hives, eczema, swelling of the face and eyelids, shortness of breath, and asthma. Rarely, royal jelly may cause severe and potentially fatal asthma attacks (*status asthmaticus*) and allergic reactions (*anaphylaxis*). Royal jelly should be avoided by those with asthma and atopy.

Practical Information

Anyone considering bee venom therapy should first discuss it with a physician. For possible allergic reactions, it is important to have a bee sting kit available and to know how to use it. The names of local beekeepers can be obtained from the U.S. Department of Agriculture. Other bee products are available in pharmacies, health food stores, and apitherapy specialty stores.

Conclusion

No well-documented benefits have been noted for the use of bee venom therapy and other bee products for people with MS. One well-designed study of bee venom therapy in MS did not find any benefits in terms of various MRI and clinical measures. In addition, this type of treatment produces rare, but potentially serious, adverse effects, which include severe allergic reactions and death with bee venom therapy, and allergic reactions and worsening of asthma with the use of other bee products.

Additional Readings

Books

Bowling AC. Complementary and alternative medicine: practical considerations. In: Rae-Grant A, Fox R, Bethoux F, eds. *Multiple Sclerosis and Related Disorders: Diagnosis, Medical Management, and Rehabilitation*. New York, NY: Demos; 2013:243–249.

Cassileth BR. *The Alternative Medicine Handbook*. New York, NY: W.W. Norton; 1998:155–158.

Fetrow CW, Avila JR. *Professional's Handbook of Complementary and Alternative Medicines*. Philadelphia, PA: Lippincott Williams & Wilkins; 2004:79–81, 718–720.

Jellin JM, Batz F, Hitchens K. *Natural Medicines Comprehensive Database*. Stockton, CA: Therapeutic Research Faculty; 2014.

Journal Articles

Alqutub AN, Masooni I, Alsayari K, Alomair A. Bee therapy-induced hepatotoxicity: a case report. *World J Hepatol.* 2011;27:268–270.

Bowling AC. Complementary and alternative medicine and multiple sclerosis. *Neurol Clin.* 2011;29:465–480.

Boz C, Velioglu S, Ozmenoglu M. Acute disseminated encephalomyelitis after bee sting. *Neurol Sci.* 2003;23:313–315.

Castro HJ, Mendez-Inocencio JI, Omidvar B, et al. A phase I study of the safety of honeybee venom extract as a possible treatment for patients with progressive forms of multiple sclerosis. *Allergy Asthma Proc.* 2005;26:470–476.

DeMatos Silva LF, DePaula Ramos ER, Ambiel CR, Correia-de-Sá P, Alves-Do-Prado W. Apamin reduces neuromuscular transmission by activating inhibitory muscarinic M(2) receptors on motor nerve terminals. *Eur J Pharmacol.* 2010;626:239–243.

Ilhan A, Akyol O, Gurel A, Armutcu F, Iraz M, Oztas E. Protective effects of caffeic phenethyl ester against experimental allergic encephalomyelitis-induced oxidative stress in rats. *Free Radic Biol Med.* 2004;37:386–394.

Karimi A, Ahmadi F, Parivar K, et al. Effect of honey bee venom on Lewis rats with experimental allergic encephalomyelitis, a model for multiple sclerosis. *Iran J Pharm Res.* 2012;11:671–678.

Kim JI, Yang EJ, Lee MS, et al. Bee venom reduces neuroinflammation in the MPTP-induced model of Parkinson's disease. *Int J Neurosci.* 2011;121: 209–217.

Lee WR, Kim SJ, Park JH, et al. Bee venom reduces atherosclerotic lesion formation via anti-inflammatory mechanism. *Am J Chin Med.* 2010;38:1077–1092.

Lublin FD, Oshinsky RJ, Perreault, M, Siebert K. Effect of honey bee venom on EAE. *Neurology.* 1998;50:A424.

Maltzman JS, Lee AG, Miller NR. Optic neuropathy occurring after bee and wasp sting. *Ophthalmol.* 2000;107:193–195.

Mirshafiey A. Venom therapy in multiple sclerosis. *Neuropharmacol.* 2007;53: 353–361.

Motamed H, Forouzan A, Rasooli F, Majidi A, Verki MM. An isolated bee sting involving multiple cranial nerves. *Case Rep Emerg Med.* 2013;2013:920928.

Nam KW, Je KH, Lee JH, et al. Inhibition of COX-2 activity and proinflammatory cytokines (TNF-alpha and IL-1beta) production by water-soluble subfractionated parts from bee (Apis mellifera) venom. *Arch Pharm Res.* 2003;26:383–388.

Reisman RE. Unusual reactions to insect stings. *Curr Opin Allergy Clin Immunol.* 2005;5:355–358.

Song H-S, Wray SH. Bee sting optic neuritis. *J Clin Neuroophthalmol.* 1991;11: 45–49.

Wesselius T, Heersema DJ, Mostert JP, et al. A randomized crossover study of bee sting therapy for multiple sclerosis. *Neurology.* 2005;65:1764–1768.

⊘ Biofeedback

Biofeedback uses the mind–body connection for therapeutic purposes. Biofeedback involves the use of machines to monitor bodily functions such as heart rate, pulse, or muscle tension. An individual undergoing biofeedback attempts to consciously alter one of these presumably "involuntary" bodily processes. The use of biofeedback has been investigated for many medical conditions.

Treatment Method

In biofeedback, monitoring equipment is used to translate the activity of specific bodily functions into images or sounds. The images may be seen on a computer screen or the sounds may be heard. The monitoring methods that are used depend on which physiologic activity is of interest:

- Electromyography (EMG) biofeedback to monitor muscle tension.
- Thermal biofeedback to monitor skin temperature.
- Electrodermal response to monitor perspiration.
- Respiration biofeedback to monitor the rate, rhythm, and volume of breathing.
- Finger pulse biofeedback to monitor pulse rate.
- Brainwave biofeedback to monitor brain electrical activity.

During a biofeedback session, a biofeedback therapist assists an individual in altering the activity of a particular body process through mental or physical exercises. The individual learns methods to produce the desired change through feedback from the monitor, input from the therapist, and experimentation. These methods eventually can be used without the use of monitoring equipment.

Studies in Multiple Sclerosis and Other Conditions

Biofeedback may have applications for multiple sclerosis (MS)-related symptoms. For anxiety and insomnia, which may be significant problems in MS, biofeedback may be beneficial by promoting relaxation. It also may be helpful in treating some types of pain, including tension headaches, migraines, and low back pain. However, the use of biofeedback to treat MS-associated pain has not been formally studied.

Some research suggests that biofeedback may be helpful for people with urinary incontinence, a problem that may occur in MS. Medications and pelvic exercises are available for incontinence. These approaches may not be fully effective, however, and the medications may have undesirable side effects. Some, but not all, studies for biofeedback treatment of urinary incontinence have reported positive results—a few of these positive studies have been in MS. Biofeedback may be especially effective for people who have difficulty knowing which muscles to contract during the performance of pelvic exercises. Studies must be done to more fully evaluate biofeedback therapy for urinary incontinence.

People with MS also may experience bowel problems, including constipation and incontinence. In studies of people with MS and other medical conditions, biofeedback has produced beneficial effects on constipation and incontinence.

Biofeedback is currently under investigation for a wide range of other symptoms, some of which may occur in people with MS. These research studies are preliminary and use specialized equipment that is not currently available for widespread use. In these studies, promising results have been obtained with depression, walking difficulties, muscle stiffness (spasticity), and cognitive function.

An interesting issue is whether biofeedback may be used to regulate the immune system and, conceivably, thereby alter immune diseases such as MS. Variable effects of biofeedback-induced relaxation on immune function have been obtained; no consistent results have been reported.

Biofeedback may be an effective treatment for many other conditions. Biofeedback may decrease blood pressure. In addition, it may be beneficial for alcoholism, drug abuse, and posttraumatic stress disorder.

Side Effects

Biofeedback is usually very well tolerated. In the case of electrodermal biofeedback, people with heart conditions and pacemakers should be cautious and should discuss the treatment with their physician. Biofeedback should be done with medical supervision in those with psychosis or severe personality disorders. Biofeedback—and other methods that may promote relaxation—may occasionally cause anxiety, dizziness, disorientation, and floating sensations.

Practical Information

Biofeedback should be obtained from a trained therapist. Self-operated biofeedback devices are available, but biofeedback monitoring is a complex process that is most likely to be helpful when it is performed by a qualified practitioner. Biofeedback sessions typically last 30 to 60 minutes. The number of sessions required ranges from a few to 30 or 40. Health insurance sometimes provides coverage for this therapy.

Many trained biofeedback therapists are psychologists. Certification is provided by the Biofeedback Certification Institute of America. A directory of biofeedback therapists is available from:

- The Biofeedback Certification International Alliance (www.bcia.org), 10200 W. 44th Avenue, Suite 310, Wheat Ridge, CO 80033 (303-420-2902)

General information and information about research in this area is available:

- The Association for Applied Psychophysiology and Biofeedback (www.aapb.org), 10200 W. 44th Avenue, Suite 304, Wheat Ridge, CO 80033 (303-422-8894)

Conclusion

Biofeedback is a low-risk, moderate-cost therapy that may be beneficial for some MS-associated conditions. It may be especially helpful in those situations in which conventional medical approaches are not fully effective or produce side effects. MS symptoms that may be responsive to biofeedback include anxiety, bladder problems (incontinence), bowel problems (constipation, incontinence), pain, and sleeping problems. Further studies are needed to fully evaluate the effectiveness of biofeedback for MS symptoms. In terms of general health, biofeedback may reduce blood pressure.

Additional Readings

Books

Bauer B, ed. *Mayo Clinic Book of Alternative Medicine and Home Remedies.* New York, NY: Time Home Entertainment; 2013:98,99.

Bowling AC. Complementary and alternative medicine in multiple sclerosis. In: Geisser B, ed. *Primer on Multiple Sclerosis.* New York, NY: Oxford University Press; 2011:369–381.

Bowling AC. Complementary and alternative medicine: practical considerations. In: Rae-Grant A, Fox R, Bethoux F, eds. *Multiple Sclerosis and Related Disorders: Diagnosis, Medical Management, and Rehabilitation.* New York, NY: Demos; 2013:243–249.

Ernst E, ed. *The Desktop Guide to Complementary and Alternative Medicine: An Evidence-Based Approach.* Edinburgh, UK: Mosby; 2001:40–142.

Fugh-Berman A. *Alternative Medicine: What Works.* Baltimore, MD: Williams & Wilkins;1997:41–46.

Jellin JM, Gregory PJ, Batz F, et al. *Pharmacist's Letter/ Prescriber's Letter Natural Medicines Comprehensive Database.* Stockton, CA: Therapeutic Research Faculty; 2014.

McGrady A. Biofeedback in the neurologic disorders. In: Weintraub MI, Micozzi MS, eds. *Alternative and Complementary Treatment in Neurologic Illness.* New York, NY: Churchill Livingstone; 2001:156–165.

Micozzi MS, ed. *Fundamentals of Complementary and Alternative Medicine.* Philadelphia, PA: Saunders Elsevier; 2011:122,123.

Synovitz LB, Larson KL. *Complementary and Alternative Medicine for Health Professionals.* Burlington, MA: Jones & Bartlett Learning; 2013:209,210.

Journal Articles

Baram Y, Miller A. Glide-symmetric locomotion reinforcement in patients with multiple sclerosis by visual feedback. *Disabil Rehab Asst Techn.* 2010;5:323–326.

Brook RD, Appel LF, Rubenfire M, et al. Beyond medications and diet: alternative approaches to lowering blood pressure: a scientific statement from the American Heart Association. *Hypertension.* 2013;61:1360–1383.

Cattaneo D, Ferrarin M, Frasson W, Casiraghi A. Head control: volitional aspects of rehabilitation training in patients with multiple sclerosis compared with healthy subjects. *Arch Phys Med Rehabil.* 2005;86:1381–1388.

Klarskov P, Heely E, Nyholdt I, Rottensten K, Nordenbo A. Biofeedback treatment of bladder dysfunction in multiple sclerosis. A randomized trial. *Scand J Urol Nephrol Suppl.* 1994;157:61–65.

McClurg D, Ashe RG, Lowe-Strong AS. Neuromuscular electrical stimulation and the treatment of lower urinary tract dysfunction in multiple sclerosis—a double-blind, placebo controlled, randomized clinical trial. *Neurourol Urodyn.* 2008;27:231–237.

Munteis E, Andreu M, Martinez-Rodriguez JE, Ois A, Bory F, Roquer J. Manometric correlations of anorectal dysfunction and biofeedback outcome in patients with multiple sclerosis. *Mult Scler.* 2008;14:237–242.

Preziosi G, Raptis DA, Storrie J, Raeburn A, Fowler CJ, Emmanuel A. Bowel biofeedback treatment in patients with multiple sclerosis and bowel symptoms. *Dis Colon Rectum.* 2011;54:1114–1121.

Prosperini L, Leonardi L, De Carli P, Mannocchi ML, Pozzilli C. Visuo-proprioceptive training reduces risk of falls in patients with multiple sclerosis. *Mult Scler.* 2010;16:491–499.

Senders A, Wahbeh H, Spain R, Shinto L. Mind-body medicine for multiple sclerosis: a systematic review. *Autoimmune Dis.* 2012;2012:12.

Wahbeh H, Elsas S-M, Oken BS. Mind-body interventions: applications in neurology. *Neurology.* 2008;70:2321–2328.

Wiesel PH, Norton C, Roy AJ, Storrie JB, Bowers J, Kamm MA. Gut focused behavioural treatment (biofeedback) for constipation and faecal incontinence in multiple sclerosis. *J Neurol Neurosurg Psychiatry.* 2000;69:240–243.

⚠ Candida Treatment

Multiple sclerosis (MS) has been associated with Candida infections, which are caused by fungal infections due to a particular species of yeast. The most common type of Candida is *Candida albicans*. Mild infections with *Candida* may involve the mouth, which is referred to as thrush, or the vagina, which is referred to as monilia. More significant infections with *Candida* usually occur in people with conditions that suppress the immune system, such as AIDS and the use of chemotherapy medications. These infections may involve the mouth, throat, eye, heart, and bloodstream.

It has been proposed that many medical conditions are associated with an "overgrowth" of *Candida,* which is known as Candidiasis hypersensitivity, polysystemic candidiasis, or chronic candidiasis syndrome. Candidiasis hypersensitivity has been specifically suggested to be involved in MS. It is claimed that it may occur with MS because of MS-associated immune system abnormalities or the use of steroids and other MS medications that may suppress the immune system. In addition to MS, candidiasis hypersensitivity has been associated with fatigue, depression, anxiety, schizophrenia, rheumatoid arthritis, AIDS, breathing problems, and bladder infections. It is claimed that 30% of people in the United States have candidiasis hypersensitivity. Demonstrating the presence of the organism is apparently not necessary to make the diagnosis. These ideas have been popularized by Drs. William Crook and Orion Truss.

Treatment Method

Several treatment measures often are recommended for people with suspected candidiasis hypersensitivity. These include avoidance of moldy environments and dietary changes to eliminate foods that might contain yeast. Therapy also may involve the use of vitamin supplements and antifungal drugs such as nystatin, ketoconazole, or amphotericin.

Studies in MS and Other Conditions

There is not scientific or clinical evidence that *Candida* plays an important role in MS or in conditions other than obvious *Candida* infections. One Italian research group has identified biochemical evidence of *Candida* organisms in people with MS. However, the significance of these findings is not clear since these biochemical markers do not necessarily indicate true infection and they may be found in the general population. No large clinical studies have shown drug or diet therapy for *Candida* to be beneficial for MS or MS-associated symptoms.

Side Effects

If *Candida* therapy is considered, it must first be discussed with a physician. The antifungal drugs used for this therapy are generally well tolerated. However, they occasionally produce liver inflammation and, in rare situations, they have caused fatal liver injury.

Conclusion

Treatment for *Candida* should be approached cautiously. There is not any clear evidence that *Candida* causes MS or that treatment for *Candida* improves the course of the disease or symptoms of MS. Rarely, toxicity is associated with the medications used for treatment.

Additional Readings

Journal Articles

Benito-Leon J, Pisa D, Alonso R, Calleja P, Díaz-Sánchez M, Carrasco L. Association between multiple sclerosis and Candida species: evidence from a case-control study. *Eur J Clin Microbiol Infect Dis.* 2010;29:1139–1145.

Bennett JE. Searching for the yeast connection. *N Engl J Med.* 1990;323:1766–1767.

Blonz ER. Is there an epidemic of chronic candidiasis in our midst? *JAMA.* 1986;256:3138–3189.

Pisa D, Alonso R, Carrasco L. Fungal infection in a patient with multiple sclerosis. *Eur J Clin Microbiol Infect Dis.* 2011;30:1173–1180.

Pisa D, Alonso R, Jimenez-Jimenez FJ, Carrasco L. Fungal infection in cerebrospinal fluid from some patients with multiple sclerosis. *Eur J Clin Microbiol Infect Dis.* 2013;32:795–801.

! Chelation Therapy

Chelation therapy is a procedure in which metal-binding chemicals are given for health reasons. This form of treatment has sometimes been claimed to be effective for multiple sclerosis (MS). Some proponents advocate for its use for heart disease. Chelation has also been recommended for people with strokes, Parkinson's disease, Alzheimer's disease, muscular dystrophy, heart disease, narrowing of peripheral blood vessels (peripheral vascular disease), cancer, and arthritis. It is estimated that chelation therapy is used by more than 100,000 people in the United States annually.

Treatment Method

In chelation therapy, ethylenediaminetetraacetic acid (EDTA) or other chelating agents are administered by injection or by mouth. These agents bind strongly to (chelate) harmful metals to form "complexes" that are then excreted in the urine. Vitamin and mineral supplements are also frequently given. A course of treatment may involve 20 to 30 infusions that are given over the course of a few months.

Studies in MS and Other Conditions

The only clear indication for chelation therapy is heavy metal poisoning. Iron chelation has produced positive results in the animal model of MS and in limited clinical trials in people with MS. However, these studies are not definitive and therefore further research is needed. In the area of heart disease, a very large clinical investigation, the Trial to Assess Chelation Therapy (*TACT*) study, evaluated the effects of chelation in people with a past history of heart attacks. This study found moderately beneficial effects of chelation, but there were flaws with the study and, as a result, additional research is needed.

Side Effects

Chelation has potential risks. Side effects include kidney injury, bone marrow damage, anemia, breathing difficulty, irregular heart rhythms, low blood pressure, low blood levels of calcium and sugar (glucose), bleeding problems, and inflammation at the sites used for intravenous lines. Rarely, fatalities may occur. Fourteen deaths were attributed to chelation therapy in one clinic.

Practical Information

Chelation therapy is expensive. A course of treatment may cost between $3,000 and $5,000.

Conclusion

At this time, there is not strong clinical or scientific evidence to support the use of chelation in MS. This therapy is very expensive and may rarely produce serious side effects.

Additional Readings

Books

Cassileth BR. *The Alternative Medicine Handbook.* New York, NY: W.W. Norton; 1998:152, 153, 176,178.

Ernst E, ed. *The Desktop Guide to Complementary and Alternative Medicine: An Evidence-Based Approach.* Edinburgh, UK: Mosby; 2001:43,44.

Jellin JM, Gregory PJ, Batz F, et al. *Pharmacist's Letter/ Prescriber's Letter Natural Medicines Comprehensive Database.* Stockton, CA: Therapeutic Research Faculty; 2014.

Spencer JW, Jacobs JJ. *Complementary and Alternative Medicine: An Evidence-Based Approach.* St. Louis, MO: Mosby; 2003:156,157, 213,214.

Journal Articles

Bauchner H, Fontanarosa PB, Golub RM. Evaluation of the Trial to Assess Chelation Therapy (TACT): the scientific process, peer review, and editorial scrutiny. *JAMA.* 2013;309:1291,1292.

Ernst E. Fatalities after CAM: an overview. *Brit J Gen Pract.* 2011;61:404,405.

Lamas GA, Goertz C, Boineau R, et al. Effect of disodium EDTA chelation regimen on cardiovascular events in patients with previous myocardial infarction. *JAMA.* 2013;309:1241–1250.

Nissen SE. Concerns about reliability in the Trial to Assess Chelation Therapy (TACT). *JAMA.* 2013;309:1293,1294.

Wax PM. Current use of chelation in American health care. *J Med Toxicol.* 2013;9:303–307.

Weigel KJ, Lynch SG, LeVine SM. Iron chelation and multiple sclerosis. *ASN Neuro.* 2014;6:e00136.

Chiropractic Medicine

✓ **Chiropractic for Low Back Pain**

? **Chiropractic for Neck Pain and Other Symptoms**

Chiropractic medicine is one of the most popular forms of complementary and alternative medicine (CAM) in the United States. Chiropractors are the largest group of alternative medicine practitioners and the third largest group of health care professionals in the United States (after physicians and dentists). Among Americans, it is estimated that chiropractic care is used by about 5% of the general population and about 25% of those with multiple sclerosis (MS).

Part of the popularity of this therapy in the United States may be due to the fact that chiropractic medicine, unlike many other forms of CAM, was founded in this country. It was developed by Daniel D. Palmer, in Iowa, in the 1890s. Some form of spinal manipulation, as used in chiropractic medicine, also has been practiced in other cultures, including ancient Egypt and ancient Greece.

Chiropractic medicine has been severely criticized by mainstream medical professionals. The American Medical Association (AMA) has long questioned the effectiveness and safety of chiropractic medicine. In the 1960s, the AMA passed a resolution banning physicians from association with chiropractors and established a board, The Committee on Quackery, to discourage the use of chiropractors. In 1990, the Supreme Court ruled that the AMA was guilty of a conspiracy to "contain and eliminate" the chiropractic profession.

Treatment Method

Chiropractors believe that mild bone abnormalities of the spine are the cause of many medical disorders. According to this theory, the function of those nerves that leave the spine is altered by *subluxations* or misalignments of the bones of the spine. As a result, these bony abnormalities may produce nerve pressure, which may then affect many different muscles and organs of the body. This is sometimes compared to the decreased flow of water caused by standing on a garden hose and the increased, normal flow of water, caused by taking one's foot off the hose. Chiropractors attempt to treat these bone abnormalities through a variety of spinal manipulation techniques or *adjustments,* which presumably normalize the bone positions. In addition to this theory of spinal manipulation, chiropractic medicine holds that the body is able to heal itself; chiropractic medicine discourages the use of drugs and surgery.

Two groups of chiropractors are recognized: "straights" and "mixers." Straights use only spinal manipulation. Mixers, who represent the majority of chiropractors in the United States, use manipulation techniques and other measures, which may include ultrasound, massage, herb or vitamin supplements, and dietary recommendations.

Studies in MS and Other Conditions

No well-documented clinical trials demonstrate that chiropractic therapy improves the course of MS or improves MS-specific symptoms. Studies of chiropractic medicine applied to MS are limited to clinical studies with significant shortcomings or to isolated reports of individual responses to this therapy.

Musculoskeletal conditions that are seen in MS may respond favorably to chiropractic therapy. Specifically, multiple studies have evaluated the chiropractic treatment of low back pain, which may occur in people with MS. Of note, besides chiropractors, physical therapists and osteopaths also perform spinal manipulation. In addition, low back pain may resolve with no therapy at all and may respond to nonmanipulative forms of therapy given by primary care doctors, orthopedic physicians, neurologists, and physical therapists. The relative effectiveness and expense of these different approaches is not clear. In 1994, the Agency for Health Care Policy and Research endorsed chiropractic therapy for low back pain that is recent and not longstanding.

Spinal manipulation may also relieve neck pain, which occurs intermittently in many people, including those with MS. Some studies have reported positive results in this area, but in general these studies are less definitive than those in low back pain.

Chiropractic therapy has been investigated in other conditions. Among neurologic disorders, small or single-case studies note beneficial responses in people with headaches and spinal cord injury. These studies are too small to be conclusive. Chiropractic therapy sometimes is recommended for many other conditions, including asthma, ear infections, and gastrointestinal disorders. No strong evidence supports its use in these conditions.

Side Effects

Chiropractic therapy usually is well tolerated. Most complications are from neck manipulation. For people with serious diseases or symptoms, it is important to be evaluated and treated fully by a physician and not to substitute chiropractic medicine for conventional medicine. This is because chiropractors are not as well trained in diagnosis as are physicians.

For people who pursue chiropractic therapy, one of the more common adverse effects is achy muscles, which may last for 1 to 2 days after therapy. Chiropractic treatment may also cause headaches and fatigue. One significant possible complication is stroke associated with neck manipulation. This is very rare (one in 20,000 to one in approximately 3,000,000), but it also may be very serious. Bone fractures and injuries to disks are also very rare. Injuries to nerves of the lower spine as a result of lower back manipulation (cauda equina syndrome) are also extremely rare.

Chiropractic manipulation should be avoided by women who are pregnant and by people with spinal-bone fractures or dislocations, spine trauma, severe disc herniations, cancer or infection of the bone, severe osteoporosis, severe arthritis, severe diabetes, and those undergoing treatment with blood-thinning medications.

Practical Information

Chiropractic treatment often is done on a weekly basis. The initial visit is 30 to 60 minutes in length and may cost from $60 to $225. Follow-up visits, which typically take 10 to 20 minutes, may cost $30 to $75. Medicare, Medicaid, and some private health insurance plans may cover the cost of chiropractic therapy.

The amount of therapy needed depends on the individual and the type of problem. The number of visits is typically two to fifteen. For low back pain, improvement typically starts within 4 weeks, and the entire therapy course generally lasts 6 to 8 weeks.

Chiropractors are licensed in all states. More information about chiropractic medicine and practitioners may be obtained from:

- The American Chiropractic Association (www.acatoday.org), 1701 Clarendon Boulevard, Arlington, VA 22209 (703-276-8800).

- International Chiropractors Association (www.chiropractic.org), 6400 Arlington Boulevard, Falls Church, VA 22042 (703-528-5000).

Conclusion

There is not strong evidence that chiropractic therapy is beneficial for MS attacks or in altering the overall course of the disease. However, low back pain, which may occur with MS, responds positively to chiropractic manipulation. There is less supportive evidence that chiropractic therapy improves neck pain and headaches. Users of chiropractic therapy should be aware of the rare side effects, including stroke, and should rely on physicians, not on chiropractors, for the diagnosis and treatment of potentially serious conditions.

Additional Readings

Books

Bauer B, ed. *Mayo Clinic Book of Alternative Medicine and Home Remedies.* New York, NY: Time Home Entertainment; 2013:138,139.

Ernst E, ed. *The Desktop Guide to Complementary and Alternative Medicine: An Evidence-Based Approach.* Edinburgh, UK: Mosby; 2001:45–48.

Haldeman S, Hooper P. Chiropractic approach to neurologic illness. In: Weintraub MI, Micozzi MS, eds. *Alternative and Complementary Treatment in Neurologic Illness.* New York, NY: Churchill Livingstone; 2001:93–108.

Jellin JM, Gregory PJ, Batz F, et al. *Pharmacist's Letter/ Prescriber's Letter Natural Medicines Comprehensive Database.* Stockton, CA: Therapeutic Research Faculty; 2014.

Micozzi MS, ed. *Fundamentals of Complementary and Alternative Medicine.* Philadelphia, PA: Saunders Elsevier; 2011:255–273.

Navarra T. *The Encyclopedia of Complementary and Alternative Medicine.* New York, NY: Checkmark Books; 2005:27–29.

Swenson RS, Haldeman S. Chiropractic. In: Oken BS, ed. *Complementary Therapies in Neurology: An Evidence-Based Approach.* London, UK: Parthenon Publishing Group; 2003:27–49.

Synovitz LB, Larson KL. *Complementary and Alternative Medicine for Health Professionals.* Burlington, MA: Jones & Bartlett Learning; 2013:179–184.

Journal Articles

Bronfort G, Evans R, Anderson AV, Svendsen KH, Bracha Y, Grimm RH. Spinal manipulation, medication, or home exercise with advice for acute and subacute neck pain: a randomized trial. *Ann Intern Med.* 2012;156:1–10.

Elster E. Eighty-one patients with multiple sclerosis and Parkinson's disease undergoing upper cervical chiropractic care to correct vertebral subluxation: a retrospective analysis. *J Vertebral Sublux Res.* 2004;23(8):1–9.

Ernst E. Chiropractic: a critical evaluation. *J Symptom Pain Man.* 2008;35:544–562.

Ernst E. Fatalities after CAM: an overview. *Brit J Gen Pract.* 2011;61:404,405.

Goertz CM, Pohlman KA, Vining RD, Brantingham JW, Long CR. Patient-centered outcomes of high-velocity, low-amplitude spinal manipulation for low back pain: a systematic review. *J Electromyogr Kinesiol.* 2012;22:670–691.

Gouveia LO, Castanho P, Ferreira JJ. Safety of chiropractic interventions: a systematic review. *Spine.* 2009;34:e405–e413.

Kaptchuk TJ, Eisenberg DM. Chiropractic—origins, controversies, and contributions. *Arch Intern Med.* 1998;158:2215–2224.

Maiers M, Bronfort G, Evans R, et al. Spinal manipulative therapy and exercise for seniors with chronic neck pain. *Spine J.* 2013;13:1630–1636.

Plastaras C, Schran S, Kim N, Darr D, Chen MS. Manipulative therapy (Feldenkrais, massage, chiropractic manipulation) for neck pain. *Curr Rheum Rep.* 2013;15:339.

Rubinstein SM, Terwee CB, Assendelft WJ, de Boer MR, van Tulder MW. Spinal manipulative therapy for acute low back pain: an update of the Cochrane review. *Spine.* 2013;38:158 177.

Smith F, Bolton PS. What are the clinical criteria justifying spinal manipulative therapy for neck pain?—a systematic review of randomized controlled trials. *Pain Med.* 2013;14:460–468.

Smith WS, Johnston SC, Skalabrin EJ, Weaver M, Azari P, Albers GW, Gress DR. Spinal manipulative therapy is an independent risk factor for vertebral artery dissection. *Neurology.* 2003;60:1424–1428.

Walker BF, French SD. Pain in the neck: many (marginally different) treatment choices. *Ann Int Med.* 2012;156:52,53.

Walker BR, French SD, Grant W, Green S. A Cochrane review of combined chiropractic interventions for low-back pain. *Spine.* 2011;36:230–242.

⊙ Chronic Cerebrospinal Venous Insufficiency

Chronic cerebrospinal venous insufficiency (CCSVI), which refers to a condition of the veins that drain blood from the brain, has been claimed to play an important role in multiple sclerosis (MS). According to the CCSVI theory, which was first proposed in 2009, MS is caused by impaired blood flow away from the brain. This concept is very different from the current understanding that immune system abnormalities are primarily involved in MS. It has been claimed that MS may be treated by correcting CCSVI with medical procedures, known as angioplasty and stenting, which improve blood flow in these abnormal veins in the head and neck.

Treatment Method

Two procedures, sometimes referred to as *liberation therapy*, have been proposed to treat CCSVI. The main procedure that has been used is *balloon angioplasty*, which refers to inserting tubes, known as catheters, into the involved veins and inflating balloons attached to the catheters to expand the veins. If this is unsuccessful, then *stent placement* may be used—this procedure involves permanently placing small tubing in the obstructed areas of the veins.

Studies in MS and Other Conditions

The three original studies of CCSVI in MS were published by an Italian group in 2009 (1,2,3). These studies proposed specific tests and criteria for diagnosing CCSVI and procedures for its treatment. It was reported that 90% to 100% of people with MS have CCSVI. Also, in the original clinical trial, which had several limitations, CCSVI treatment was associated with significant improvement in function and decreased risk for MS attacks and new MRI lesions.

Since 2009, CCSVI in MS has been studied in many different research centers in multiple countries (4–9). The results of these studies do not provide support for the original claims about CCSVI. It has been difficult to diagnose the condition, since different diagnostic tests may produce conflicting results in the same individual. Also, many studies show that possible abnormalities in the veins are actually uncommon in people with MS and that the prevalence of abnormalities in those with MS is no different than that in the general population (4–9). For example, one high quality study used two different diagnostic procedures, catheter venography and ultrasound (5). With catheter venography, only 2% of people with MS were diagnosed with CCSVI, while 3% of those in a *control group*, who had no neurological condition, met the diagnostic criteria. When ultrasound was used in the same two groups, CCSVI was diagnosed in 44% of people with MS and 45% of those in the control group.

Side Effects

The procedures that are used to treat CCSVI may produce significant side effects (4,5). In 2012, the Food and Drug Administration (FDA) issued an alert about the potential dangers of CCSVI (10). This alert states that CCSVI procedures may produce serious and sometimes fatal complications. The FDA has received reports of one person with MS who died from bleeding in the brain and another who had a stroke after CCSVI treatment. Other side effects described in the FDA report include movement of stents from the vein to the heart, injury to veins, blood clots in the veins or stents, blood clots in the brain, damage to the nerves that travel from the brain to the facial area (*cranial nerves*), and abdominal bleeding.

Conclusion

There are not any studies that demonstrate that CCSVI is the cause of MS. The criteria for diagnosing CCSVI have not been established. CCSVI procedures do not produce any definite improvement in those with MS, and these procedures may cause significant adverse events, including death.

Additional Readings

Journal Articles

Anon. *FDA Safety Communication: Chronic Cerebrospinal Venous Insufficiency Treatment in Multiple Sclerosis Patients*. http://www.fda.gov/MedicalDevices/Safety/AlertsandNotices/ucm303318.htm. Updated 2012.

Comi G, Battaglia MA, Bertolotto A, et al. Observational case-control study of the prevalence of chronic cerebrospinal venous insufficiency in multiple sclerosis: results from the CoSMo study. *Mult Scler.* 2013;19:1508–1517.

Diuaconu CI, Conway D, Fox RJ, Rae-Grant A. Chronic cerebrospinal venous insufficiency as a cause of multiple sclerosis: controversy and reality. *Curr Treatment Opt Cardiovasc Med.* 2012;14:203–214.

Paul F, Wattjes MP. Chronic cerebrospinal venous insufficiency in multiple sclerosis: the final curtain. *Lancet.* 2014;383:106–108.

Rodger IW, Dilar D, Dwyer J, et al. Evidence against the involvement of chronic cerebrospinal venous abnormalities in multiple sclerosis. A case-control study. *PLoS One.* 2013;8:e72495.

Traboulsee AL, Knox KB, Machan L, et al. Prevalence of extracranial venous narrowing on catheter venography in people with multiple sclerosis, their siblings, and unrelated healthy controls: a blinded, case-control study. *Lancet.* 2014;383:138–145.

Tsivgoulis G, Sergentanis TN, Chan A, et al. Chronic cerebrospinal venous insufficiency and multiple sclerosis: a comprehensive meta-analysis of case-control studies. *Ther Adv Neurol Disord.* 2014;7:114–136.

Zamboni P, Galeotti R, Menegatti E, et al. Chronic cerebrospinal venous insufficiency in patients with multiple sclerosis. *J Neurol Neurosurg Psych.* 2009;80:392–399.

Zamboni P, Galeotti R, Menegatti E, et al. A prospective open-label study of endovascular treatment of chronic cerebrospinal venous insufficiency. *J Vasc Surg.* 2009;50:1348–1358.

Zamboni P, Menegatti E, Galeotti R, et al. The value of cerebral Doppler venous hemodynamics in the assessment of multiple sclerosis. *J Neurol Sci.* 2009;282:21–27.

ⓘ Colon Therapy, Detoxification, and Enemas

Colon therapy has been practiced for thousands of years. It was used in ancient Egypt and ancient Greece. The use of colon therapy in the United States began in the 1890s. At that time, it was often part of the therapy provided at health spas. One of the most well-known colonic therapists was John Harvey Kellogg, who, after treating thousands of people with colon therapy, went on to found the Kellogg cereal company. The popularity of colon therapy waned during the 1940s but has grown significantly since that time. It is estimated that tens of thousands of Americans are currently treated using colon therapy. Colon therapy sometimes is suggested for people with multiple sclerosis (MS) and also as a component of preventive health care.

Treatment Method

In colon therapy, the large intestine, or colon, is cleansed with liquid. Plastic tubes are placed in the rectum, and a solution, which may be water or water mixed with herbs, coffee, or enzymes, is then passed through the tubing and into the colon. The solution is eventually passed out through one of the tubes in the rectum. Although an ordinary enema generally uses about 1 quart of water, a session of colon therapy may use 20 or more gallons of water. Colon therapy sessions last approximately 1 hour.

Colon therapy is claimed to be beneficial because it involves "detoxification." It is believed that waste material on the walls of the intestine is toxic and that this material is absorbed into the bloodstream and produces disease. This toxic material is removed through colonic irrigation, and beneficial effects are allegedly produced.

Studies in MS and Other Conditions

No studies document that colon therapy is beneficial for MS. Colon therapy does not appear to be effective for any other medical condition or for improving or promoting general health. Standard enemas are effective for constipation.

Side Effects

It is important to be aware of possible serious side effects from colon therapy. Intestinal infections may develop if sanitary procedures are not used. In some well-known cases from the 1980s, people died from severe intestinal infections following colon therapy. Colon therapy also may produce generalized weakness, worsen hemorrhoids, cause chemical imbalances, and produce perforations, or holes, in the intestine. Colon therapy may be more dangerous in people with known diseases of the intestine, such as Crohn's disease, colon cancer, ulcerative colitis, and diverticulitis.

Conclusion

Colon therapy should be discussed with a physician. This therapy has no known beneficial effects for people with MS or any other medical condition and it may produce serious side effects.

Additional Readings
Books

Ernst E, ed. *The Desktop Guide to Complementary and Alternative Medicine: An Evidence-Based Approach*. Edinburgh, UK: Mosby; 2001:79.

Jellin JM, Gregory PJ, Batz F, et al. *Pharmacist's Letter/ Prescriber's Letter Natural Medicines Comprehensive Database*. Stockton, CA: Therapeutic Research Faculty; 2014.

Navarra T. *The Encyclopedia of Complementary and Alternative Medicine*. New York, NY: Checkmark Books; 2005:29–30.

Journal Articles

Acosta RD, Cash BD. Clinical effects of colonic cleansing for general health promotion: a systematic review. *Am J Gastroenterol.* 2009;104:2830–2936.

Ernst E. Colonic irrigation and the theory of autointoxication: a triumph of ignorance over science. *J Clin Gastroenterol.* 1997;24:196–198.

Ernst E. Colonic irrigation: therapeutic claims by professional organisations, a review. *Int J Clin Pract.* 2010;64:429–431.

Handley DV, Rieger NA, Rodda DJ. Rectal perforation from colonic irrigation administered by alternative practitioners. *Med J Austral.* 2004;181:575–576.

Mishori R, Otubu A, Jones AA. The dangers of colon cleansing. *J Fam Pract.* 2011;60:454–457.

Noriela S, Izham C, Khalid BAK. Colonic irrigation-induced hyponatremia. *Malaysian J Pathol.* 2004;26:117,118.

Preziosi G, Gosling J, Raeburn A, Storrie J, Panicker J, Emmanuel A. Transanal irrigation for bowel symptoms in patients with multiple sclerosis. *Dis Colon Rectum.* 2012;55:1066–1073.

Richards DG, McMillin DL, Mein EA, Nelson CD. Colonic irrigations: a review of the historical controversy and the potential for adverse effects. *J Altern Compl Med.* 2006;12:389–393.

Seow-Choen F. The physiology of colonic hydrotherapy. *Colorectal Dis.* 2009;11:686–688.

⊘Cooling Therapy

Cooling therapy is a unique form of therapy used by people with multiple sclerosis (MS). Small decreases in body temperature may lead to relief of some MS-related symptoms. Cooling methods range from the simple to the complex. The use of cooling suits for MS was introduced in the United States in the early 1990s.

The effect of heat on MS symptoms has been known for years. Worsening of symptoms with small increases in body temperature, which occurs in 60% to 80% of people with MS, was first described in the late 1800s by Dr. Wilhelm Uhthoff. The "hot bath test," developed in the 1960s, was one of the earliest methods for diagnosing MS. With this test, which is no longer used, people suspected of having MS were placed in a hot bath and assessed for any worsening of symptoms. A similar process may be observed early in the course of MS when the only noticeable manifestation of the disease is a symptom, such as weakness, numbness, or visual blurring, which occurs only in situations that increase body temperature, such as exercise, sunbathing, fever, or warm showers or baths.

Although warming may produce a worsening of symptoms, cooling may lead to improvement in symptoms. This cooling effect has been observed with cold baths or exposure to cold air. This beneficial response to cooling is the basis of cooling therapy.

Cooling therapy has a scientific basis. Nerve fibers (axons) that have damage to their insulating layer (myelin), as occurs in MS, exhibit slowing or blocking of nerve signal conduction with small increases in temperature. Thus, small decreases in temperature may facilitate transmission of nerve signals.

Treatment Method

Different techniques may be used to elicit cooling. Simple measures include taking cool showers or baths, sitting near a fan or air conditioner, using an ice pack, wearing cotton clothing, avoiding warm environments, and drinking cold liquids. More sophisticated approaches utilize garments, such as vests, that produce body cooling. Cooling garments may be "passive" or "active." Passive garments, which use ice packs or evaporation for cooling, are simpler and more portable, while active garments, which actively circulate coolants, appear to produce more effective cooling.

More sophisticated cooling methods are currently under investigation. Specialized "heat extraction devices" involve placement of one hand on a cold surface within a chamber that is under a vacuum. These devices take advantage of the large volume of blood that circulates just under the skin on the palm of the hand.

Studies in MS and Other Conditions

Small research studies indicate that cooling produces improvement in MS symptoms. One of the older studies, reported in the late 1950s, showed that a temperature reduction of as little as 1°F led to noticeable benefits. A 1995 investigation of six people with MS showed that cooling primarily improved fatigue and leg strength (1).

A rigorous study of cooling in MS was reported in 2003 (2). In this relatively large study, 84 people with MS and heat sensitivity were evaluated for both the short- and long-term effects of cooling. The cooling apparatus used in this research involved technology developed at the National Aeronautics and Space Administration (NASA). For the short-term component of the study, low-dose and high-dose cooling were administered for 1 hour. For the group that received high-dose cooling, a small amount of improvement was noted in multiple objectively measured parameters, including walking speed and visual abilities. Less notable changes were observed with low-dose cooling. In the long-term portion of the study, the effects of daily cooling over 1 month were examined. By self-assessment, people believed they improved in fatigue, strength, and thinking processes during this time.

Many other studies have yielded positive results for cooling in MS. Taken together, these various studies indicate cooling may produce improvement in a wide range of MS symptoms, including bladder dysfunction, cognitive problems, incoordination, fatigue, sexual difficulties, spasticity, speech problems, tremor, visual difficulties, walking, and leg weakness.

Side Effects

In general, the use of cooling garments is well tolerated. However, there may be a feeling of discomfort when cooling begins. Some people report that handling the garments is cumbersome.

It is important to keep in mind that individual variation occurs in the amount of cooling and the extent of benefit. Some people exhibit little or no reduction in body temperature with cooling. In approximately 10% of people with MS, a *paradoxical response* may occur, and symptoms may actually worsen with cooling therapy.

Practical Information

Cooling garments are available from several sources and are manufactured by:

- Body Cooler & Warmer (www.bodycooler.com), 1795 N. Fry Rd., Ste. 281, Katy, TX 77449 (832-422-7449 or 800-209-2665)

- Polar Products, Inc. (www.polarsoftice.com), 3380 Cavalier Trail, Stow, OH 44224 (330-253-9973 or 800-763-8423)

- Shafer Enterprises, L.L.C. (www.coolshirt.net), 10 Andrew Drive, Suite 200, Stockbridge GA 30281 (800-345-3176)
- Steele Incorporated (www.steelevest.com), P.O. Box 7304, Kingston WA 98346 (888-783-3538)

Health insurance coverage for cooling garments may be available.

Conclusion

Limited research studies have found that cooling produces improvement in multiple MS-associated symptoms, including bladder dysfunction, cognitive problems, fatigue, incoordination, sexual difficulties, spasticity, speech problems, tremor, visual difficulties, walking, and leg weakness. This therapy is usually well tolerated.

Additional Readings

Journal Articles

Brenakker EA, Oparina TI, Hartgring A, Teelken A, Arutjunyan AV, De Keyser J. Cooling garment treatment in MS: clinical improvement and decrease in leukocyte NO production. *Neurology.* 2001;57:892–894.

Capell E, Gardella M, Leandri M, et al. Lowering body temperature with a cooling suit as symptomatic treatment for thermosensitive multiple sclerosis patients. *Ital J Neurol Sci.* 1995;16:533–539.

Feys P, Helsen W, Liu X, et al. Effect of peripheral cooling on intention tremor in multiple sclerosis. *J Neurol Neurosurg Psych.* 2005;76:373–379.

Flensner G, Lindencrona C. The cooling-suit: a study of ten multiple sclerosis patients' experience in daily life. *J Adv Nursing.* 1999;29:1444–1453.

Grahn DA, Cao VH, Nguyen CM, Liu MT, Heller HC. Work volume and strength training responses to resistive exercise improve with periodic heat extraction from the palm. *J Strength Cond Res.* 2012;26:2558–2569.

Grahn DA, Murray J, Heller HC. Cooling via one hand improves physical performance in heat-sensitive individuals with multiple sclerosis: a preliminary study. *BMC Neurol.* 2008;8:14.

Guthrie TC, Nelson DA. Influence of temperature changes on multiple sclerosis: critical review of mechanisms and research potential. *J Neurol Sci.* 1995;29:1–8.

Ku Y-T, Montgomery LD, Lee HC, Luna B, Webbon BW. Physiologic and functional responses of MS patients to body cooling. *Am J Phys Med Rehabil.* 2000;79:427–434.

Ku Y-T, Montgomery LD, Webbon BW. Hemodynamic and thermal responses to head and neck cooling in men and women. *Am J Phys Med Rehab.* 1996;75:443–450.

Ku YT, Montgomery LD, Wenzel KC, Webbon BW, Burks JS. Physiologic and thermal responses of male and female patients with multiple sclerosis to head and neck cooling. *Am J Phys Med Rehab.* 1999;8:447–456.

Meyer-Heim A, Rothmaier M, Weder M, Kool J, Schenk P, Kesselring J. Advanced lightweight cooling-garment technology: functional improvements in thermosensitive patients with multiple sclerosis. *Mult Scler.* 2007;13: 232–237.

NASA/MS Cooling Study Group. A randomized controlled study of the acute and chronic effects of cooling therapy for MS. *Neurology.* 2003;60:1955–1960.

Nilsagard Y, Denison E, Gunnarsson LG. Evaluation of a single session with cooling garment for persons with multiple sclerosis—a randomized trial. *Disabil Rehabil Assist Technol.* 2006;1:225–233.

Poyraz T, Idiman E, Uysal S, et al. The cooling effect on proinflammatory cytokines interferon-gamma, tumor necrosis factor-alpha, and nitric oxide in patients with multiple sclerosis. *ISRN Neurol.* 2013;2013:964572.

Reynolds LF, Short CA, Westwood DA, Cheung SS. Head pre-cooling improves symptoms of heat-sensitive multiple sclerosis patients. *Can J Neurol Sci.* 2011;38:106–111.

White AT, Wilson TE, Davis SL, Petajan JH. Effect of precooling on physical performance in multiple sclerosis. *Mult Scler.* 2000;6:176–180.

⑦ Craniosacral Therapy

Craniosacral therapy, also known as cranial therapy, cranial osteopathy, and craniopathy, is a form of bone manipulation derived from chiropractic and osteopathic medicine. Dr. William G. Sutherland initially developed the technique in the United States in the early 1900s. A modified version was developed by Dr. John Upledger in the 1970s. Dr. Upledger currently provides instruction in this therapy to large numbers of health care providers through the Upledger Institute in Florida.

Treatment Method

Craniosacral therapy focuses on the bones of the skull, spine, and pelvis. Through massage, craniosacral therapy presumably facilitates the smooth flow of the cerebrospinal fluid (CSF), a watery liquid that surrounds the brain and spinal cord. According to the theory, more freely flowing CSF results in improved functioning of the central nervous system, immune system, and other bodily processes. Craniosacral therapists claim that they can detect the rhythmic movements of the skull bones.

Studies in Multiple Sclerosis and Other Conditions

The basic ideas that underlie craniosacral therapy are not consistent with the conventional understanding of skeletal anatomy or nervous-system functioning.

There is no clear evidence that impaired CSF flow is a common cause of disease or that craniosacral massage significantly alters CSF flow. Also, it is not clear that craniosacral therapy rhythm is a meaningful measurement or that it can be reliably detected.

In addition to the lack of scientific rationale for craniosacral therapy, there is a paucity of clinical research. Craniosacral therapy has not been specifically investigated in MS. Dr. Upledger writes: "We have treated a large number of multiple sclerosis patients with only moderate success. We often find a rather significant emotional component along with multiple sclerosis. Most often the emotional resistance is such that we have been unable to achieve optimal results with craniosacral therapy" (1).

Beneficial effects are claimed for many disorders. There are reports in the medical literature of improvement in anxiety, depression, MS-associated bladder difficulties, various types of pain, and sleeping difficulties. However, these studies have significant limitations.

Craniosacral therapy should be avoided in infants and children because the skull bones are not stable at a young age and manipulation could produce injury. Adverse effects of craniosacral therapy have been described in adults. Mild headaches were reported in one study of 55 people with mild head injury (2). In addition, three people, or approximately 5%, reported more serious side effects. These included dizziness and body stiffness (spasticity), both of which may be present in MS. Craniosacral therapy should be avoided by those with brain aneurysms (outpouching of blood vessels in the brain), bleeding in the brain, and increased pressure within the brain (increased intracranial pressure). Practitioners of craniosacral therapy state that the therapy may increase the effects of psychiatric, epileptic, and diabetic medications.

Practical Information

Craniosacral therapy sessions generally last from 30 to 60 minutes and cost between $50 and $250. For short-term conditions, one to three sessions over 1 to 3 weeks may be recommended. Long-term conditions may require weekly treatment for several months. The number of treatment sessions needed varies. Therapy may be performed by chiropractors, osteopaths, naturopaths, physical therapists, nurses, massage therapists, and physicians.

Conclusion

Most claims about the effectiveness of craniosacral therapy are not supported by well-designed clinical studies. Side effects may occur in 5% of people who are treated. The theoretical basis for the therapy is not consistent with the current understanding of the nervous system.

Additional Readings

Books

Ernst E, ed. *The Desktop Guide to Complementary and Alternative Medicine: An Evidence-Based Approach.* Edinburgh, UK: Mosby; 2001:48–50.

Jellin JM, Gregory PJ, Batz F, et al. *Pharmacist's Letter/ Prescriber's Letter Natural Medicines Comprehensive Database.* Stockton, CA: Therapeutic Research Faculty; 2014.

Micozzi MS, ed. *Fundamentals of Complementary and Alternative Medicine.* Philadelphia, PA: Saunders Elsevier; 2011:229,230.

Navarra T. *The Encyclopedia of Complementary and Alternative Medicine.* New York, NY: Checkmark Books; 2005:31.

Upledger JE. *Craniosacral Therapy.* Berkeley, CA: North Atlantic Books; 2001.

Journal Articles

Arnadottir TS, Sigurdardottir AK. Is craniosacral therapy effective for migraine? Tested with HIT-6 questionnaire. *Compl Ther Clin Pract.* 2013;19:11–14.

Castro-Sanchez AM, Mataran-Penarroche GA, Sanchez-Labraca N, et al. A randomized controlled trial investigating the effects of craniosacral therapy on pain and heart rate variability in fibromyalgia patients. *Clin Rehabil.* 2011;25: 25–35.

Elden H, Ostgaard HC, Glantz A, Marciniak P, Linnér AC, Olsén MF. Effects of craniosacral therapy as adjunct to standard treatment for pelvic girdle pain in pregnant women: a multicenter, single blind, randomized controlled trial. *Acta Obstet Gynecol Scand.* 2013;92:775–782.

Fernandez-de-Las-Penas C, Alonso-Blanco C, Cuadrado ML, Miangolarra JC, Barriga FJ, Pareja JA. Are manual therapies effective in reducing pain from tension-type headaches?: a systematic review. *Clin J Pain.* 2006;22:278–285.

Green C, Martin CW, Bassett K, Kazanjian A. A systematic review of craniosacral therapy: biological plausibility, assessment reliability and clinical effectiveness. *Compl Ther Med.* 1999;7:201–207.

Greenman PE, McPartland JM. Cranial findings and iatrogenesis from craniosacral manipulation in patients with traumatic brain syndrome. *J Am Osteopath Assoc.* 1995;95:182–188, 191–192.

Hanten WP, Dawson DD, Iwata M, Seiden M, Whitten FG, Zink T. Craniosacral rhythm: reliability and relationships with cardiac and respiratory rates. *J Orthoped Sports Phys Ther.* 1998;27:213–218.

Hartman SE, Norton JM. Craniosacral therapy is not medicine. *Phys Ther.* 2002;82:1146–1147.

Jakel A, von Hauenschild P. A systematic review to evaluate the clinical benefits of craniosacral therapy. *Compl Ther Med.* 2012;20:456–465.

Mataran-Penarroacha GA, Castro-Sanchez AM, Garcia GC, Moreno-Lorenzo C, Carreño TP, Zafra MD. Influence of craniosacral therapy on anxiety, depression and quality of life in patients with fibromyalgia. *Evid Based Complement Alternat Med.* 2011;2011:178769.

Moran RW, Gibbons P. Intraexaminer and interexaminer reliability for palpation of the cranial rhythmic impulse at the head and sacrum. *J Manipulative Physiol Ther.* 2001;24:183–190.

Raviv G, Shefi S, Nizani D, Achiron A. Effect of craniosacral therapy on lower urinary tract signs and symptoms in multiple sclerosis. *Complem Ther Clin Pract.* 2009;15:72–75.

Rogers JS, Witt PL, Gross MT, Hacke JD, Genova PA. Simultaneous palpation for the cranialsacral rate at the head and feet: intrarater and interrater reliability and rate comparisons. *Phys Ther.* 1998;78:1175–1185.

Wirth-Pattullo V, Hayes KW. Interrater reliability of craniosacral rate measurements and their relationship with subjects' and examiners' heart and respiratory rate measurements. *Phys Ther.* 1994;74:917–920.

① Dental Amalgam Removal

The removal of dental amalgam has been proposed as a therapy for multiple sclerosis (MS). This treatment is based on the idea that metal in amalgam is slowly released and causes or worsens MS.

Dental amalgam is composed of mercury as well as silver, copper, tin, and zinc. Amalgam has been used for more than 150 years to fill cavities and is used currently for 80% to 90% of tooth restorations.

Very small amounts of mercury are released from amalgam in teeth in the form of solid mercury and mercury vapor. It is claimed that the mercury released from amalgam damages the immune system and nervous system and thereby causes MS and other diseases. In addition, it has been proposed that disease is caused by harmful allergic reactions to the mercury or to the electrical currents generated by mercury. The presumed mercury toxicity is termed *mercury hyper-sensitivity, mercury sensitivity, mercury toxicity,* or *micromercurialism*. Electricity generated by mercury is called *electrogalvinism* or *oral galvanism*.

Treatment Method

A specific procedure often is used when amalgam removal is considered. Questionnaires about symptoms may be administered. The evaluation may include electrical readings of restorations, skin-patch allergy testing, mercury-vapor tests, and hair analysis. Amalgam removal may be done by removing a few fillings at a time; this technique is claimed to release "locked mercury." Gold or plastic fillings are used after amalgam removal.

Studies in MS and Other Conditions

Dental amalgam has been implicated in MS on the basis of several claims and observations. Anecdotal reports exist of people with MS benefiting from amalgam removal. Also, MS has been associated with both dental caries—the bacterial disease of teeth that produces cavities—and dental treatment. Finally, it has been proposed that MS is caused by exposure to mercury or other heavy metals.

Dental amalgam has been implicated in many other diseases. These include diseases that may have an immunologic basis, such as arthritis, lupus, and chronic fatigue syndrome, as well as other neurologic diseases, such as headache, epilepsy, brain tumor, and Parkinson's disease. Amalgam also has been implicated in depression, cancer, and heart disease.

Contrary to what sometimes is claimed, no evidence demonstrates that mercury causes MS or that the removal of dental amalgam improves the course of MS. Although mercury toxicity may produce symptoms that resemble those of MS, the underlying damage to the nervous system with mercury toxicity is quite different from that of MS. The levels of mercury in the brain are similar for people with MS and the general population. In addition, some people with MS have no dental amalgam, and MS was recognized as a disease before amalgam was used routinely in dental practice. Some studies of large populations have shown a trend for people with MS to have more dental caries or more dental amalgam than the general population—these trends, however, have not been statistically significant. Finally, the amount of mercury released from amalgam is very low. Studies in the early 1980s first indicated that relatively high levels of mercury are released, but subsequent studies demonstrated low levels of mercury release.

It is estimated that mercury from amalgam constitutes 10% or less of all the mercury consumed by an individual; other sources of mercury are food (especially fish), pollution, medications, paints, and disinfectants. For dental amalgam to produce mercury levels that are associated with even minimal toxic effects, it has been calculated that an individual would need approximately 500 amalgam surfaces or approximately 200 dental fillings.

Although some anecdotal reports document benefit from amalgam removal, no well-designed studies demonstrate that amalgam removal improves the course of MS. Studies of large numbers of people with MS have not shown any association between dental treatment and MS attacks. Dentists and dental staffs are exposed to relatively high doses of mercury and have blood mercury levels that are three to five times higher than the general population, yet MS is no more common in the dental profession than in the general population.

Professional guidelines do not recommend amalgam removal for MS. The medical advisory board of the National Multiple Sclerosis Society of the United States, the Public Health Service, and the National Institutes of Health (NIH) do not support this treatment. In 1987, the American Dental Association (ADA) determined that unnecessary amalgam removal is improper and unethical. In 1996, a Colorado dentist who actively performed amalgam removal on people with MS had his dentist's license revoked by the Colorado State Board of Medical Examiners.

No evidence demonstrates that significant allergies to mercury cause disease. Allergy to mercury actually is extremely rare and, when it does occur, it produces swelling of the tissues around an amalgam-filled tooth—it has not been associated with other diseases or conditions.

No large, well-documented studies have formally evaluated this treatment. In other words, no large group of people with MS has been studied to determine if removing amalgam produces a statistically better clinical course than not removing amalgam. Although the ideal clinical study has not been conducted, it is not clear that enough suggestive evidence warrants the time, resources, and expense of such a study.

Side Effects

In general, dental amalgam removal is well tolerated. Rarely, it can damage nerves or tooth structure. For a short time, removal of amalgam may actually *increase* blood levels of mercury.

Conclusion

It is very difficult to determine with absolute certainty whether a compound such as dental amalgam is completely safe. The ideal clinical studies in MS have not been conducted. However, based on available evidence, there is no strong indication that dental amalgam causes or worsens MS or that amalgam removal has a beneficial effect on MS. Amalgam removal is usually well tolerated, but it may be very expensive.

Additional Readings

Journal Articles

Aminzadeh KK, Etminan M. Dental amalgam and multiple sclerosis: a systematic review and meta-analysis. *J Public Health Dent.* 2007;67:64–66.

Attar MA, Kharkhanch A, Etemadifar M, Keyhanian K, Davoudi V, Saadatnia M. Serum mercury level and multiple sclerosis. *Biol Trace Elem Res.* 2012;146:150–153.

Bates MN, Fawcett J, Garrett N, Cutress T, Kjellstrom T. Health effects of dental amalgam exposure: a retrospective cohort study. *Int J Epidemiol.* 2004;33:1–9.

Casetta I, Invernizzi M, Granieri E. Multiple sclerosis and dental amalgam: case control study in Ferrara, Italy. *Neuroepidemiology.* 2001;20:134–137.

Clarkson TW, Magos L. The toxicology of mercury and its chemical compounds. *Crit Rev Toxicol.* 2006;36:609–662.

Ekstrand J, Bjorkman L, Edlund C, Sandborgh-Englund G. Toxicological aspects on the release and systemic uptake of mercury from dental amalgam. *Eur J Oral Sci.* 1998;106:678–686.

Eley BM, Cox SW. The release, absorption, and possible health effects of mercury from dental amalgam: a review of recent findings. *Brit Dental J.* 1993;175: 355–362.

Eulalia-Troisfontaines ES, Martinez-Perez E-M, Miegimolle-Herrero M, Planells-Del Pozo P. Oral health status of a population with multiple sclerosis. *Med Oral Patol Oral Cir Buccal.* 2012;17:223–227.

Eyeson J, House I, Yang YH, Warnakulasuriya KA. Summary of relationship between mercury levels in blood and urine and complaints of chronic mercury toxicity from amalgam restorations. *Brit Dental J.* 2010;208:162,163.

Fung YK, Meade AG, Rack EP, Blotcky AJ. Brain mercury in neurodegenerative disorders. *J Toxicol Clin Toxicol.* 1997;35:49–54.

Mackert JR, Berglund A. Mercury exposure from dental amalgam fillings: absorbed dose and the potential for adverse health effects. *Crit Rev Oral Biol Med.* 1997;8:410–436.

McGrother CW, Dugmore C, Phillips MJ, Raymond NT, Garrick P, Baird WO. Multiple sclerosis, dental caries and fillings: a case-control study. *Brit Dent J.* 1999;187:261–264.

NIH Conference Assessment. Effects and side-effects of dental restorative materials. *Adv Dental Res.* 1992;6:1–144.

Sheridan P. Amalgam restorations and multiple sclerosis. *MS Management.* 1997;4:21–40.

! Enzyme Therapy

Enzymes are a type of protein used by the body to perform chemical reactions. Enzymes break down food in the digestive tract and carry out essential chemical functions in the rest of the body. It is claimed that treatment with enzymes is beneficial for many diseases, including multiple sclerosis (MS).

Enzyme therapy has a long history. In one form of possible enzyme therapy, the Indians of Central America and South America traditionally use the leaves and fruit of papaya trees and the fruit of pineapples to treat inflammatory conditions. John Beard, a Scottish embryologist, first used enzyme therapy for cancer treatment in 1902. During the 1920s, Dr. Edward Howell claimed that consuming large amounts of enzymes prevented the body from depleting its own natural enzyme supply. In Germany, during the 1960s and 1970s, enzyme treatment was recommended for MS, cancer, viral infections, and a variety of inflammatory conditions. Enzyme therapy was promoted by Drs. Max Wolf and Karl Ransberger.

Two major types of enzyme therapy are used. In *digestive enzyme* therapy, advocates claim that digestive enzyme supplements improve the breakdown of food, increase nutrient absorption, and decrease the accumulation of toxins. Through these mechanisms, enzyme therapy is believed to effectively treat hundreds of diseases and maintain health. With the other type of enzyme therapy, *systemic enzyme therapy*, it is believed that special enzyme preparations pass through the stomach undigested and then are absorbed into the bloodstream from the intestines. Whether this process occurs, and whether it offers any benefit, is unproven. It is claimed that enzyme therapy has been used by many well-known public figures, including Charlie Chaplin, Marlene Dietrich, J. Edgar

Hoover, Aldous Huxley, members of the Kennedy family, Marilyn Monroe, and Pablo Picasso.

Enzyme therapy was under much scrutiny in the United States during the 1980s. In 1986, the U.S. Food and Drug Administration (FDA) ordered one company, Enzymatic Therapy, Inc., to discontinue its published research bulletins because of false claims. Subsequently, the FDA continued to monitor informational seminars and material produced by the company. In 1992, the use of false claims by the company was prohibited by a court order.

Treatment Method

Most enzyme therapy involves taking supplements that contain enzymes obtained from animals or plants. Digestive enzymes from animal sources include proteases (chymotrypsin and trypsin), amylases, and lipases. Examples of plant-derived enzymes are bromelain from pineapples, papain from papaya, and ficin from figs. In Europe, intravenous infusions of enzymes or enemas of enzyme-containing solutions are also sometimes recommended.

Rare situations occur in which enzyme therapy is used in conventional medicine. These conditions include pancreatitis, cystic fibrosis, and Gaucher disease. An enzyme known as *lactase* is given for people who cannot tolerate dairy products (lactose-intolerance). People with excessive gas may find relief from Beano, an enzyme (alpha-galactosidase) that improves the digestion of high-fiber foods, such as beans, peas, and whole grains.

Studies in MS

Specific enzyme treatment regimens, along with vitamin and mineral supplements, are sometimes recommended for people with MS. Surprisingly, some of these enzymes and other supplements are suggested because they stimulate the immune system. Despite the detailed and lengthy recommendations offered for MS, there is not any clinical research evidence that supports the use of this therapy in MS.

A form of enzyme treatment known as *oral hydrolytic enzyme therapy* has been studied in MS. Some early reports in the German medical literature suggested that this type of enzyme therapy may be helpful for MS. Also, this therapy was reported to be beneficial in the animal model of MS and to produce immune-system changes in humans that, in theory, would be beneficial for MS. Due to these observations, a study of oral hydrolytic enzyme therapy was conducted (1). This 2-year study, which included more than 300 people with relapsing MS at 22 MS clinics in Europe, compared the clinical and magnetic resonance imaging (MRI) effects of an enzyme therapy (bromelain, trypsin, rutoside) with placebo. This study met the criteria for a well-conducted clinical trial—it involved multiple clinics (*multicenter*), placebo treatment (*placebo-controlled*), the random assignment of enzyme treatment or placebo to patients (*randomized*), and patients and clinicians who were unaware of who received enzyme therapy or placebo (*double-blinded*). Unfortunately, enzyme therapy did not produce therapeutic effects on the basis of progression of disability, number of attacks, or multiple MRI criteria.

Intravenous enzyme therapy also has been proposed for MS and other immune system diseases. It is claimed that intravenous enzymes may help break down harmful "immune complexes." A preliminary study in Austria reported some beneficial effects for this therapy in MS. Enzyme-containing enemas also have been recommended for MS, but no research evidence supports their use.

Side Effects

Oral enzyme therapy is generally well tolerated. There may be changes in the color, consistency, and odor of the stools when starting treatment. Excessive gas, nausea, diarrhea, and minor allergic reactions also may occur. Ulcers may be worsened by the use of one class of enzymes known as proteases. People with hypersensitivity to pork may not tolerate pork-derived pancreatic enzymes. No significant side effects were reported in the large study of enzyme therapy in MS (1). The safety of long-term enzyme therapy has not been investigated. There is a theoretical possibility that long-term use could decrease the ability of the digestive system to secrete its own enzymes. Enzyme therapy should be avoided by women who are pregnant or breastfeeding, people who take blood-thinning medications, and people who have blood-clotting disorders, severe kidney disease, protein allergies, and recent surgical procedures. With intravenous enzyme therapy, rare but serious adverse effects are possible, including infections and severe allergic reactions.

Conclusion

In the medical literature published in English, no well-documented benefits of enzyme therapy have been noted for people with MS. A well-designed European clinical trial did not demonstrate any therapeutic effects of enzyme therapy in MS. Claims about this therapy may be exaggerated. The long-term safety of enzyme therapy has not been determined. Intravenous enzyme therapy may produce rare, but serious, side effects.

Additional Readings

Books

Cassileth BR. *The Alternative Medicine Handbook.* New York, NY: W.W. Norton & Company, Inc.; 1998:183–185.

Kowalak JP, Mills EJ, eds. *Professional Guide to Complementary and Alternative Therapies.* Springhouse, PA: Springhouse Publishing; 2001:193–194.

Journal Articles

Baumhackl U, Kappos L, Radue EW, et al. A randomized, double-blind, placebo-controlled study of oral hydrolytic enzymes in relapsing multiple sclerosis. *Mult Scler.* 2005;11:166–168.

Desser L, Rehberger A, Kokron E. Cytokine synthesis in human peripheral blood mononuclear cells after oral administration of polyenzyme preparations. *Oncology.* 1993;50:403–407.

Taragoni OS, Tary-Lehmann M, Lehmann PV. Prevention of murine EAE by oral hydrolytic enzyme treatment. J *Autoimmunol.* 1999;12:191–198.

⊛ Exercise

Exercise has been categorized in many different ways over the years. In the past, exercise and other lifestyle approaches were actually sometimes classified as forms of complementary and alternative medicine (CAM). More recently, exercise has been viewed as conventional medicine or entirely out of the realm of medicine, as a type of self-care or as a component of one's lifestyle. Some forms of *unconventional* exercise, such as tai chi and yoga, are still often regarded as forms of CAM. Regardless of its formal classification, it is important to consider exercise because it has significant health implications for people with multiple sclerosis (MS) and it is not always fully discussed or monitored on an ongoing basis during conventional medical office visits.

Attitudes about exercise and MS have changed dramatically. In the past, regular exercise was not generally recommended for people with MS. However, more recent research indicates that exercise produces multiple beneficial effects and may actually be one of the best nonpharmacologic strategies for alleviating multiple MS symptoms. Appropriate forms of regular exercise are now routinely recommended for people with MS. In this book, additional information about exercise and MS may be found in the *Step 4—Physical Activity* chapter of *Part 2*.

Treatment Method

Many exercise programs are possible for people with MS. Conventional exercise programs typically include aerobic exercise and strengthening. A comprehensive program also includes stretching and balance exercises, two areas that may be particularly beneficial for those with MS and are often absent from standard exercise programs. Many exercise regimens may be modified so they are appropriate for all levels of physical functioning.

The absolute *best* exercise program for people with MS has not been established. A Canadian committee of experts methodically reviewed the large number of clinical studies of exercise and MS and developed guidelines based on these studies (1). The guidelines, which are for people with mild to moderate disability, state that "important fitness benefits" can be obtained with the following regimen:

- Aerobic activity: at least 30 minutes of moderate intensity activity twice weekly

- Muscle strengthening: at least twice weekly strengthening of all major muscle groups

Of note, these exercise recommendations are based only on MS studies. Studies of other conditions, such as heart disease, indicate that more exercise should be done on a weekly basis. For example, for overall heart health, the American Heart Association (AHA) recommends:

- Aerobic: at least 30 minutes of moderate intensity activity for at least 5 d/wk for a total of 150 minutes weekly or at least 25 minutes of vigorous, or a combination of moderate and vigorous, activity for at least 3 d/wk for a total of 75 minutes weekly

- Muscle strengthening: at least 2 d/wk of moderate- to high-intensity of strengthening

Exercise programs must be tailored to the interests and needs of the individual. Each person with MS has individualized exercise preferences and, due to the diverse effects of MS, specific physical strengths and weaknesses. These must be taken into account in order to develop a program that is safe and effective. Also, the program should be enjoyable and rewarding so that one is motivated to do it regularly and on a long-term basis. An individualized exercise program for a person with MS is typically developed by a physical therapist.

In addition to conventional exercise programs, there are *unconventional* exercise programs, some of which may be particularly well-suited to those with MS. *Hydrotherapy*, or *aquatic therapy*, refers to exercising in water. This form of exercise is especially appropriate for those with MS because water makes one feel lighter and eliminates the risk of injuries from falling. Also, cool water may prevent body warming while exercising. People with MS may benefit from a wide range of other unconventional exercise approaches, especially those that emphasize stretching or balance, such as yoga, tai chi, and Pilates—all of these approaches are discussed in detail elsewhere in this book (see chapters on *Yoga, Tai Chi, and Qigong,* and *Pilates Method and PhysicalMind Method.*

Studies in MS and Other Conditions

Exercise produces a remarkable array of preventive and therapeutic health effects. These range from very specific neurological and psychological benefits to more general effects on conditions such as heart disease, stroke, diabetes, cancer, and osteoporosis.

In the area of MS and exercise, a landmark study was published in 1996 (2). This study significantly changed the attitudes and approaches of health professionals toward exercise in MS. This study of 54 people with MS evaluated the effects of 40 minutes of aerobic exercise that was done three times weekly for 15 weeks. Exercise produced benefits for physical as well as mental symptoms, including weakness, impaired bowel and bladder function, fatigue, depression, and anger.

There have been many subsequent studies that have shown beneficial effects of exercise for many MS symptoms (3–14). It is important to note that these studies have been in people with a wide range of disabilities and also in people with relapsing as well as progressive forms of MS. It is also important to recognize that this is an evolving area of research. There are now a large number of studies in this area, but there limitations with some of the studies and challenges with interpreting the diverse results of the studies.

There are many MS symptoms that have shown improvement with exercise. The most consistent results have been with muscle strength. Many studies have also reported improvement with walking and balance. One of the more paradoxical findings has been improvement in fatigue, the most common disabling MS symptom. While exercise is a *physical* activity, studies in MS and other conditions indicate that exercise alleviates *mental* symptoms, such as depression, anxiety, and anger. In fact, when considering depression therapies other than medications and psychotherapy, exercise is probably the most effective treatment. Perhaps related to this effect on mood, exercise has been associated with improved sleep. In addition, several studies on MS and other neurological conditions indicate that aerobic exercise may improve cognitive function. Stretching exercises, which may be part of a conventional exercise program or a component of unconventional exercise programs such as tai chi, Pilates, and yoga, may decrease muscle stiffness (spasticity).

Pain is a common MS symptom and, on the basis of scientific studies and animal model evidence, exercise has the potential to alleviate many different types of pain. In clinical studies on exercise and pain, beneficial effects have been reported for various types of pain—the most consistent findings have been with musculoskeletal conditions, such as neck and low back pain.

A general exercise program may be beneficial for bladder and bowel function. Also, a specific type of exercise called *Kegel exercises* or pelvic-floor muscle exercises may be especially helpful. With these exercises, the pelvic muscles that are used to voluntarily stop urination are flexed on a regular basis. It often is recommended that these muscles be exercised 60 to 80 times daily.

Some studies indicate that Kegel exercises improve urinary function in both women and men by decreasing incontinence, urgency, and frequency. In some of these studies, the exercises have been combined with electrical stimulation or biofeedback (see *Biofeedback* chapter). For bowel function, pelvic-floor exercises may improve incontinence and constipation.

MS may impair sexual function in men and women, and various forms of exercise may improve sexual function. For example, in the general population, limited studies indicate that increased exercise levels improve sexual function in men as well as women. In men, pelvic-floor exercise may improve erectile dysfunction. Finally, among unconventional exercise programs, it is plausible that Pilates and yoga could produce beneficial effects (see *Pilates* and *Yoga* chapters). There are anecdotal claims that Pilates and yoga greatly enhance sexual function and satisfaction. These approaches could increase pelvic awareness and muscle strength in a way that could improve sexual function. However, there is very little formal research in this area.

The range of MS-associated symptoms that may potentially improve with exercise is remarkable. To summarize, exercise may improve:

- Strength, walking, and spasticity

- Anxiety, depression, and anger

- Bowel, bladder, and sexual function

- Cognitive function

- Sleep

- Fatigue

- Pain

In addition to its effects on MS symptoms, exercise has other significant general health benefits. The list of exercise effects in this area is long and wide-ranging:

- Reduces the risk of heart disease and stroke

- Lowers blood pressure and improves blood lipids (cholesterol)

- Helps with weight management and decreases the risk of obesity and obesity-related diseases

- Decreases the risk of diabetes and helps with diabetes control

- Decreases the risk of some forms of cancer, including colon, breast, prostate, and uterine lining (endometrium)

- Prevents and treats osteoporosis, which may occur in MS

- Reduces overall risk of death

As can be seen, many of the general health effects of exercise are on typical *lifestyle diseases* that are not directly related to the nervous system, such as heart disease, high blood pressure, diabetes, and obesity. However, studies indicate that having one of these lifestyle diseases along with MS is associated with a higher level of neurological disability and lower overall quality of life.

In order to obtain the full benefits of physical activity, it is important for one to have a sense of the *physicality* of one's body. Many people who are diagnosed with MS may not already have this sense. In this situation, there may be a type of *physical education* that is needed, and this may take months or even years to develop. This education may be obtained through physical and occupational therapy, *mindful* exercising on one's own, or unconventional exercise programs that focus on slow, mindful movements, including tai chi, yoga, and Pilates as well as less well-known approaches such as Feldenkrais and Tragerwork (see individual chapters on these therapies).

Physical activity, like other lifestyle approaches such as nutrition, is a "two-edged sword." Regular exercise may produce wide-ranging emotional, physical, and general health benefits. On the flip side, lack of exercise, which is also referred to as *physical deconditioning* or a *sedentary lifestyle*, may have wide-ranging negative health effects. Specifically, physical inactivity may *worsen* multiple MS-associated symptoms and *increase* the risk for lifestyle diseases, which, as noted, have been associated with *lower* overall quality of life and *higher* level of disability in people with MS. Several studies indicate that, relative to the general population, people with MS are less physically active.

Exercise has multiple actions on the immune system, many of which are not fully understood. The effect that these immune system changes might have on MS has not been well studied. Moderate levels of exercise have been associated with immune system activation and a decreased risk of viral infections, while strenuous exercise appears to produce mild immune suppression and an increased risk of viral infections. Because exercise has so many clear beneficial effects, the uncertain immune-system changes associated with exercise should not factor strongly into decision making about exercise.

An exciting area of exercise research involves proteins known as *growth factors*. A variety of these growth factors occur in the central nervous system—these usually are referred to by acronyms such as BDNF (brain-derived neurotrophic factor) and NGF (nerve growth factor). Animal studies demonstrate that regular exercise increases the brain levels of several growth factors. Growth factors have multiple effects that could be therapeutic for MS:

- Anti-inflammatory effects: May decrease the risk of inflammation-related MS attacks

- Nerve-protecting effects: May decrease the risk of injury to nerve fibers (*axonal injury*)

- Nerve-regenerating effects: May help injured nerves grow new nerve fibers

The diverse and potentially therapeutic biological effects of growth factors make it possible that exercise, like the Food and Drug Administration (FDA)-approved drugs for MS, could slow down the underlying disease process of MS and perhaps even have nerve-regenerating effects. This possible "disease-modifying effect" of exercise is currently an active area of research. Studies at this point indicate that exercise may have disease-modifying effects in experimental autoimmune encephalomyelitis (EAE), the animal model of MS. In clinical studies in people with MS, some, but not all, studies also suggest that there may be disease-modifying effects. Possible disease-modifying effects of exercise have also been noted in other neurological conditions, including Parkinson's disease and Alzheimer's disease. Further research is needed in this area in MS and other neurological conditions.

Side Effects

The risks of exercise depend on the type of exercise. Increased body temperature associated with exercise may provoke neurologic symptoms in some people with MS. In this situation, known as *Uhthoff's phenomenon,* resistance exercises may be tolerated better than aerobic exercises and hydrotherapy (aquatic exercise) and various cooling strategies may be used to limit the elevation of body temperature during exercise (see *Cooling Therapy*). Musculoskeletal pain or injury may occur with overuse or trauma. The risk of exercise-induced injury is greater in those who are overweight, are older, or have had previous injuries. Finally, asthma may be provoked by exercise.

Practical Information

People with MS should develop an exercise program with the guidance of a physical therapist. This is especially important for those with significant physical disabilities or heart or lung conditions. Although information on exercise is readily available from popular books and recreation centers, this information should not be used instead of consulting with a professional.

Conclusion

Exercise is a simple, safe, low-cost approach that may produce many health benefits and may be modified for those with disability. Exercise studies in MS indicate improvement in walking, weakness, and fatigue. In addition, exercise may alleviate a wide range of other MS symptoms, including anxiety, anger, depression, bowel and bladder difficulties, pain, sleeping difficulties, muscle stiffness (spasticity), and cognitive problems. General health benefits of exercise include reduction of risk for heart disease and stroke, lowering of blood pressure, improved blood lipids (cholesterol), weight reduction, prevention and treatment of diabetes and osteoporosis, decreased risk of multiple cancers, and overall decreased risk of death.

Additional Readings

Books

Bauer B, ed. *Mayo Clinic Book of Alternative Medicine and Home Remedies.* New York, NY: Time Home Entertainment; 2013:26–29.

Blech J. *Healing Through Exercise.* Cambridge, MA: Da Capo Press; 2009.

Jackson K, Mulcare JA. Multiple sclerosis. In: Durstine JL, Moore GE, Painter PL, et al., eds. *ACSMs Exercise Management for Persons with Chronic Diseases and Disabilities.* Champaign, IL: Human Kinetics; 2009:321–326.

Ratey JJ. *Spark: The Revolutionary New Science of Exercise and the Brain.* New York, NY: Little, Brown and Company; 2008.

Salem Y, Csiza L, Harrison M, et al. *Aquatic Exercise and Multiple Sclerosis: A Healthcare Professional's Guide.* Cherry Hill, NJ: MS Association of America; 2013. [available from the MS Association of America]

Journal Articles

Adlard PA, Perreau VM, Engesser-Cesar C, Cotman CW. The timecourse of induction of brain-derived neurotrophic factor mRNA and protein in the rat hippocampus following voluntary exercise. *Neurosci Lett.* 2004;363:43–48.

Asmundson GJ, Fetzner MG, Deboer LB, Powers MB, Otto MW, Smits JA. Let's get physical: a contemporary review of the anxiolytic effects of exercise and its disorders. *Depress Anxiety.* 2013;30:362–373.

Blumenthal JA, Smith PJ, Hoffman BM. Is exercise a viable treatment for depression? *ACSMs Health Fit J.* 2012;16:14–21.

Booth FW, Roberts CK, Laye MJ. Lack of exercise is a major cause of chronic diseases. *Compr Physiol.* 2012;2:1143–1211.

Brown TR, Kraft GH. Exercise and rehabilitation for individuals with multiple sclerosis. *Phys Med Rehab Clin N Am.* 2005;16:513–555.

Castro-Sanchez AM, Mataran-Penarrocha GA, Lara-Palomo I, Saavedra-Hernández M, Arroyo-Morales M, Moreno-Lorenzo C. Hydrotherapy for the treatment of pain in people with multiple sclerosis: a randomized controlled trial. *Evid Based Complement Altern Med.* 2012;2012:473963.

Chen H, Zhang SM, Schwarzschild MA, Hernán MA, Ascherio A. Physical activity and the risk of Parkinson disease. *Neurology.* 2005;64:664–669.

Cooney GM, Dwan K, Greig CA, et al. Exercise for depression. *Cochrane Database Syst Rev.* 2013;9:CD004366.

Dalgas U, Stenager E. Exercise and disease progression in multiple sclerosis: can exercise slow down the progression of multiple sclerosis? *Ther Adv Neurol Disord.* 2012;5:81–95.

Ernst E, Rand JI, Stevinson C. Complementary therapies for depression: an overview. *Arch Gen Psych.* 1998;55:1026–1032.

Fragala MS, Kraemer WJ, Denegar DR, Maresh CM, Mastro AM, Volek JS. Neuroendocrine-immune interactions and responses to exercise. *Sports Med.* 2011;41:621–639.

Karpatkin HI. Multiple sclerosis and exercise: a review of the evidence. *Int J MS Care.* 2005;7:36–41.

Khoo J, Tian HH, Tan B, et al. Comparing effects of low- and high-volume moderate-intensity exercise on sexual function and testosterone in obese men. *J Sex Med.* 2013;10:1823–1832.

Kjolhede T, Vissing K, Dalgas U. Multiple sclerosis and progressive resistance training: a systematic review. *Mult Scler J.* 2012;18:1215–1228.

Latimer-Cheung AE, Martin Ginis KA, Hicks AL, et al. Development of evidence-informed physical activity guidelines for adults with multiple sclerosis. *Arch Phys Med Rehabil.* 2013;94:1829–1836.

Latimer-Cheung AE, Pilutti LA, Hicks AL, et al. Effects of exercise training on fitness, mobility, fatigue, and health-related quality of life among adults with multiple sclerosis: a systematic review to inform guideline development. *Arch Phys Med Rehabil.* 2013;94:1800–1828.

Leung L, Riutta T, Kotecha J, Rosser W. Chronic constipation: an evidence-based review. *J Amer Board Fam Med.* 2011;24:436–451.

Lorenz TA, Meston CM. Acute exercise improves physical sexual arousal in women taking antidepressants. *Ann Behav Med.* 2012;43:352–361.

Lucio AC, Perissinoto MC, Natalin RA, Prudente A, Damasceno BP, D'ancona CA. A comparative study of pelvic floor muscle training in women with multiple sclerosis: its impact on lower urinary tract symptoms and quality of life. *Clinics (Sao Paolo).* 2011;66:1563–1568.

McDonnell MN, Smith AE, Mackintosh SF. Aerobic exercise to improve cognitive function in adults with neurological disorders. *Arch Phys Med Rehabil.* 2011;92:1044–1052.

Motl RW, Pilutti LA. The benefits of exercise training in multiple sclerosis. *Nat Rev Neurol.* 2012;8:487–497.

Petajan JH, Gappmaier E, White AT, Spencer MK, Mino L, Hicks RW. Impact of aerobic training on fitness and quality of life in multiple sclerosis. *Ann Neurol.* 1996;39:432–441.

Rietberg MB, Brooks D, Uitdehaag BM, et al. Exercise therapy for multiple sclerosis. *Cochrane Database Syst Rev.* 2005;1:CD003980.

Romberg A, Virtanen A, Ruutiainen J, Suh Y, Balantrapu S, Motl RW. Effects of a 6-month exercise program on patients with multiple sclerosis: a randomized study. *Neurology.* 2004;63:2034–2038.

Sandroff BM, Dlugonski D, Weikert M, Suh Y, Balantrapu S, Motl RW. Physical activity and multiple sclerosis: new insights regarding inactivity. *Acta Neurol Scand.* 2012;126:256–262.

Scully D, Kremer J, Meade MM, Graham R, Dudgeon K. Physical exercise and psychological well being: a critical review. *Br J Sports Med.* 1998;32:111–120.

Skjerbaek AB, Moller AB, Jensen E, et al. Heat sensitive persons with multiple sclerosis are more tolerant to resistance exercise than to endurance exercise. *Mult Scler J.* 2013;19:932–940.

Solari A, Filippini G, Gasco P, et al. Physical rehabilitation has a positive effect on disability in multiple sclerosis patients. *Neurology.* 1999;52:57–62.

Sullivan AB, Schemen J, Venesy D, Davin S. The role of exercise and types of exercise in the rehabilitation of chronic pain: specific and nonspecific effects. *Curr Pain Headache Rep.* 2012;16:153–161.

Yang PY, Ho KH, Chen HC, Chien MY. Exercise training improves sleep quality in middle-aged and older adults with sleep problems: a systematic review. *J Physiother.* 2012;58:157–163.

Zhao G, Zhou S, Davie A, Su Q. Effects of moderate and high intensity exercise on T1/T2 balance. *Exerc Immunol Rev.* 2012;18:98–114.

Fats: Fish Oil and Polyunsaturated Fatty Acids*

☑ **"Healthful Diet"**

❓ **Swank Diet**

❓ **Fish Oil**

❗ **Other Fatty Acid Supplements**

For more than 50 years, it has been proposed that multiple sclerosis (MS) is associated with the intake of fish and other sources of dietary fat. Over the years, scientific and epidemiological studies, animal model experiments, and human clinical trials have explored this dietary aspect of MS and have generated significant controversy and confusion. While these studies have advanced our understanding in this area, the exact role of dietary fats in causing and treating MS remains unclear.

In the body, fats, which are stored in fatty tissue, are important for producing energy and providing the necessary chemical structure for the outer surfaces or membranes of all cells in the body. Fats are made up of *fatty acids,* long chains of carbon atoms attached to each other. Hydrogen and oxygen atoms are attached to these chains.

Two types of fats exist. One is *saturated fat,* which is hard at room temperature and is what we generally think of as "fat." The fat on meat is one of the most important forms of this type of fat. Saturated fat also is present in butter and hard cheese. The fatty acids in saturated fats will not allow any more hydrogen atoms to attach to them. In other words, the fatty acids are already "saturated" with hydrogen.

---

*This chapter is in greater depth than other chapters. As a result, for those wanting a more concise approach, italicized summaries are provided at the end of some chapter sections.

Another type of fat is *unsaturated fat* or unsaturated fatty acids. Unsaturated fat is soft or liquid at room temperature and is frequently referred to as "oil." Examples of unsaturated fat include margarine and oils from vegetables, seeds, and fish.

The fatty acids in unsaturated fats exist in two forms. *Monounsaturated fatty acids*, which are present in olive oil, have one position at which hydrogen atoms may attach. *Polyunsaturated fatty acids* have two or more positions at which hydrogen atoms may attach. The body is not able to make polyunsaturated fatty acids. As a result, polyunsaturated fatty acids are essential in the diet and are referred to as *essential fatty acids*.

Polyunsaturated fatty acids have been the subject of most dietary studies in MS. Two important forms of polyunsaturated fatty acids exist. One type is known as *omega-6* (or ω-6), a term that relates to the chemical structure of these fatty acids. Different forms of omega-6 fatty acids exist, and these different forms may be converted into each other by a pathway of chemical reactions (Figure 3.1).

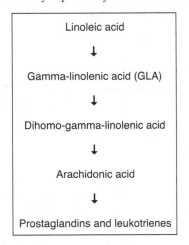

FIGURE 3.1 BIOCHEMICAL PATHWAY OF OMEGA-6 FATTY ACIDS

The first fatty acid in the omega-6 pathway is *linoleic acid*. Linoleic acid is present in a variety of foods, especially the oils of seeds and nuts. It is converted to gamma-linolenic acid (GLA). GLA is not nearly as common in food as linoleic acid. Relatively high levels of GLA are only present in unusual sources such as evening primrose oil. Further chemical reactions convert GLA to dihomo-gamma-linolenic acid and then to arachidonic acid. Finally, arachidonic acid is converted to prostaglandins and other chemicals that may be important for regulating the immune system and other body processes.

The other important polyunsaturated fatty acid is known as omega-3 (or ω-3) fatty acid. Fish and other seafood are the most well-known sources of this fatty acid. Once again, there is a pathway of different omega-3 fatty acids (Figure 3.2). The first fatty acid in this pathway is alpha-linolenic acid, which is

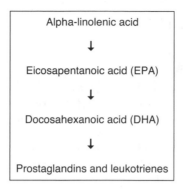

FIGURE 3.2 BIOCHEMICAL PATHWAY OF OMEGA-3 FATTY ACIDS

present in green leafy vegetables and flaxseed (or linseed) oil. Alpha-linolenic acid is then converted to eicosapentanoic acid (EPA) and docosahexanoic acid (DHA). Both of these fatty acids are present in fish and fish oils. DHA is converted to prostaglandins and leukotrienes, which are the same types of chemicals found at the end of the omega-6 pathway.

For years, MS has been associated with polyunsaturated fatty acids. In the early 1950s, studies were conducted in several countries to evaluate the possible impact of food intake on MS. Some of these studies suggested that MS was more common in areas where the consumption of saturated fat, especially animal fat, was relatively high. Some research also associated MS with a high intake of dairy products. In contrast, in some studies, populations with a relatively high intake of polyunsaturated fatty acids, including vegetable oil and fish, appeared to have lower rates of MS.

As a result of the studies of polyunsaturated fatty acids in the diet of different populations, the actual levels of polyunsaturated fatty acids were determined in people with MS. Some, but not all, blood studies found decreased levels of polyunsaturated fatty acids, especially omega-6 fatty acids such as linoleic acid. A few studies also reported decreased levels of omega-3 fatty acids.

How could fatty acids have anything to do with MS? When the original fatty-acid studies were conducted, it was claimed that people with MS may have blood that is too thick and, as a result, flows slowly or "sludges." This idea is not consistent with our current scientific understanding of MS. It also has been proposed that, because polyunsaturated fatty acids are an important component of the lining of nerve cells (myelin), an abnormality of polyunsaturated fatty acids could produce abnormalities in the myelin, as is observed in MS. A more current idea is that prostaglandins and other chemicals in the pathway of the omega-6 and omega-3 fatty acids (Figures 3.1 and 3.2) decrease or alter the activity of the immune system. This suppressing or "modulating" effect may be beneficial because the immune system is excessively active in MS.

Treatment Methods
The Swank Diet

Some of the original studies on MS and dietary fat were done by Dr. Roy Swank. Because of the apparent association of dietary fat with MS, in 1948, he began treating people with MS with a specific diet. The diet involves a very low intake of saturated fat and a high intake of polyunsaturated fatty acids:

- Saturated fat is decreased to 15 g/d
- No red meat is allowed in the first year—thereafter, 3 oz of red meat per week are permitted
- No high-fat dairy products or processed foods that contain saturated fats are allowed
- A high intake of polyunsaturated fatty acids, cod-liver oil supplements, frequent meals with fish, and a multivitamin are recommended

Healthful Diets That Include Relatively Low Saturated Fat and High Polyunsaturated Fat

Many other low saturated fat diets have been proposed for MS as well as for other medical conditions and for general health promotion. A diet that is relatively low in saturated fat and high in polyunsaturated fat is recommended by the American Heart Association and the U.S. Dietary Guidelines (developed by the U.S. Department of Agriculture and the U.S. Department of Health and Human Services). General dietary approaches that are consistent with these recommendations about fats, emphasize other healthful eating habits, and help maintain a well-balanced diet are as follows:

- Decrease total fat in diet to 20% to 35% of calories
  - Most of the fat should come from plant oils such as sunflower, safflower, canola, olive, and soybean
- Limit saturated fat intake to 10% or less of calories
  - Decrease animal-based food, such as full fat cheese, processed meats, and dairy desserts like ice cream
  - Decrease highly processed snack food, such as cakes and cookies
  - Fill most of the plate with fruits and vegetables
- Decrease *trans fats*, which are also known as "partially hydrogenated oils"
  - Limit intake of fried food and baked goods that contain these fats
- Eat fish at least two times per week
- Eat lean meats and poultry
- Eat whole-grain, high fiber foods
- Limit salt intake
- Consume appropriate number of daily calories

Linoleic Acid

Good sources of linoleic acid are the oils of seeds and nuts, such as safflower oil, sunflower oil, and sesame seed oil. Flaxseed (or linseed) oil contains linoleic acid as well as omega-3 fatty acids (see section on omega-3 fatty acids). Seeds and nuts themselves also contain linoleic acid.

A simple measure to increase linoleic acid intake is to increase the consumption of linoleic acid-containing foods, including oils. A more aggressive approach is to take oil supplements. The optimal dosage of linoleic acid is not known. In addition, the amount of omega-6 fatty acids relative to the amount of omega-3 fatty acids (the omega-6:omega-3 ratio) is probably important, but the most desirable ratio of these fatty acids has not been established.

It is sometimes recommended that approximately four teaspoons of linoleic acid-containing oils be taken daily. The oil may be used in salad dressings or mixed in with vegetables, yogurt, or soft cheese. It should not be heated and should be stored under cool and dark conditions.

Gamma-Linolenic Acid

Very few sources of GLA exist. Evening primrose oil is one of the most commonly recommended sources. It contains 8% to 10% GLA and approximately 70% linoleic acid. A single evening primrose oil capsule generally contains about 40 mg of GLA. Some capsules of evening primrose oil also contain vitamin E in low levels, such as 10 international units (IU) per capsule.

An Australian study evaluated the consistency of evening primrose oil preparations (1). Fourteen of 16 different preparations contained reasonable amounts (7%–10%) of GLA. Because of the presence of other fatty acids in some of the capsules, it was proposed that *borage seed oil*, another source of GLA, may have been added to these preparations.

If evening primrose oil is taken, approximately six capsules daily are often recommended. It should be kept in mind that GLA is present in low levels—six capsules daily result in a daily dose of only approximately 240 mg. As a result, other omega-6 fatty acids (see the earlier sections) may need to be taken as well if one is attempting to significantly increase the total intake of omega-6 fatty acids.

GLA is found in several other sources. *Borage seed oil*, which is sometimes recommended, is a rich source of GLA. It contains 18% to 26% GLA, more than twice the amount in evening primrose oil. However, borage seed oil may contain chemicals (pyrrolizidine alkaloids) that are toxic to the liver. As a result, it is safest to avoid borage seed oil. Some borage seed oil preparations claim to be free of pyrrolizidine alkaloids.

Like borage seed oil, *black currant seed oil* contains a higher concentration of GLA (6%–19%) than does evening primrose oil. However, this oil has not been extensively studied with regard to adverse effects, especially with long-term use. *Spirulina*, or blue-green algae, may contain high concentrations of GLA, but the amount of GLA in a given spirulina product usually is not specified and may be negligible (see *Herbs* chapter).

> *In conclusion, evening primrose oil generally is preferred over other products for supplementation with GLA. Borage seed oil, black currant seed oil, and spirulina are of uncertain safety or contain variable and uncertain amounts of GLA.*

Omega-3 Fatty Acids

Fish is a common food source of omega-3 fatty acids. Thus, a simple approach to increase omega-3 fatty-acid intake is to increase the consumption of fish, especially fatty fish such as salmon, Atlantic herring, sardines, Atlantic mackerel, and bluefin tuna. Two to three servings of fish weekly are sometimes recommended.

Omega-3 fatty acids also may be consumed as supplements. The optimal dose of omega-3 fatty acids is not known. Also, the amount of omega-3 fatty acids relative to that of omega-6 fatty acids (omega-6:omega-3 ratio) may be important, but currently not enough information is known to make specific recommendations.

Fish oil and cod-liver oil supplements are available as liquid oil or as capsules. Concentrated EPA and DHA also are available. Total daily doses of 3 g or less are believed to be safe. One tablespoon of fish oil contains approximately 140 cal and 14 g of fat.

A unique source of omega-3 fatty acids is flaxseed (or linseed) oil, which contains both omega-3 and omega-6 fatty acids. The omega-3 fatty acids are in the form of alpha-linolenic acid (see Figure 3.2), as opposed to EPA and DHA, which are present in fish oil and cod-liver oil. Of note, alpha-linolenic acid may not produce as potent effects as do EPA and DHA. (Of note, walnuts are also a source of alpha-linolenic acid.) Linoleic acid is the omega-6 fatty acids in flaxseed oil. Consuming flaxseed oil is a way to obtain both omega-3 and omega-6 fatty acids from a single source. One tablespoon of flaxseed oil daily sometimes is recommended.

Vitamin E and Other Supplements Sometimes Recommended With Polyunsaturated Fatty Acids

Polyunsaturated fatty acids may decrease vitamin E levels. As a result, if high levels of polyunsaturated fatty acids are consumed in the diet or through the use of supplements, vitamin E intake must be increased. However, *high doses* of vitamin E do not appear to be necessary. According to many recommendations, the ratio of vitamin E (in IU) to polyunsaturated fatty acids (in grams) should be about 0.9 to

1.3. This means that, on a daily basis, 0.9 to 1.3 IU of vitamin E are needed for each gram of polyunsaturated fatty acids. Consequently, given an intake of about 25 g of polyunsaturated fatty acids, only 20 to 30 IU of vitamin E would be required. It is sometimes stated that hundreds of IU of supplemental vitamin E are needed if polyunsaturated fatty-acid supplements are taken. This does not appear to be true. In fact, because it may be best to avoid high doses of vitamin E and other antioxidants in MS, as discussed elsewhere in the chapter on vitamins, lower doses of vitamin E, such as 100 IU, may be adequate and may actually be more appropriate. Some omega-3 fatty-acid supplements, such as evening primrose oil capsules, contain vitamin E, in which case additional vitamin E may not be necessary.

In addition to vitamin E, several other supplements sometimes are recommended with the use of polyunsaturated fatty acids. Vitamin B_6 (pyridoxine) and zinc are recommended by some because the fatty-acid chemical pathway uses vitamin B_6 and zinc. In fact, the intake of these micronutrients from the diet is probably adequate and, in the case of zinc, supplements pose a theoretic risk because they may stimulate the immune system (see *Vitamins, Minerals, and Other Nonherbal Supplements*). If these supplements are taken, the daily dose of vitamin B_6 should not exceed 50 mg, and low doses of zinc should be taken (see *Vitamins, Minerals, and Other Nonherbal Supplements*).

For antioxidant supplementation, vitamin C and beta-carotene sometimes are recommended in addition to vitamin E. As noted, only low doses of additional vitamin E appear to be needed, and there is no strong evidence that additional antioxidant vitamins are required. Because the benefits and risks of antioxidant vitamins in MS are not known, as discussed in the section on vitamins, it is not clear that vitamin C and beta-carotene supplements are beneficial. In fact, it is possible that, in higher doses, they may be immune-stimulating and therefore may negatively affect the course of MS. If vitamin C and beta-carotene supplements are used, they probably should be taken in moderation (see *Vitamins, Minerals, and Other Nonherbal Supplements*).

> *In summary, low doses of supplemental vitamin E may be required when high levels of polyunsaturated fatty acids are consumed. It is not clear that a need exists for any other supplements, including vitamin B_6, zinc, vitamin C, and beta-carotene.*

Studies in MS and Other Conditions
Specific Diets
The Swank Diet

In 1970, Dr. Swank reported the results of his diet in people with MS (2). On average, he observed patients over a 17-year period. People on the diet had less frequent and less severe attacks, less worsening of their overall neurologic condition, and a decreased death rate. The diet was reported to be most beneficial when it was started in people who were early in the disease course or who had mild disability. Some of the results were dramatic. For example, he described a 95% reduction in the frequency of MS attacks.

A follow-up report was published in 1990 (3). In this report, 144 patients were monitored over 34 years. Once again, the diet produced significant benefits and appeared to be especially effective when started in people who were mildly affected or were early in the disease course.

In 2003, Dr. Swank published another follow-up to his initial clinical trial (4). This report described people who had been on his diet for 50 years. Of the 15 people who were examined, only two had significant disability. The other 13 people had done well neurologically, had "joyful laughter," and "appeared youthful." Although these findings are impressive, no description of standard neurologic test results was given, and the examined group represented only a small subgroup of the 144 people who were originally enrolled in the study.

As noted, this diet is strict. Saturated fat intake is very low and polyunsaturated fat intake is high. Because of the decreased intake of meat, people who follow this diet should be certain that protein intake is adequate.

Most physicians and other health care professionals have a reserved approach to the Swank diet because the study was not carried out by guidelines that are now traditionally used in trials of new medical therapies. In particular, patients were not randomly given a specific therapy (randomization), the clinician who examined the patients was aware of their treatment (in other words, the clinician was not "blinded"), and no placebo-treated group was used.

The Swank diet is a fairly extreme dietary approach without strong clinical studies to support its use. More details and specific recipes are provided in a book by Dr. Swank and Barbara Dugan, *The Multiple Sclerosis Diet Book*.

Other Low Saturated Fat Diets

Other diets that are low in saturated fats have been proposed for MS and other medical conditions. No MS clinical studies have compared the Swank diet with a less strict low saturated fat diet, and therefore it is not clear which dietary approach might be most beneficial to those with MS.

Other Health Effects

The effect of dietary fat on diseases other than MS also has been examined. Saturated fat, especially animal fat, increases cholesterol levels. High cholesterol levels are associated with heart disease and stroke. A diet that is relatively low in saturated fat may have beneficial effects on heart disease and stroke as well as diabetes and obesity. Importantly, when other medical conditions, such as heart disease, stroke, and obesity, occur in combination with MS, they may worsen the quality of life and increase the level of disability.

Supplements of Polyunsaturated Fatty Acids

In addition to modifying the diet, the intake of polyunsaturated fatty acids may be increased by taking supplements. Some of these supplements actually have been studied in clinical trials of people with MS.

Omega-6 Polyunsaturated Fatty Acids

Linoleic Acid

Supplementation with linoleic acid, the first chemical in the omega-6 fatty-acid pathway (see Figure 3.1), has been extensively studied. In experimental autoimmune encephalomyelitis (EAE), an animal model of MS, supplements of linoleic acid are beneficial, whereas deficiencies of linoleic acid are harmful. Three studies have been undertaken of linoleic acid supplements in people with relapsing MS. Linoleic acid was given as some form of sunflower seed oil in these studies. All three studies meet the formal clinical research criteria of being randomized, blinded, and placebo-controlled.

The first study was reported in 1973 (5). Seventy-five people were studied over 2 years, and the daily dose of linoleic acid was 2 g. Treatment produced decreased duration and severity of attacks. No effect was noted on the frequency of attacks or the progression of the disease.

The second study was published in 1978 (6). Over a 2-year period, 116 people were studied. As in the first study, the severity and duration of attacks were significantly improved, but there was no change in the frequency of attacks or the progression of disability.

The third study also was reported in 1978 (7). Seventy-six people with MS were monitored over 2.5 years. In contrast to the two other studies, no benefit was found in this investigation.

In summary, two studies produced limited positive results and one study found no benefit. To attempt to clarify the mixed results of these studies, a combined analysis was published in 1984 (8). The information on a total of 172 people from all three studies was pooled. It was noted that, in the third study, which did not report any benefit, the people had more severe MS and had MS for a longer time than did people in the other two studies. Using the combined analysis, linoleic acid treatment slowed the progression of disability in people with little or no disability at the start of the treatment. Regardless of the duration or severity of the disease, linoleic acid treatment was associated with reduced length and severity of attacks. The statistical methods used in this combined analysis have been questioned. Overall, the effects of linoleic acid supplements on MS are suggestive but not definitive.

Gamma-Linolenic Acid

Evening primrose oil is a popular supplement sometimes recommended for MS because it contains GLA, which is one step beyond linoleic acid in the omega-6 biochemical pathway (see Figure 3.1).

There are some theoretical reasons why GLA may be better than linoleic acid, but scant clinical information exists in this area. A preparation of evening primrose oil (Naudicelle) was used in one of the linoleic acid trials in 1978. Eight capsules daily were not effective. In the same trial, linoleic acid alone was somewhat beneficial for relapsing MS. It should be noted that low doses of GLA (340 mg daily) were used in this trial, and it is possible that higher doses could have produced a benefit. However, this would have meant consuming up to 40 evening primrose oil capsules daily!

Two other limited studies have been undertaken of evening primrose oil in relapsing MS. One of these studies also used a drug known as *colchicine*. Both studies produced some positive results. However, they involved a small number of people and did not include a placebo-treated group. Consequently, it is difficult to be confident about the results. A 1977 study of people with progressive MS found no benefit for evening primrose oil (9).

Scientific studies indicate that GLA suppresses immune system activity. In rats, evening primrose oil decreases the activity of *T cells,* a type of immune cell. GLA supplementation decreases the severity of disease in mice and rats with EAE, an animal model of MS.

Evening primrose oil has been claimed to be effective for many other conditions. Conflicting results have been obtained in studies of other immune diseases, such as rheumatoid arthritis. Evening primrose oil may decrease breast pain (mastalgia), increase bone density in those with osteoporosis, and be helpful for two skin conditions—eczema and atopic dermatitis.

In summary, the limited clinical information about GLA supplementation in MS does not strongly support its use. However, only low doses have been studied clinically, and scientific studies and clinical studies in other diseases suggest that it may be effective. In theory, GLA could provide the same benefits as linoleic acid, but high doses may be necessary, and such high doses may not be practical on a regular basis because of its cost.

Omega-3 Fatty Acids

There are multiple studies of omega-3 fatty-acid supplement use in MS. Early studies suggested beneficial effects with these supplements. However, questions about the effectiveness of these supplements have been raised by more recent research in this area.

Studies of immunologic function indicate that, in laboratory animals and in humans, omega-3 fatty-acid supplementation decreases the activity of several components of the immune system. In limited studies of EAE, omega-3 fatty acids have produced variable effects. Some studies actually indicate that omega-3 fatty acids worsen the disease, but others indicate beneficial effects.

There are multiple past MS studies of omega-3 fatty acids with suggestive, but not definitive, results:

- One study (10), conducted over 2 years and reported in 1989, involved 312 people and daily treatment with 10 g of fish oil. The daily doses of specific fatty acids were 1.7 g of EPA and 1.1 g of DHA (see Figure 3.2). People in this study also were instructed to increase omega-6 fatty-acid intake and to decrease animal fat intake. In the untreated group, 52% worsened, whereas in the treated group, 43% worsened. A trend was noted toward a beneficial effect, but formal analysis showed that this effect was not quite statistically significant.

- A small 1986 study evaluated the effect of cod-liver oil supplements, which contain omega-3 fatty acids, on the MS attack rate in 10 people with MS (11). A beneficial effect of treatment was noted, but this study is limited by several factors, including the absence of a placebo-treated group and treatment that involved vitamin D, calcium, and magnesium in addition to cod-liver oil.

- Another study of 16 people with MS evaluated the effects of omega-3 fatty-acid supplements, other dietary supplements (vitamins A, B, C, D, and E), and dietary advice (including decreased saturated fat and increased fish intake) over 2 years (12). Compared with clinical status before the study, treatment was associated with a significant decrease in the attack rate and improvement in the level of disability. No placebo group was used in this small study.

- A study of 31 people with MS assessed the effects of omega-3 fatty-acid supplements in combination with glatiramer acetate (Copaxone) or interferons (Avonex, Betaseron, Rebif) (13). People were treated with the conventional MS medications along with either fish oil and a very low-fat diet or with olive oil and a low-fat diet. A trend for improved emotional and physical functioning was found in those taking fish oil—these results were not statistically significant. Both dietary approaches were associated with a decrease in attack rate.

All of these past studies have significant limitations and have produced inconsistent results. To address these issues and inconsistencies, a large, rigorous clinical trial of fish oil in MS, known as the "OFAMS Study," was conducted in Norway. This is the highest quality clinical trial of fish oil in MS. The results of this study were published in 2012 (14). In this study, which involved 92 people with MS, people were treated for 6 months with a single treatment, known as "monotherapy," of fish oil or placebo. They then continued on fish oil or placebo but also started on treatment with an interferon MS medication (interferon-beta-1a, Rebif) and were monitored on this "combination treatment" for another 18 months. Many measures of disease activity were used during this study. The main measure was MRI activity—other measures included attacks, disability progression, fatigue, and quality of life. With these multiple measures, this study found that fish oil alone was no better than placebo as a monotherapy or as a combination therapy with interferon. This study has raised significant concerns about the effectiveness of fish oil in MS. It should be noted that, although this study is the most rigorous thus far, it does have limitations. It was relatively short and included only a modest number of people with MS. In addition, people in the study were not instructed to make dietary changes, such as increasing fish intake and decreasing saturated fat intake, which could have beneficial effects.

Another recent MS study did evaluate food intake as well as omega-3 supplement use (15). This international study was an Internet-based survey in which nearly 2,500 people with relapsing and progressive MS were asked questions about their MS and their diet and supplement use. Increased fish consumption and omega-3 supplement use was associated with lower disability level and higher quality of life. In addition, among those with relapsing MS, the rate of attacks was significantly decreased in those taking flaxseed oil supplements, which contain omega-3 as well as omega-6 fatty acids. There was a "trend," which was not "statistically significant," for decreased attack rate in those taking fish oil. A strength of this study is the large number of people with MS and the large amount of data that were collected. A significant limitation is that it was not a rigorous clinical trial. Rather, it relied on people to "self-report" on the condition of their MS and their diet and supplement use. The findings of this study warrant further research.

Studies of immune diseases other than MS have indicated a possible therapeutic effect with the use of omega-3 fatty acids. Omega-3 fatty-acid supplements may decrease joint stiffness and joint swelling in rheumatoid arthritis. These supplements may be helpful for another immune condition known as *antiphospholipid antibody syndrome.*

Omega-3 fatty acids may have other important health benefits. They have the potential to prevent and treat heart disease, but the findings in this area are not definitive. Fish oil and cod-liver oil appear to reduce elevated blood levels of triglycerides, which have been associated with heart disease.

Combinations of Omega-3 and Omega-6 Fatty Acids

Two recent small studies have produced promising findings with combinations of omega-3 and omega-6 fatty acids in MS:

- An Iranian study, reported in 2013, evaluated the effects of evening primrose oil and also hemp seed oil (which contains both omega-3 and omega-6 fatty acids) and a diet used in traditional Iranian medicine known as the "hot-nature diet," which is relatively low in saturated fat, sugar, and refined carbohydrates and high in fish, fruits, and vegetables (16–18). This 6-month study of 65 people with MS found that people who were treated with the oils or the oils combined with the diet had less disability progression and lower attack rates than those treated with olive oil. Due to the limitations of this study, including small numbers of people with MS and short duration of the study, further research is needed on this novel, multimodal dietary approach.

■ A study reported from Greece and Cyprus in 2013 evaluated various dietary supplements in MS, including a combination of omega-3 and omega-6 fatty acids known as "PLP10" (19). In this study, those treated with PLP10 had lower attack rates and less disability progression than those treated with placebo. This study also has limitations—it was small and nearly half of the participants dropped out of the study before it was completed.

Side Effects
The Swank Diet

The food component of the Swank diet does not have any adverse effects if the diet remains well balanced. Cod-liver supplements that are used in the Swank diet may have side effects and their safety for long-term use has not been established (see following under *Omega-3 Fatty Acids*.).

Linoleic Acid

Linoleic acid is generally well tolerated. The oily taste may be unpleasant, and diarrhea may occur in some people. Omega-6 fatty-acid supplements may increase triglyceride levels in those with elevated triglyceride levels. Polyunsaturated fatty acids in general may produce vitamin E deficiency—low doses of vitamin E supplements may be indicated (see the next section). The possible adverse effects of long-term supplementation have not been studied formally and consequently are not known.

GLA In general, evening primrose oil is well tolerated. Because sources of GLA usually contain linoleic acid, the adverse effects and risks of linoleic acid are present. These include an unpleasant taste and soft stools or diarrhea. Additional concerns with evening primrose oil include the expense, as well as nausea and headache. Evening primrose oil, borage seed oil, and black currant seed oil may provoke seizures in people taking antipsychotic medications. In addition, evening primrose oil, borage seed oil, and black currant seed oil may affect blood clotting and thus probably should be avoided by people who take blood-thinning medications or high doses of aspirin, people who have blood-clotting disorders, and people who are undergoing surgery. Borage seed oil may contain liver toxins. Spirulina may actually stimulate the immune system and thus could worsen MS or inhibit the therapeutic effects of disease-modifying MS medications. In general, the safety of black currant seed oil and Spirulina has not been well studied.

All supplements containing polyunsaturated fatty acids may produce vitamin E deficiency. Consequently, low doses of vitamin E supplements should be taken if vitamin E is not already present in the fatty-acid supplement.

Omega-3 Fatty Acids

Omega-3 fatty acids may be obtained through food, such as fish, or supplements. For fish, a very high intake raises concerns about mercury toxicity, especially among women who are pregnant or may become pregnant. Fish with relatively high mercury levels include shark, swordfish, and king mackerel.

With regard to supplements, the U.S. Food and Drug Administration (FDA) determined that fish oil supplements were generally safe when the total daily intake of EPA and DHA was less than 3 g. In one long-term study of 295 people, no serious adverse effects were observed with 7 years of fish oil use. Multiple fish oil products have been analyzed and have generally not been found to contain significant mercury.

Cod-liver oil has a fishy taste, and flaxseed oil has a bitter taste. These unpleasant tastes may be lessened by cooling the oils. Daily doses greater than 45 g of flaxseed oil may have a laxative effect, and daily doses greater than 60 g may theoretically increase blood levels of cyanide-containing compounds. Vitamin E deficiency may potentially develop when taking omega-3 fatty acids. Thus, supplemental vitamin E should be taken.

Most commercial fish oil products do not contain vitamin A. However, halibut, shark, and cod-liver oils contain relatively high levels of vitamin A. Excessive doses of these oils should be avoided because high levels of vitamin A may be toxic, especially during pregnancy (see chapter on *Vitamins, Minerals, and Other Nonherbal Supplements*).

Omega-3 fatty-acids may increase blood sugar levels in diabetic patients and produce excessive mental and physical activity, a condition known as *hypomania*, in people with depression or manic-depressive illness. It is not known if omega-3 fatty-acid supplements are safe in women who are pregnant or breastfeeding.

Finally, omega-3 fatty acids may inhibit blood clotting. These oils should be used with caution by people who are undergoing surgery, people who have blood-clotting disorders, and people who take blood-thinning medication or high doses of aspirin.

Conclusion

The area of fatty acids and MS is controversial. This review of the evidence shows that positive as well as negative studies exist. All of the studies have limitations and thus none of these studies are definitive. At this time, most of the studies have been done with *either* omega-3 or omega-6 fatty acid supplements. However, some studies suggest that *combinations* of omega-3 and omega-6 fatty acids may have beneficial effects. Also, there is emerging evidence in other medical conditions that changing overall food intake may have more beneficial health effects than taking specific dietary supplements. Overall, the findings in this area indicate that further research is needed, especially with studies that are more rigorous and also perhaps with dietary approaches that are more complex, such as combinations of fatty acid supplements or changes in overall food intake rather than simply taking dietary supplements.

With the limited and inconsistent information in this area, it is not possible to be definitive about a specific dietary approach with fatty acids and MS. One option is to wait until more information is available. Another approach is to use a dietary strategy. With the Swank diet, there are no clear risks and it may have beneficial effects on MS and other conditions, but it has not been rigorously studied and may be challenging for many to comply with over the long term. Another dietary approach that is simpler than the Swank diet and perhaps just as beneficial is the "Healthful Diet" that was outlined earlier in the chapter. This diet is well balanced and relatively easy to follow, does not have any risks, and may produce beneficial effects on MS. Also, this diet may help prevent other medical conditions, such as heart disease, stroke, diabetes, and obesity, that may secondarily worsen disability and quality of life in people with MS.

If fatty acid supplements are taken, this should be done with consideration of the limited effectiveness and safety information regarding these supplements. Long-term safety information is available for fish oil but not for other fatty acid supplements, including evening primrose oil, black currant seed oil, borage seed oil, spirulina, and cod-liver oil. Also, there are potential side effects with all of these supplements, and uncertainties about the quality of some products. Taking all of this information into account, a modest supplement approach is to take fish oil at a dose that provides 1 to 2 g of EPA and DHA daily and, to avoid possible vitamin E deficiency, to take modest doses of vitamin E, such as 100 IU daily.

Additional Readings

Books

Bowling AC. Complementary and alternative medicine: practical considerations. In: Rae-Grant A, Fox R, Bethoux F, eds. *Multiple Sclerosis and Related Disorders: Diagnosis, Medical Management, and Rehabilitation.* New York, NY: Demos; 2013: 243–249.

Bowling AC, Stewart TS. *Dietary Supplements and Multiple Sclerosis: A Health Professional's Guide.* New York, NY: Demos Medical Publishing; 2004.

Campbell TC. *Whole: Rethinking the Science of Nutrition.* Dallas, TX: BenBella Books; 2013.

Duyff RL. *American Dietetic Association Complete Food and Nutrition Guide.* Boston, MA: Houghton Mifflin Harcourt; 2012.

Fragakis AS. *The Health Professional's Guide to Popular Dietary Supplements.* Chicago, IL: The American Dietetic Association; 2003.

Jellin JM, Batz F, Hitchens K. *Natural Medicines Comprehensive Database.* Stockton, CA: Therapeutic Research Faculty; 2014.

Katz DL. *Nutrition in Clinical Practice.* Philadelphia, PA: Lippincott Williams & Wilkins; 2008.

Polman CH, Thompson AJ, Murray TJ, Bowling AC, Noseworthy JH. *Multiple Sclerosis: The Guide to Treatment and Management.* New York, NY: Demos Medical Publishing; 2006.

Swank RL, Dugan BB. *The Multiple Sclerosis Diet Book.* New York, NY: Doubleday; 1987.

Ulbricht CE, Basch EM, eds. *Natural Standard Herb and Supplement Reference: Evidence-Based Clinical Reviews.* St. Louis, MO: Elsevier-Mosby; 2005.

U.S. Dept. of Agriculture and U.S. Dept. of Health and Human Services. *Dietary Guidelines for Americans, 2010.* Washington, DC: US Govt. Printing Office; 2010.

Journal Articles

Anon. Omega-3 oil: fish or pills? *Consum Rep.* 2003;68:30–33.

Anon. Fat facts and fat fiction. *Consum Rep Health.* 2013;1:4–5.

Bates D, Cartlidge NEF, French JM, et al. A double-blind controlled trial of long chain n-3 polyunsaturated fatty acids in the treatment of multiple sclerosis. *J Neurol Neurosurg Psychiatry.* 1989;52:18–22.

Bates D, Fawcett PRW, Shaw DA, Weightman D. Polyunsaturated fatty acids in treatment of acute remitting multiple sclerosis. *Br Med J.* 1978;2:1390–1391.

Bates D, Fawcett PRW, Shaw DA, Weightman D. Trial of polyunsaturated fatty acids in nonrelapsing multiple sclerosis. *Br Med J.* 1977;10:932–933.

Bowling AC. Complementary and alternative medicine and multiple sclerosis. *Neurol Clin N Am.* 2011;29:465–480.

Bowling AC, Stewart TM. Current complementary and alternative therapies of multiple sclerosis. *Curr Treat Opt Neurol* 2003;5:55–68.

Chowdhury R, Warnakula S, Kunutsor S, et al. Association of dietary, circulating, and supplement fatty acids with coronary risk. *Ann Intern Med.* 2014;160:398–406.

Dworkin RH, Bates D, Millar JHD, Paty DW. Linoleic acid and multiple sclerosis: a reanalysis of three double-blind trials. *Neurology.* 1984;34:1441–1445.

Farinotti M, Vacchi L, Simi S, et al. Dietary interventions for multiple sclerosis. *Cochrane Database Syst Rev.* 2012;12:CD004192.

Horrobin DF. Multiple sclerosis: the rational basis for treatment with colchicine and evening primrose oil. *Med Hyp.* 1979;5:365–378.

Jelinek GA, Hadgkiss EJ, Weiland TJ, Pereira NG, Marck CH, van der Meer DM. Association of fish consumption and omega 3 supplementation with quality of life, disability and disease activity in an international cohort of people with multiple sclerosis. *Int J Neurosci.* 2013;123:792–801.

Lauer K. Diet and multiple sclerosis. *Neurology.* 1997;49:S55–S61.

Mehta LR, Dworkin RH, Schwid SR. Polyunsaturated fatty acids and their potential therapeutic role in multiple sclerosis. *Nat Clin Pract.* 2009;5:82–92.

Meyer-Reinecker HJ, Jenssen HL, Kohler H, Field EJ, Shenton BK. Effect of gamma-linolenate in multiple sclerosis. *Lancet.* 1976;10:966.

Miller JHD, Zilkha KJ, Langman MJS, et al. Double-blind trial of linoleate supplementation of the diet in multiple sclerosis. *Br Med J.* 1973;1:765–768.

Nordvik I, Myhr KM, Nyland H, Bjerve KS. Effects of dietary advice and Q-3 supplementation in newly diagnosed MS patients. *Acta Neurol Scand.* 2000;102:143–149.

Pantzaris MC, Loukaides GN, Ntzani EE, Patrikios IS. A novel oral nutraceutical formula of omega-3 and omega-6 fatty acids with vitamins (PLP10) in relapsing remitting multiple sclerosis: a randomized, double-blind, placebo-controlled proof-of-concept clinical trial. *BMJ Open.* 2013;3(4). pii: e002170.

Paty DW, Cousin I IK, Read S, Adlakha K. Linoleic acid in multiple sclerosis: failure to show any therapeutic benefit. *Acta Neurol Scand.* 1978;58:53–58.

Rezapour-Firouzi S, Arefhosseini SR, Ebrahimi-Mamaghani M, et al. Erythrocyte membrane fatty acids in multiple sclerosis patients and hot-nature dietary intervention with co-supplemented hemp-seed and evening-primrose oils. *Afr J Trad Complem Altern Med.* 2013;10:519–527.

Rezapour-Firouzi S, Arefhosseini SR, Farhoudi M, et al. Association of expanded disability status scale and cytokines after intervention with co-supplemented hemp seed, evening primrose oils and hot-natured diet in multiple sclerosis patients. *Bioimpacts.* 2013;3:43–47.

Rezapour-Firouzi S, Arefhosseini SR, Mehdi F, et al. Immunomodulatory and therapeutic effects of hot-nature diet and co-supplemented hemp seed, evening primrose oils intervention in multiple sclerosis. *Complement Ther Med.* 2013;21:473–480.

Stewart TM, Bowling AC. Polyunsaturated fatty acid supplementation in MS. *Int MSJ.* 2005;12:88–93.

Swank RL. Multiple sclerosis: twenty years on low fat diet. *Arch Neurol.* 1970;23:460–474.

Swank RL, Dugan BB. Effect of low saturated fat diet in early and late cases of multiple sclerosis. *Lancet.* 1990;336:37–39.

Swank RL, Goodwin J. Review of MS patient survival on a Swank low saturated fat diet. *Nutrition.* 2003;16:161–162.

Torkildsen O, Wegeland S, Bakke S, et al. Omega-3 fatty acid treatment in multiple sclerosis (OFAMS Study). *Arch Neurol.* 2012;69:1044–1051.

Valk EE, Hornstra G. Relationship between vitamin E requirement and poly-unsaturated fatty acid intake in man: a review. *Int J Vitamin Nutr Res.* 2000;70: 31–42.

Weinstock-Guttnam B, Baier M, Park Y, et al. Low fat dietary intervention with omega-3 fatty acid supplementation in multiple sclerosis patients. *Prostaglandins Leukot Essent Fatty Acids.* 2005;73:392–404.

Wergeland S, Torkildsen O, Bo L, Myhr KM. Polyunsaturated fatty acids in multiple sclerosis therapy. *Acta Neurol Scand. Suppl.* 2012;126:70–75.

⑦ Feldenkrais

Feldenkrais is a type of *bodywork* that focuses on efficient and comfortable body movements. It was developed by Moshe Feldenkrais, a Russian-born physicist. Feldenkrais is claimed to decrease stress, relieve pain, and improve balance and coordination.

Treatment Method

Feldenkrais uses very structured body movements. The position of the head is of particular importance. Feldenkrais is usually initially learned with lessons known as Awareness Through Movement (ATM), in which attention is focused on the motion of specific body parts during simple movements, such as walking or bending. In another type of Feldenkrais, Functional Integration (FI), more efficient movements are developed by a teacher who manipulates one's joints and muscles during movement. It is possible for people with significant disabilities to do Feldenkrais.

Unlike some conventional exercise programs, Feldenkrais aims to enhance body awareness. This may provide a form of *physical education* to those who do not already have a strong sense of the physicality of their bodies. Other unconventional therapies that focus on body awareness and thus may provide similar benefits include Pilates, tai chi, yoga, and Tragerwork.

Studies in Multiple Sclerosis and Other Conditions

Multiple sclerosis (MS) may limit body movement and function due to nervous system injury. Various forms of physical activity may improve body movement. However, people with MS who do not have a high level of awareness of their body movement may find it difficult to take full advantage of physical activity. Thus, approaches such as Feldenkrais have the potential to improve body function by improving body awareness.

At this time, only limited studies have formally evaluated Feldenkrais therapy. In a small study in MS conducted at the University of North Carolina, 20 people with MS received Feldenkrais or a "sham" therapy for 8 weeks (1). Some of the participants had significant walking difficulties and required the use of a cane or walker. Feldenkrais did not improve arm function, multiple MS symptoms, or overall level of function. It decreased stress and may have reduced anxiety.

Feldenkrais has undergone limited study in other conditions. Preliminary studies indicate that Feldenkrais may relieve depression, fatigue, sleeping problems, walking difficulties, and neck pain and stiffness.

Side Effects

Feldenkrais generally is regarded as a safe therapy.

Practical Information

The cost of Feldenkrais depends on the type of therapy. ATM classes cost $15 to $30, whereas FI sessions are about $50 to $100. Feldenkrais usually is not covered by insurance. However, insurance coverage may be available if Feldenkrais is provided by a physical therapist or occupational therapist.

Feldenkrais may be offered at local health clubs and recreation centers. More information and a list of certified practitioners may be obtained from:

- The Feldenkrais Guild of North America (www.feldenkrais.com), 401 Edgewater Place, Ste. 600, Wakefield, MA 01880 (781-876-8935)

Conclusion

In summary, Feldenkrais is a safe, low- to moderate-cost therapy. This therapy's focus on body movement could play an important role in optimizing body function in those with MS, but only limited studies have been conducted at this time. One small study in MS indicated that Feldenkrais decreased stress and possibly reduced anxiety. Limited studies in other conditions have shown improvement in depression, fatigue, neck pain, sleep, and walking. Further studies are needed to determine whether it has definite therapeutic effects.

Additional Readings

Books

Bauer B, ed. *Mayo Clinic Book of Alternative Medicine and Home Remedies.* New York, NY: Time Home Entertainment; 2013:130.

Kowalak JP, Mills EJ, eds. *Professional Guide to Complementary and Alternative Therapies.* Springhouse, PA: Springhouse Publishing; 2001:203–205.

Micozzi MS, ed. *Fundamentals of Complementary and Alternative Medicine.* Philadelphia, PA: Saunders Elsevier; 2011:221.

Journal Articles

Connors KA, Galea MP, Said CM. Feldenkrais method balance classes improve balance in older adults: a controlled trial. *Evid Based Complem Altern Med.* 2011;2011:873672.

Connors KA, Galea MP, Said CM, Remedios LJ. Feldenkrais Method balance classes are based on principles of motor learning and postural control retraining: a qualitative research study. *Physiother.* 2010;96(4):324–336.

Connors KA, Pile CP, Nichols ME. Does the Feldenkrais Method make a difference: an investigation into the use of outcome measurement tools for evaluating changes in clients. *J Bodywork Movement Ther.* 2011;15:446–452.

Jain S, Janssen K, DeCelle S. Alexander technique and Feldenkrais method: a critical overview. *Phys Med Rehabil Clin.* 2004;15:811–825.

Johnson SK, Frederick J, Kaufman M, Mountjoy B. A controlled investigation of bodywork in multiple sclerosis. *J Alt Complem Med.* 1999;5:237–243.

Mehling WE, Wrubel J, Daubenmier JJ, et al. Body awareness: a phenomenological inquiry into the common ground of mind-body therapies. *Philos Ethics Human Med.* 2011;6:6.

Netz Y, Lidor R. Mood alterations in mindful versus aerobic exercise modes. *J Psychol.* 2003;137:405–419.

Ohman A, Astrom L, Malmgren-Olsson E-B. Feldenkrais therapy as group treatment for chronic pain—a qualitative evaluation. *J Bodywork Movement Ther.* 2011;15:153–161.

Plastaras CT, Schran S, Kim N, et al. Complementary and alternative treatment for neck pain: chiropractic, acupuncture, TENS, massage, yoga, tai chi, and Feldenkrais. *Phys Med Rehabil Clin N Am.* 2011;22:521–537.

Plastaras C, Schran S, Kim N, Darr D, Chen MS. Manipulative therapy (Feldenkrais, massage, chiropractic manipulation) for neck pain. *Curr Rheum Rep.* 2013;15:339.

Ullmann G, Williams HG. Can Feldenkrais exercises ameliorate subclinical depressive symptoms in older adults? A pilot study. *J S Carolina Med Assoc.* 2011;107:7–10.

Ullmann G, Williams HG, Hussey J, Durstine JL, McClenaghan BA. Effects of Feldenkrais exercises on balance, mobility, balance confidence, and gait performance in community dwelling adults age 65 and older. *J Altern Compl Med.* 2010;16:97–105.

Webb R, Cofre Lizama LE, Galea MP. Moving with ease: Feldenkrais Method classes for people with arthritis. *Evid Based Complement Alternat Med.* 2013;2013:479142.

⭐ Fiber

Dietary fiber, also known as roughage, is a form of carbohydrate. Fiber provides many important health benefits even though it passes through the gut undigested and does not provide energy or essential nutrients for the body. In the general population and in those with multiple sclerosis (MS), fiber intake may be inadequate and thus many people may not be obtaining the diverse health benefits of this important component of the diet.

There are two forms of fiber:

- Insoluble dietary fiber: This type of fiber, which includes compounds known as cellulose and lignins, acts as a natural laxative and stool softener. Insoluble fiber stimulates the intestinal wall to contract and relax, which facilitates the movement of solid materials through the digestive tract and may relieve constipation. Also, this form of fiber absorbs water and makes one feel full after eating. The absorption of water softens stools and reduces the risk of hemorrhoids.

- Soluble dietary fiber: This form of fiber includes pectins, which are in fruit, and beta-glucans, which are in oats and barley. This form of fiber lowers cholesterol and thus may provide protection against heart disease.

Treatment Method

Fiber is found in a wide range of foods. It is present in all plant foods, including fruits, vegetables, grains, and nuts. However, there is not any fiber in foods from animals, such as meat, fish, poultry, eggs, and milk.

Diets that are generally rich in fruits, vegetables, and grains provide adequate dietary intake of fiber. Insoluble fiber may be obtained from leaves (such as cabbage), roots (such as carrots and beets), grains, and beans. Sources of soluble fiber include fruits, grains, beans, cereals, and seeds. Attempts to increase fiber intake should be done on a gradual basis (as is true for many lifestyle changes) since rapid increases in fiber intake may produce diarrhea and gas.

The current recommendations for daily fiber intake are as follows:

- Women
  - 19 to 50 years old: 25 g
  - Over 50: 21 g
- Men
  - 19 to 50 years old: 38 g
  - Over 50: 30 g

Daily fiber intake may be calculated by examining one's diet. As noted, animal-derived foods do not contain any fiber. Among the fiber-containing foods, there are large differences in fiber content. Generally, there is more fiber in foods that are less processed, such as whole grains and cooked (as opposed to canned) vegetables, fruits, and beans. Table 3.4 provides the fiber content of one serving of various food types. As can be seen, a general rule is that one serving of fruits, vegetables, grains, and breads provides 2 to 6 g of fiber, while nuts are somewhat lower than this (1–2 g) and beans are higher (5–20 g). An "herbal" strategy to increase fiber intake is psyllium (see *Herbs* chapter).

TABLE 3.4 FIBER CONTENT OF ONE SERVING OF DIFFERENT FOODS

FOOD	AVERAGE SERVING	FIBER CONTENT PER SERVING
Nuts	One tablespoon	1–2 g
Fruits, vegetables, grains	One-half cup	2–6 g
Cereals	One-half to one cup	2–6 g
Bread	Two slices	2–6 g
Beans	One-half to one cup	5–20 g

Studies in MS and Other Conditions

There are extensive studies of fiber in the general population and in those with many different medical conditions. However, studies of fiber specifically in MS are extremely limited. Several studies have evaluated the food intake of those with MS, but these have generally not measured fiber intake. The few studies that have measured fiber intake have found that it is significantly below the recommended daily amount (1,2). One MS study found that higher intake of whole-grain foods was associated with less difficulty with bowel movements (3).

Studies in the general population demonstrate that fiber provides many health benefits yet fiber intake is generally inadequate. In the United States, the average intake of fiber is only about 50% of the recommended amount. In terms of health benefits, fiber relieves constipation—this is very relevant to MS because 30% to 40% of those with MS experience constipation. Other potential health benefits of fiber intake include reduction of cholesterol levels, improved control of blood sugar levels in diabetics, and reduced risk of heart disease, cancer, and obesity. The presence of some of these conditions, such as heart disease and diabetes, may decrease quality of life and worsen neurological disability in those with MS. Thus, preventing these "nonneurological conditions" through adequate fiber intake, as well as other lifestyle-based approaches, may help optimize neurological function and quality of life in those with MS.

Side Effects

Moderate intake of fiber is well tolerated. Excessive intake of fiber, such as 50 to 60 g/d, may irritate the gut, cause gas and diarrhea, and interfere with the absorption of vitamins and minerals, including calcium, iron, magnesium, and zinc. Similar symptoms may develop if the intake of fiber is increased too rapidly. Fiber that is consumed without adequate amounts of water may lead to masses of fiber that obstruct the intestines.

Conclusion

For people with MS, adequate fiber intake may provide many health benefits. In contrast, inadequate fiber intake may produce a variety of adverse effects. Many people consume inadequate amounts of fiber, which may cause multiple health problems, one of which is constipation, a common symptom in MS. Constipation in those with MS may be due to the disease process itself but it may also be due to inadequate fiber intake. Likewise, adequate fiber intake in those with MS may help prevent or manage constipation.

Low fiber intake increases the risk or severity of many other conditions, such as heart disease, diabetes, cancer, and obesity, which do not generally have direct effects on the nervous system. However, the presence of some of these conditions in combination with MS may increase neurological disability and lower one's overall quality of life. Preventing or managing these conditions through adequate fiber intake, as well as other lifestyle-based approaches, may secondarily help optimize neurological function and quality of life in those with MS.

Additional Readings

Books

Duyff RL. *American Dietetic Association Complete Food and Nutrition Guide*. Boston, MA: Houghton Mifflin Harcourt; 2012.

Jellin JM, Batz F, Hitchens K. *Natural Medicines Comprehensive Database*. Stockton, CA: Therapeutic Research Faculty; 2014.

Katz DL. *Nutrition in Clinical Practice*. Philadelphia, PA: Lippincott Williams & Wilkins; 2008.

Journal Articles

Goodman S, Gulick E. Dietary practices of people with multiple sclerosis. *Int J MS Care*. 2008;10:47–57.

Hewson DC, Phillips MA, Simpson KE, Drury P, Crawford MA. Food intake in multiple sclerosis. *Human Nutr Appl Nutr*. 1984;38A:355–367.

King DE, Mainous AG, Lambourne CA. Trends in dietary fiber intake in the United States, 1999-2008. *J Acad Nutr Diet*. 2012;112:642–648.

Timmerman GM, Stuifbergen AK. Eating patterns of women with multiple sclerosis. *J Neurosci Nurs*. 1999;31:152–158.

Gluten Sensitivity and Celiac Disease

 Gluten Restriction Generally

⭐ **Gluten Restriction in Celiac Disease**

Interest in gluten sensitivity has grown dramatically in the United States. There are high levels of interest in the general public and also in the medical as well as business communities. Gluten sensitivity may cause multiple medical conditions, and, for decades, there have been claims about possible connections between multiple sclerosis (MS) and gluten sensitivity.

Gluten refers to proteins in specific grains, including wheat, barley, and rye. Although oats are naturally gluten free, they may still contain small amounts of gluten due to cross-contamination. Gluten is present in foods that are made from gluten-containing grains.

There are two forms of gluten sensitivity:

- Celiac disease. This condition is a severe form of gluten sensitivity and affects about 1% of the population. It is also known as *celiac sprue, non-tropical sprue,* and *gluten-sensitive enteropathy.* In people with celiac disease, gluten causes abdominal discomfort, bloating, and diarrhea. Like MS, celiac disease is autoimmune. In celiac disease, the immune system is activated in a way that it attacks the intestines and ultimately impairs the ability of the intestine to absorb nutrients. As a result, celiac disease may lead to conditions associated with nutrient deficiencies, including osteoporosis due to vitamin D deficiency and anemia due to iron deficiency. Celiac disease is also associated with other conditions, such as diabetes, cancer, and thyroid and liver disease.

- Non-celiac gluten sensitivity. This is a controversial condition that, relative to celiac disease, is thought to be less severe but more common. It is sometimes referred to as *gluten sensitivity* or *celiac lite* and is claimed to affect 10% to 25% of the population. This condition does not necessarily produce gastrointestinal symptoms. Instead, it is claimed to produce a wide range of symptoms, including fatigue and headache. Individuals with the conditions may have very different collections of symptoms.

Treatment Method

In the case of celiac disease, diagnostic tests are administered prior to treatment. There are specific criteria that must be met in order to make a diagnosis of celiac disease. An important component of these criteria are the results of various blood tests and biopsy of the intestine. The main treatment approach for celiac disease is a gluten-free diet. In addition, nutrient deficiencies, such as vitamin D deficiency and iron deficiency, may need to be treated, and there should be ongoing monitoring for other conditions that may develop in association with celiac disease.

The diagnostic approach for gluten sensitivity may be challenging and ambiguous. Unlike celiac disease, gluten sensitivity does not currently have specific objective criteria or tests to assist in making the diagnosis. Rather, the diagnosis is based on subjective information about how an individual feels after eating gluten. For those who are thought have gluten sensitivity, the treatment is a diet that has low levels of gluten or is completely gluten free.

Studies in MS

There are multiple studies of gluten and MS. The results of these studies have not been entirely consistent with each other, and thus it is not possible to make definitive conclusions. However, the majority of the studies do not indicate a clear association of MS with gluten sensitivity. In studies of the blood test markers and intestinal biopsy indicators of celiac disease, most (1–3), but not all (4), studies have *not* found abnormalities that are any higher than would be expected in the general population. The largest study of celiac disease in MS did not find that celiac disease was more common in MS than the general population (5), but a smaller study did (6). In the animal model of MS, gluten-free diets have *worsened* the disease (7). One study of people with MS found that gluten-free diets did not produce beneficial effects (8).

There are not any studies in MS of gluten sensitivity, the condition that appears to be different from celiac disease. Some people with MS report that their chronic symptoms are improved with a gluten-free diet, which could be an indicator of gluten sensitivity. The lack of clear diagnostic criteria for gluten sensitivity makes it difficult to conduct formal studies of this condition in MS or any other disease.

Side Effects

Gluten-free diets are generally well tolerated. However, they may be expensive and laborious. For those interested in experimenting with gluten-free diets on their own, it is important to keep in mind that celiac disease is a serious condition that requires ongoing medical monitoring and treatment. As a result, those who feel significantly improved on gluten-free diets, especially with regard to gastrointestinal symptoms, should discuss this situation with health professionals in order to be certain that they do not have celiac disease.

Conclusion

There are not clear associations of MS with celiac disease or gluten sensitivity. The studies in this area are limited and inconsistent. Gluten-free diets are generally well tolerated. However, due to the potential serious complications of celiac disease, people should not diagnose and treat this condition on their own.

Additional Readings

Books

Duyff RL. *American Dietetic Association Complete Food and Nutrition Guide.* Boston, MA: Houghton Mifflin Harcourt; 2012.

Journal Articles

DiMarco R, Mangano K, Quattrocchi C, et al. Exacerbation of protracted-relapsing experimental allergic encephalomyelitis in DA rats by gluten-free diets. *APMIS.* 2004;112:651–655.

Di Sabatino A, Corazza GR. Nonceliac gluten sensitivity: sense or sensibility? *Ann Intern Med.* 2012;156:309–311.

Hadjivassiliou M, Sanders DS, Grunewald RA, et al. Gluten sensitivity: from gut to brain. *Lancet Neurol.* 2010;9:318–330.

Haghighi AB, Ansari N, Mokhtari M, et al. Multiple sclerosis and gluten sensitivity. *Clin Neurol Neurosurg.* 2007;109:651–653.

Hunter AL, Rees BW, Jones LT. Gluten antibodies in patients with multiple sclerosis. *Human Nutr Appl Nutr.* 1984;38:142–143.

Jones PE, Pallis C, Peters TJ. Morphological and biochemical findings in jejunal biopsies from patients with multiple sclerosis. *J Neurol Psych.* 1979;42:402–406.

Murray J. Gluten-free confusion: separating fact from fiction. *Nutr Action Healthletter.* 2011;38:9.

Nicoletti A, Patti F, Lo Fermo S, et al. Frequency of celiac disease is not increased among multiple sclerosis patients. *Mult Scler.* 2008;14:698–700.

Rodrigo L, Hernandez-Lahoz C, Fuentes D, et al. Prevalence of celiac disease in multiple sclerosis. *BMC Neurol.* 2011;11:31.

Sapone A, Bai JC, Ciacci C, et al. Spectrum of gluten-related disorders: consensus on new nomenclature and classification. *BMC Med.* 2012;10:13.

Shor D B-A, Barzilai O, Ram M, et al. Gluten sensitivity in multiple sclerosis: experimental myth or clinical truth? *Contemp Chall Autoimmun.* 2009;1173: 343–349.

Tengah CP, Lock RJ, Unsworth J, et al. Multiple sclerosis and occult gluten sensitivity. *Neurology.* 2004;62:2326–2327.

Troncone R, Jabri B. Coeliac disease and gluten sensitivity. *J Intern Med.* 2011;296:582–590.

Volta U, De Giorgio R. Gluten sensitivity: an emerging issue behind neurological impairment? *Lancet Neurol.* 2010;9:233–235.

✓ Guided Imagery

Guided imagery is a technique frequently used in hypnosis as well as in meditation and other relaxation therapies. Although it generally is used to produce relaxation, guided imagery may be used for other purposes.

Treatment Method

In guided imagery, an individual creates images that have specific effects on the mind and body. For example, to produce a state of relaxation, one may imagine sitting in a tranquil location such as a beach or a mountain. These images may be visual but may also involve sounds, taste, and smells associated with a particular setting. A very different type of imagery that is under active investigation in multiple sclerosis (MS), other neurological conditions, and sports is *motor imagery*. This novel technique involves imagining body movement in order to ultimately improve actual body movement.

Studies in MS and Other Conditions

Guided imagery has not undergone extensive investigation in MS. One study conducted in Pennsylvania evaluated the effects of imagery and relaxation techniques in 33 people with MS (1). For imagery, people were instructed to imagine the repair of injured myelin and beneficial immune system activity. People who practiced daily imagery along with relaxation experienced less anxiety and produced more active and powerful images of their disease process. No effect of imagery and relaxation was noted on depression or specific MS-associated symptoms.

Guided imagery has been investigated in other medical conditions. Some, but not all, studies indicate that imagery may relieve fatigue. Other studies suggest that imagery may improve anxiety, depression, pain, and sleeping difficulties. One study in Parkinson's disease found that guided imagery improved tremor. However, the relevance of this finding to MS-associated tremor is not clear since the underlying basis for the tremors of MS and Parkinson's disease are different. Imagery is sometimes used to assist in managing heart disease because of its relaxation effect and ability to decrease blood pressure.

Studies are currently underway to investigate how motor imagery might be used to improve walking and other neurological functions in MS and other conditions. Motor imagery is sometimes used by athletes to enhance physical performance.

Imagery could conceivably be used to alter immune system function. Limited studies in this area have produced mixed results.

Side Effects

Imagery generally is well tolerated. It should not be used instead of conventional medication for serious conditions, such as modifying the course of MS. People with psychiatric conditions, including severe depression, should use caution with imagery. Rarely, imagery-induced relaxation may paradoxically *increase* anxiety. Imagery may also cause disturbing thoughts and fear of losing control.

Practical Information

Most imagery sessions last 20 to 30 minutes. Books and audiotapes are available for additional instruction. Alternatively, a trained therapist may be used. More information about guided imagery may be obtained from:

- The Academy of Guided Imagery (www.acadgi.com), 30765 Pacific Coast Highway, Ste. 355, Malibu, CA 90265 (424-242-6369).

Conclusion

Guided imagery is inexpensive and generally safe. Limited studies in MS and other conditions indicate that it may improve anxiety, depression, fatigue, pain, and sleeping difficulties. Further studies are needed to examine its effectiveness.

Additional Readings

Books

Bauer B, ed. *Mayo Clinic Book of Alternative Medicine and Home Remedies.* New York, NY: Time Home Entertainment; 2013:100–101.

Cassileth BR. *The Alternative Medicine Handbook.* New York, NY: W.W. Norton; 1998:122–130.

Ernst E, ed. *The Desktop Guide to Complementary and Alternative Medicine: An Evidence-Based Approach.* Edinburgh, UK: Mosby; 2001.

Jellin JM, Gregory PJ, Batz F, et al. *Pharmacist's Letter/ Prescriber's Letter Natural Medicines Comprehensive Database.* Stockton, CA: Therapeutic Research Faculty; 2014.

Micozzi MS, ed. *Fundamentals of Complementary and Alternative Medicine.* Philadelphia, PA: Saunders Elsevier; 2011:123–126.

Journal Articles

Apostolo JL, Kolcaba K. The effects of guided imagery on comfort, depression, anxiety, and stress of psychiatric inpatients with depressive disorders. *Arch Psych Nurs.* 2009;23:403–411.

Dickstein R, Deutsch JE, Yoeli Y, et al. Effects of integrated motor imagery practice on gait of individuals with chronic stroke: a half-crossover randomized study. *Arch Phys Med Rehabil.* 2013;94:2119–2125.

Freeman L, Cohen L, Stewart M, et al. Imagery intervention for recovering breast cancer patients: clinical trial of safety and efficacy. *J Soc Integr Oncol.* 2008;6:67–75.

Hall H, Minnes L, Olness K. The psychophysiology of voluntary immunomodulation. *Int J Neurosci.* 1993;69:221–234.

Heremans E, Nieuwboer A, Spildooren J, et al. Cued motor imagery in patients with multiple sclerosis. *Neurosci.* 2012;206:115–121.

Lazarus AA, Mayne TJ. Relaxation: some limitations, side effects, and proposed solutions. *Psychotherapy.* 1990;27:261–266.

Lee MH, Kim DH, Yu HS. The effect of guided imagery on stress and fatigue in patients with thyroid cancer undergoing radioactive iodine therapy. *Evid Based Complem Altern Med.* 2013;2013:130324.

Lengacher CA, Bennett MP, Gonzalez L, et al. Immune responses to guided imagery during breast cancer treatment. *Biol Res Nurs.* 2008;9:205–214.

Maguire BL. The effects of imagery on attitudes and moods in multiple sclerosis patients. *Alt Ther.* 1996;2:75–79.

Menzies V, Jallo N. Guided imagery as a treatment option for fatigue: a literature review. *J Holist Nurs.* 2011;29:279–286.

Mizrahi MC, Reicher-Atir R, Levy S, et al. Effects of guided imagery with relaxation training on anxiety and quality of life among patients with inflammatory bowel disease. *Psychol Health.* 2012;27:1463–1479.

Posadzki P, Ernst E. Guided imagery for musculoskeletal pain: a systematic review. *Clin J Pain.* 2011;27:648–653.

Posadzki P, Lewandowski W, Terry R, et al. Guided imagery for non-musculoskeletal pain: a systematic review of randomized clinical trials. *J Pain Symptom Manage.* 2012;44:95–104.

Schaffer L, Jallo N, Howland L, et al. Guided imagery: an innovative approach to improving maternal sleep quality. *J Perinat Neonatal Nurs.* 2013;27:151–159.

Schlesinger I, Benyakov O, Erikh I, et al. Parkinson's disease tremor is diminished with relaxation guided imagery. *Mov Disord.* 2009;24:2059–2062.

Smith GR, McKenzie JM, Marmer DJ, et al. Psychologic modulation of the human immune response to *Varicella zoster. Arch Intern Med.* 1985;145:221–235.

Tabrizi YM, Mazhari S, Nazari MA, et al. Compromised motor imagery ability in individuals with multiple sclerosis and mild physical disability: an ERP study. *Clin Neurol Neurosurg.* 2013;115:1738–1744.

Torem MS. Mind-body hypnotic imagery in the treatment of auto-immune disorders. *Am J Clin Hypn.* 2007;50:157–170.

Trakhtenberg E. The effects of guided imagery on the immune system: a critical review. *Int J Neurosci.* 2008;118:839–855.

Van Fleet S. Relaxation and imagery for symptom management: improving patient assessment and individualizing treatment. *Oncol Nurs Forum.* 2000;27:501–510.

Herbs

✓ Coffee

✓ Cranberry

! Echinacea

? Garlic

? Ginkgo

? Ginseng

? Goldenseal

? Grape Seed Extract

! Kava Kava

? Padma 28

! Protandim

✓ Psyllium

(?) Pycnogenol

(?) St. John's Wort

(!) Spirulina

(?) Stinging Nettle

(✓) Valerian

(!) Yohimbe and Yohimbine

Herbal medicine has been used for tens of thousands of years. About 60,000 BCE, Neanderthals apparently used two herbs, yarrow and marshmallow, for therapeutic purposes. Within traditional Chinese medicine, herbal therapies were initially developed around 3000 BCE and, ultimately, more than 10,000 different Chinese herbal formulas were compiled.

Herbal medicine was popular in the United States from 1820 to 1920. After 1920, herbal therapies were replaced by conventional medications. A recent resurgence of interest in herbal medicine has occurred, and herbs are currently one of the most frequently used forms of complementary and alternative medicine (CAM). The use of herbs by Americans nearly quadrupled between 1990 and 1997. One U.S. study of dietary supplement and herb use in people with multiple sclerosis (MS) found that about one-quarter of those with MS used some form of herbal therapy.

Much of the popularity of herbs probably is related to the ease with which they can be used. There is no need to make an appointment with a practitioner to get started on herbal therapy. Rather, one can simply buy the herb at the local grocery store or health food store.

Herbs also became popular in the United States after the passage in 1994 of the Dietary Supplements Health and Education Act (DSHEA), which loosened the regulations for dietary supplements such as herbs. In fact, the regulations became so relaxed that few standards for safety, effectiveness, or quality exist. To counter some of the laxity of DSHEA, new directions for the U.S. market were developed in the *Consumer Health Information for Better Nutrition Initiative*. Through this program, the Food and Drug Administration (FDA) announced several objectives, including collaboration to improve the evidence base for safety and enforcement decisions, implementation of a process to evaluate safety concerns and improve the quality and consistency of products (Good

Manufacturing Practices), and the mandated creation of documents with the evidence needed to make claims of effectiveness.

Herbs Contain Many Different Chemicals

An important distinction between drugs and herbs is that most drugs consist of a single chemical compound, whereas herbs consist of many different ones. Of all the chemicals in herbs, some may be beneficial, some may be harmful, and a large number have unknown effects on the human body. Fortunately, most of the chemicals are not toxic, and most are present in small enough quantities that significant harmful effects are unlikely.

Many chemicals with beneficial activity against disease have been identified in herbs. It is estimated that 25% of prescription drugs and 60% of over-the-counter drugs are derived from plants. Well-known examples of these drugs are digitalis, which is derived from the foxglove plant, and quinine, which is derived from South American Peruvian bark. Steroids, which are used to treat MS attacks, have a very specific chemical structure. Chemicals with steroid-like structures and biologic effects have been identified in Asian ginseng (ginsenoside) and in licorice (glycyrrhizic acid).

Herbs may contain chemicals that have harmful effects. Naturally occurring chemicals in some herbs have toxic effects. For example, the lily-of-the-valley plant is known to contain potent heart toxins. Also, multiple studies indicate that herb products may be contaminated with toxic ingredients, such as heavy metals, or may be prepared with herbs that are incorrectly identified and have serious side effects, such as severe liver toxicity. Some herbs, such as chaparral and comfrey (or contaminants mixed in with the herbs), have been associated with a severe liver toxicity that has led to death or the need for liver transplantation. There is a case report in the medical literature of a 28-year-old man with mild MS who was treating his disease with zinc and two herbal medicines, skullcap and pau d'arco. He died from severe liver injury that was probably caused by a chemical contaminant in the skullcap.

Fortunately, most of the chemicals in herbs do not have toxic effects. For most herbs, the majority of the chemicals probably have neither beneficial nor harmful properties—if demonstrated beneficial effects of an herb exist, they probably are due to one or several of the many chemicals present. Thus, for many herbs, it is likely that one or a few chemicals could be producing a beneficial effect and that the remaining chemicals do not have any beneficial or harmful effects.

It is sometimes claimed that herbs cannot have harmful effects because the chemicals in them are present in such small quantities. It is also claimed that herbs have beneficial qualities. These two statements are not consistent with each other. *If a therapy is strong enough to produce beneficial effects, it usually is also strong enough to produce harmful effects.* As more research is conducted, it may indeed be found that, relative to prescription medications, herbs generally have fewer side effects, but are also somewhat less effective.

Important Features of Herbs

Most herbs have not been studied as extensively as have drugs. As a result, it is often not known exactly which chemicals in herbs are the active ingredients. Similarly, the side effects of herbs and their interactions with drugs are not fully understood. In summary, even for well-studied herbs, the full range of effectiveness and the full range of side effects are not completely known.

Another important aspect of herbs is their variability. Because of the current lack of strict regulation in the United States, there is much variability in the quantity of the presumed active ingredient present in different herbal preparations. For example, one study of ginseng found 50 times as much of the active ingredient in some products as in others. This situation is similar to a physician telling a patient to take somewhere between one and 50 pills for a medical condition. Other reports have found no active ingredient in some ginseng preparations.

Finally, herbs should be avoided in certain circumstances. People should avoid herbs if they have multiple medical problems or are taking multiple medications. Women who are pregnant or breastfeeding and children also should avoid herbs. Some medications have a very specific range in which they are effective and in which they do not have side effects. These include anticonvulsant medications, blood-thinning medications, and some heart medications. Herbs should not be taken with these drugs because it is not known if herbs could have dangerous interactions with the drugs.

Herbal Therapy Guidelines

The most conservative approach to the use of herbs in MS is to state that they should be avoided entirely. The basis for this argument is that the effects of herbs have not been directly studied in MS, and it is therefore possible that an herb now thought to be safe could through future research be found to adversely affect the MS disease process.

For those interested in considering herb use, guidelines can make decisionmaking easier. These guidelines are outlined in Table 3.5.

TABLE 3.5 HERBAL THERAPY GUIDELINES

- Herbs are often used as drugs.
- Herbs contain many different compounds, some of which may be toxic or interact with drugs.
- Herbs may contain compounds that have not yet been identified or characterized.
- The quality and composition of herbal preparations are variable.
- Herbs should generally be used for a short time for benign, self-limited conditions.
- Herbs should be avoided in women who are pregnant or breastfeeding.
- Herbs should be avoided or used with caution by people who have multiple medical problems or are taking multiple medications.
- Use caution and discuss herbal use with a physician before starting.

Choose Reliable Herb Suppliers

When using herbs, it is important to purchase them from companies that produce high-quality, consistent preparations. Some of the highest quality preparations are produced in Europe. Brands chosen should be standardized and contain specified amounts of active ingredients. The product also should list other specific information: common and scientific name of the herb, the manufacturer's name and address, batch and lot number, expiration date, dose recommendations, potential side effects, and quality control information. Higher-quality herbal products in the United States have the symbols for the U.S. Pharmacopeia (USP) or the National Formulary (NF). To evaluate the quality of some herbs and other dietary supplement products, independent laboratory evaluations of products have been done by *Consumer Reports* and by an organization known as *Consumerlab.com* (www .consumerlab.com). The results of these evaluations are available from these sources.

Consideration of Specific Herbs

Many different herbal preparations are available. To provide practical information in this area, this section reviews some of the most popular herbs in the United States. Herbs with particular relevance to MS also are reviewed. These herbs are presented in alphabetical order. Following this section, both common and uncommon herbs are discussed in terms of their possible effects on MS and possible interactions with medications frequently used to manage MS.

Herbs Commonly Used in the General Population and Herbs That Are Relevant to MS

✅ Coffee and Other Caffeine-Containing Herbs and Supplements

Coffee, perhaps not generally thought of as an herb, is in fact one of the most popular herbs in the world. Its effects on mental alertness and fatigue are well known to those who drink their regular morning cup of coffee. The effects of coffee are due to one of its chemical constituents, caffeine. In addition to coffee, other herbs and supplements contain caffeine.

Coffee is of interest for people with MS because of its possible effects on fatigue. No systematic approaches exist to using coffee or other caffeine-containing herbs in people with MS. Despite the fairly widespread use of caffeine products by people with MS, very little research has been done in this area. One published Internet-based research study of more than 2,000 people with MS, of which I was a co-author, found that 47% of people with MS reported that caffeine improved fatigue (1). Another MS study that included caffeine involved a therapy known as *Prokarin*—the results of this study are difficult to interpret for several reasons, including the fact that Prokarin contains caffeine as well as histamine (see *Prokarin* chapter).

In the general population, strong evidence indicates that coffee improves mental alertness, thereby potentially improving mental fatigue. In contrast, coffee does not appear to improve physical power or endurance and therefore probably does not have a beneficial effect on physical fatigue.

Another area of possible relevance to MS is immune system alteration by caffeine. Some studies indicate that caffeine may decrease the activity of lymphocytes, a type of immune system cell, and produce changes in a protein in the brain known as the *adenosine receptor*. In theory, these effects could be beneficial for MS. Limited studies in the animal model of MS indicate that caffeine decreases disease severity.

Other herbal sources of caffeine exist. Tea contains a significant amount of caffeine. In the United States, black tea, derived from the leaves of *Camellia sinensis*, is the most popular form. Green tea is prepared from the same plant, but the leaves are processed differently. "Energy drinks," which are rising in popularity in the United States, come in a variety of flavors and contain caffeine as well as other ingredients. Another well-known source of caffeine is chocolate and other food products derived from the cacao plant. Cola nut, also known as kola nut and bissy nut, contains caffeine. Guarana is a South American caffeine-containing herb that may be consumed as a tea or in tablet form. Another South American herb that contains caffeine, mate or yerba mate, is not especially popular in the United States but is popular in some South American countries. Finally, the most direct approach is to take caffeine itself, which is available in tablet form as a dietary supplement.

The amount of caffeine available from these products is variable. A convenient reference point to start with is a 6-ounce cup of percolated coffee, which contains approximately 100 mg of caffeine. It is important to note that less caffeine is present in instant coffee and darker roast coffees, including latte, cappuccino, and other popular espresso-based coffees. In comparison to a typical cup of coffee, approximately one-half the amount of caffeine (30–60 mg) may be obtained from a 12-ounce bottle of a cola drink, an 800-milligram tablet of guarana, or a cup of tea, cocoa, or mate. Relatively low amounts of caffeine (5–10 mg) typically are contained in a cup of "decaffeinated" coffee or a chocolate bar. Caffeine tablets often contain 100 or 200 mg of caffeine and are roughly equivalent to one or two cups of coffee.

The frequency with which one ingests caffeine may influence the herb's ability to improve mental alertness. With high levels of fatigue in the morning, people often drink extra cups of coffee at that time. However, research indicates that this may not be the most effective approach. It has been reported that small amounts of caffeine (about 20 mg or about one-fifth of a cup of coffee) taken on an hourly basis may be especially effective for promoting wakefulness.

The FDA regards the consumption of moderate amounts of coffee and other caffeine-containing herbs as generally safe. The effects of caffeine on pregnancy and breastfeeding are not clear. Thus, pregnant and breastfeeding women should avoid or limit caffeine consumption. Mate is an herb that has raised concern. Studies indicate that mate, especially in high doses, may increase the risk of cancers of the mouth, throat, kidney, bladder, and lung.

Some specific concerns exist about MS and caffeine-containing products. Caffeine use may worsen MS-associated bladder problems because it increases urination and may irritate the urinary tract. Caffeine use may increase the risk of osteoporosis, a condition to which people with MS may be especially prone. In addition, theoretical risks are associated with the use of high doses of green tea. This form of tea contains relatively high levels of antioxidants, which, in theory, may stimulate the immune system (see the *Vitamins, Minerals, and Other Nonherbal Supplements* chapter)—this effect poses a theoretical risk for people with MS.

Doses of caffeine in excess of 600 mg daily may produce multiple side effects, including anxiety, confusion, insomnia, heart palpitations, upset stomach, nausea, vomiting, high blood pressure, tremors, muscle twitching, and increased cholesterol levels. The long-term use of large doses of caffeine may lead to an addiction-type situation in which higher and higher doses are required for the same effect and in which abrupt discontinuation causes mild withdrawal symptoms such as headache, irritability, dizziness, and anxiety.

Caffeine-containing preparations also interact with other supplements and medications. Simultaneously taking moderate doses of two or three caffeine-containing supplements may lead to excessive levels of caffeine. Also, both the stimulant actions and the adverse effects of caffeine may be accentuated when it is consumed with *ma huang* (ephedra) or with grapefruit juice.

The blood levels of caffeine may be increased by multiple medications, including oral contraceptives, cimetidine (Tagamet), and verapamil (Calan).

The usual maximum daily dose of caffeine is 250 to 300 mg. This is equivalent to two to three cups of coffee or four to five cups of tea. The optimal timing and dosing of caffeine for MS-related fatigue has not been studied.

✅ Cranberry and Other Herbal Therapies for Urinary Tract Infections

Cranberry juice, obtained from the fruit of the cranberry or *Vaccinium macrocarpon* plant, is of relevance to MS because urinary tract infections (UTIs) are common with MS, and cranberry juice has a long history of use in their prevention and treatment. From the 1920s to the 1970s, it was believed that the acid from cranberry juice makes the urine acidic and that this increase in acidity prevents and treats UTIs. However, subsequent studies showed that the effect of cranberry juice was probably due to the presence of two types of compounds, fructose and a class of chemicals known as proanthocyanidins. These chemicals do not destroy bacteria. Instead, they appear to keep bacteria from attaching to the walls of the urinary tract. As a result, it is believed that bacteria present in the urinary tract are unable to cause an infection and are simply passed in the urine. In addition to these effects, cranberry juice, like antibiotic medications, also may kill some bacteria.

Limited clinical studies indicate that cranberry may prevent UTIs in some people. A beneficial effect has been reported in studies of UTI prevention in women who have normal bladder function. However, limited studies of people with abnormal bladder function, which may occur in MS, indicate that cranberry is *not* effective for UTI prevention. A rigorous, well-designed study of cranberry use for the prevention or treatment of UTIs has not been done yet. Also, it is not known how the effectiveness of cranberry compares with that of prescription antibiotics, the more conventional method for preventing UTIs.

Because UTIs in people with MS may lead to serious complications, including worsening of neurologic difficulties, cranberry juice should not be used to treat infections. On the other hand, for people interested in an herbal approach, it may be reasonable to attempt to *prevent* infections using cranberry juice. The exact doses that should be used have not been established. Doses sometimes recommended for prevention are 1 to 10 ounces of juice daily. Six capsules of dried powder or 1.5 ounces of frozen or fresh cranberries may be equivalent to 3 ounces of juice. If cranberry capsules are used, it may be best to use products that have been found to be effective in clinical trials, such as *Cran-Max* (Buckton Scott Health Products) or *Natural Cranberry With Vitamin C* (Solgar). The use of frozen or fresh cranberries may not be possible because of the sour taste of the berries. Of note, cranberry juice cocktail is 26% to 33% juice.

Cranberry generally is well tolerated. Cranberry may interact with blood-thinning medications, including warfarin (Coumadin). The chronic use of high doses may increase the risk of developing kidney stones and may cause stomach discomfort, loose stools, and nausea. The safety of cranberry use in women who are pregnant or breastfeeding is not known.

Another herb sometimes recommended for UTIs is bearberry, also known as uva ursi. Some concerns about this herb exist. Specifically, it is not clearly effective for UTI prevention, it appears to be less effective with acidic urine, it may cause nausea and vomiting, and it contains chemicals that may cause cancer and eye problems.

Several other herbs, supplements, and other strategies are sometimes recommended for preventing and treating UTIs. Vitamin C is sometimes recommended, but clinical studies do not support its use for preventing or treating UTIs. Also, vitamin C may increase the risk of kidney stones in those with a history of kidney stones, and a theoretical risk exists that high doses of vitamin C may stimulate the immune system and possibly worsen MS. Many other UTI strategies are sometimes recommended. However, there is not adequate safety or effectiveness evidence for these approaches, which include asparagus root, blackberry, echinacea, garlic, goldenrod, goldenseal, java tea, lovage, parsley, stinging nettle, and probiotics (bifidobacteria, lactobacillus, yogurt).

⚠ Echinacea

Echinacea, which is usually obtained from the *Echinacea purpurea* plant, is one of the most popular and well-studied herbs. A long history of echinacea use exists for the treatment of medical conditions, especially infections. North American Indians used echinacea medicinally, and it was the primary herbal therapy for infections in the early 1900s. Echinacea poses a theoretical risk for people with MS, yet, surprisingly, it is sometimes recommended for MS and is used by some people with the disease.

Echinacea is of interest to people with MS because it may prevent or reduce the severity of viral infections. Because viral infections may, in some instances, provoke an MS attack, their reduction has obvious potential benefit. Also, popular books on alternative medicine sometimes specifically recommend echinacea as a treatment for MS, possibly because of echinacea's effects on the immune system.

Many scientific and clinical studies have evaluated echinacea. Some, but not all, studies suggest that echinacea limits the duration and severity of infections, especially the common cold.

The important point for people with MS is that echinacea may act by stimulating two components of the immune system, *macrophages* and *T cells*. Macrophages and T cells are already excessively active in MS, and many disease-modifying MS medications generally decrease their activity.

Thus, consuming echinacea may conceivably worsen MS by further stimulating these immune cells, and this may decrease the effectiveness of MS medications. One case report documents a person who developed an MS-like condition known as *acute disseminated encephalomyelitis* (ADEM) after being treated with an herbal muscle injection that included echinacea. Theoretical concerns exist that echinacea may produce liver injury. This effect could be increased if echinacea is taken with those MS medications having possible toxic effects on the liver, including interferons (Avonex, Betaseron, Extavia, and Rebif), fingolimod (Gilenya), teriflunomide (Aubagio), and natalizumab (Tysabri). *In summary, it is safest for people with MS to avoid echinacea.*

What about other measures to prevent or treat the common cold or other minor infections? Goldenseal and garlic (see subsequent sections) have not been shown to have definite effects on infections, and the scientific basis for their use is unclear. Also, vitamin C and zinc, which are discussed in detail elsewhere in this book, sometimes are used for infections. However, both of these compounds also have unclear effects on infections and may activate the immune system.

People with MS may take several safe measures to prevent and treat viral infections such as the flu and common cold. First, the flu vaccine is readily available. The "shot" form of the vaccine, which contains *inactivated* virus, appears to be safe for people with MS and helps prevent the flu. The nasal form of the vaccine is *live* and should be avoided by those with MS. Prescription medications (oseltamivir [Tamiflu], zanamivir [Relenza]) also decrease the severity of the flu. Finally, viral infections may be prevented by simple hygiene measures such as avoiding contact with people with viral infections, frequent hand-washing, and not touching the eyes, nose, or mouth with one's fingers.

Evening Primrose Oil

See *Fats: Fish Oil and Polyunsaturated Fatty Acids* chapter.

⑦ Garlic

Over the past 25 years, more than 1,000 studies have evaluated the possible therapeutic effects of garlic (*Allium sativum*). Suggestive, but not conclusive, results have been obtained in studies of the effectiveness of garlic in treating atherosclerosis ("hardening of the arteries"), high blood pressure, and some forms of cancer. On the basis of limited scientific studies, garlic sometimes is recommended as a treatment for the common cold.

With regard to MS, some research has shown that garlic may stimulate two types of immune cells, macrophages and lymphocytes. No clinical studies have directly evaluated the effect of garlic on MS or other autoimmune diseases. However, the immune-stimulating activity of garlic could, on a theoretical basis, adversely affect the course of MS or inhibit the therapeutic effects of MS disease-modifying drugs.

Controversy exists regarding the best form and dose of garlic. Some commercial preparations actually contain none of the presumed active chemical, *allicin*. Garlic may inhibit blood clotting and thus should be avoided in people with blood-clotting disorders, people undergoing surgery, and people taking blood-thinning medications or aspirin.

(?) Ginkgo Biloba

Ginkgo biloba, often referred to simply as "Ginkgo," is one of the most extensively studied herbal therapies and is sometimes recommended for MS. Ginkgo usually refers to the extract derived from the leaf of the *Ginkgo biloba* tree, one of the oldest living species of trees.

Some of the more recent popularity of Ginkgo may be due to an investigation published in 1997 in the *Journal of the American Medical Association (JAMA)*. In this study, Ginkgo extract was found to be effective in treating cognitive difficulties in the elderly.

Several biological effects have been associated with Ginkgo. Some of its chemical constituents act as antioxidants. Other constituents inhibit the effects of platelet-activating factor (PAF), a compound in the body that plays a role in inflammation and blood clotting.

Because of the inflammatory effect of PAF, it and Ginkgo have been studied in MS. In animals with EAE, an experimental model of MS, PAF worsens the disease, whereas Ginkgo, in some but not all studies, produces improvement. On the basis of these findings in animals, a small study, reported in 1992, examined the effects of Ginkgo on MS attacks and found that 8 of 10 people improved using Ginkgo treatment (2). Some herbal medicine and CAM books recommend Ginkgo for MS because of the results of this study. It is sometimes not mentioned that this encouraging 1992 study was, unfortunately, followed by a 1995 study that found Ginkgo ineffective for treating MS attacks. The 1995 study (3), which involved 104 people, was better designed and involved a larger number of patients than did the 1992 study. *Thus, Ginkgo does not appear to be effective for the short-term treatment of MS attacks*. It is not known whether Ginkgo decreases MS disease activity when it is used on a long-term, as opposed to short-term, basis.

Several studies have evaluated the effects of Ginkgo on MS symptoms. In terms of MS-associated cognitive difficulties, smaller studies indicate possible beneficial effects (4, 5), but a large, rigorous, well-conducted study did not find any significant improvement in multiple areas of cognitive function (6). For MS-associated fatigue, one study found improvement after four weeks of treatment with Ginkgo (7).

Ginkgo usually is well tolerated. If this herb is used, it is important to keep in mind that it has a tendency to increase bleeding. Spontaneous bleeding in the eye or around or in the brain has been described in a few patients taking this herb.

It probably should be avoided by people who take blood-thinning medications (warfarin or Coumadin) or aspirin, people who have bleeding disorders, and people who are undergoing surgery. Ginkgo may increase the risk of seizures and thus should be used with caution by those with seizures. Ginkgo may also cause rashes, dizziness, headache, and gastrointestinal symptoms, including nausea, vomiting, diarrhea, and flatulence. In experimental animals, high doses of Ginkgo administered for 2 years have been associated with liver and thyroid cancer. It is not known if Ginkgo is safe in women who are pregnant or breastfeeding.

Clinical studies of Ginkgo generally use standardized leaf extracts. In these preparations, known in Germany as EGb 761 and LI 1370, a specific content of certain chemicals (24%–25% flavone glycosides and 6% terpene lactones) is present. Commercially available products that are similar to EGb 761 and LI 1370 include *Ginkai* (Lichtwer Pharma), *Ginkgo 5* (Pharmline), *Ginkgold* and *Ginkgo* (Nature's Way), and *Quanterra Mental Sharpness* (Warner-Lambert).

⑦ Ginseng

Three main types of ginseng are available for herbal therapy. Ginseng usually refers to two similar species of the plant, Asian ginseng (*Panax ginseng*) and American ginseng (*Panax* quinquefolius). Siberian ginseng (*Eleutherococcus senticosus* or simply *eleuthero*) is a different type of plant with chemical constituents that differ significantly from those of Asian and Siberian ginseng.

All three forms of ginseng are derived from roots. Some ginseng products are referred to as *adaptogens*, which means that they are believed to increase resistance to stress and increase energy levels. Although the effects of these herbs may be desired by many people with MS, it is not clear that consuming either of them is the best way to produce these effects.

Asian ginseng has been associated with many different biological actions. *Ginsenosides*, which may be the active constituents in Asian ginseng as well as American ginseng, have a chemical structure similar to that of steroids, which are used to treat MS attacks and *suppress* the immune system. In the animal model of MS, one study found decreased disease severity with Asian ginseng. A small study of Asian ginseng in MS reported improvement in fatigue (8). However, of concern for MS, *activation* of the immune system also has been associated with Asian ginseng. Multiple studies have shown that the herb stimulates immune system cells, including T cells and macrophages and, on the basis of these immune-system effects, Asian ginseng has been investigated as a possible treatment for cancer and AIDS. Clinical studies of the effects of Asian ginseng on stress, fatigue, and other medical conditions have yielded mixed results.

American ginseng has undergone limited investigation in MS and other medical conditions. Chemical components of American ginseng, like those of Asian ginseng, have been associated with immune-stimulating effects. One well-designed study of American ginseng in MS did not find any beneficial effects on fatigue (9). American ginseng does not have clear therapeutic effects for any other medical condition.

Siberian ginseng is an entirely different herb from Asian and American ginseng, but the research results thus far have been similar. Specifically, Siberian ginseng may have immune-stimulating properties, and clinical studies do not definitely show beneficial effects on stress, fatigue, and other medical conditions. Siberian ginseng has not been specifically studied in the animal model of MS or in people with MS.

Side effects and drug interactions are possible with the various forms of ginseng. As noted, all three forms of ginseng may activate the immune system. This effect could, in theory, worsen the disease process of MS or decrease the therapeutic effects of MS disease-modifying medications. Also, all three forms of ginseng may increase bleeding tendency and thus should be avoided by people who are undergoing surgery, people who have blood-clotting disorders, and people who take blood-thinning medications or aspirin. Siberian ginseng may produce sedation, while Asian ginseng may cause insomnia.

Asian, American, and Siberian ginseng do not have clear therapeutic effects on MS or any other medical condition. In addition, all three herbs have possible side effects, including immune-stimulating activity which may, in theory, be harmful to those with MS. It is reasonable for people with MS to avoid high doses and regular use of these herbs.

⑦ Goldenseal

Goldenseal (*Hydrastis canadensis*) has been used medicinally for at least 200 years. This herb is taken alone or in combination with echinacea for a variety of infections, including the common cold. Unlike echinacea, which has been investigated extensively, little information is available about the biological effects, clinical effectiveness, or safety of goldenseal or its chemical constituents, berberine and hydrastine. There are no studies of goldenseal in MS. Because of the extremely limited information, it is not possible to make any definite conclusions about the safety or effectiveness of this herb for MS or any other medical condition. The clinical studies to date do not support its use for infections.

⑦ Grape Seed Extract

Grape seed extract use has grown in popularity recently. It is sold for its antioxidant activity. Grape seed extract contains complex mixtures of chemicals known as *oligomeric proanthocyanidins* or *OPCs*. The chemicals that are present in grape seed extract are similar to those in pycnogenol (see *Pycnogenol* section below) and act as antioxidants. Another dietary supplement that is related to grapes is *resveratrol,* a chemical that is present in red grapes (see chapter on *Vitamins, Minerals, and Other Nonherbal Supplements*).

The safety and clinical use of grape seed extract has not been studied extensively in MS or any other medical condition that is of relevance to MS. As a result, there is not any MS-relevant safety and effectiveness information available. For people with MS who want to take antioxidants, it may be best to take low doses of inexpensive antioxidant vitamins, such as vitamin A (beta-carotene), vitamin C, and vitamin E (see the chapter on *Vitamins, Minerals, and Other Nonherbal Supplements*).

⚠️ Kava Kava

Kava kava (*Piper methysticum*) is an herb that has been used in the Pacific islands for hundreds of years for its purported relaxant effects. It is one of the few herbs for which the active chemicals have been identified. These chemicals, known as *kavalactones* or *kavapyrones,* interact with proteins in the central nervous system that are known as *GABA-A receptors.* These are the same proteins that mediate the effects of diazepam (Valium) and related antianxiety drugs. Several studies indicate that kava kava decreases mild anxiety. It does not appear to be effective for more severe forms of anxiety.

Kava kava sometimes is recommended for insomnia. However, its effects on insomnia have not been well studied. Another herb, valerian, has been more extensively studied for insomnia than kava kava (see the following section on *Valerian*).

Kava kava may increase the sedating effects of alcohol and several medications that are frequently used in MS, including lioresal (Baclofen), tizanidine (Zanaflex), and diazepam (Valium). The effects of kava kava on MS fatigue are not known. Heavy use of kava kava over months may produce skin problems, red eyes, itching, and other difficulties.

The greatest concern with kava kava is liver toxicity. In 2001, several reports surfaced of liver toxicity in association with kava kava use. Subsequently, there have been more than 100 reports of liver toxicity, which in some cases occurred after just 1 to 3 months of kava kava use. In some cases, people have died or required liver transplants. Kava kava is now banned in Switzerland, Germany, Canada, and several other countries. In the United States, the FDA has issued warnings about the herb but has not banned it. Due to these safety issues, kava kava should not be used.

❓ Padma 28

Padma 28, also known as Badmaev 28 and Gabyr-Nirynga, is a complex mixture of herbs sometimes recommended for MS. This herbal combination was developed in the late 19th century in the Buryat region of the Russian Empire by two physicians, Sul-Tim-Badma and Zham-Saram-Badma, also known as Dr. Alexander Badmaev and Dr. Peter Badmaev. The practices of these physicians were influenced by traditions of Ayurvedic and Tibetan medicine.

Padma 28 is taken by mouth and contains more than 20 different herbs and calcium. It appears to have antioxidant effects and may mildly decrease immune system activity.

Padma 28 has been claimed to be effective for MS and other conditions, including heart disease, peripheral vascular disease, and asthma. In mice with EAE, an animal form of MS, consuming water that contains Padma 28 is associated with longer survival times and decreased death rates. A 1992 study in Poland evaluated Padma 28 treatment in 100 people with a progressive form of MS (10). Over the course of a year, one group of people received Padma 28 and the other group received no herbal treatment. In the treated group, 44% had some type of clinical improvement; none of the untreated people improved. This study is promising, but because specific details of its design are not available, the strength of the effect is not entirely clear.

The 1992 Polish study of 100 people reported no side effects. No other detailed safety information about Padma 28 is available.

Limited studies with Padma 28 suggest that it may be beneficial for MS. However, these studies are by no means conclusive, and limited information is available on the safety of this herbal preparation, especially for long-term use.

⊘ Protandim

Protandim is a complex mixture of herbs that has antioxidant effects. It is sometimes claimed to be effective for MS. Protandim contains several herbs, including Ashwagandha, bacopa (brahmi), milk thistle, green tea, and turmeric. This herbal mixture has not been studied in people with MS. Also, it has not been studied in the animal model of MS. The safety and effectiveness of antioxidants in general in MS has not been established. One of the herbs in Protandim, Ashwagandha, is an Ayurvedic herb that has immune-stimulating effects (see *Ayurveda* chapter) which could, in theory, worsen MS or inhibit the therapeutic effects of MS disease-modifying medications. Also, another herb, bacopa, may potentially slow the heart rate, which could accentuate the heart-rate lowering effect of fingolimod (Gilenya), one of the MS disease-modifying medications.

⊘ Psyllium, Bran, and Other Herbs for Constipation

Psyllium, obtained from the seed of the *Psyllium plantago* plant, is an herb used to relieve constipation. It is of potential importance to people with MS because about one-half of people with MS experience constipation. Psyllium is an ingredient in many commercially available products for constipation, including *Metamucil*.

Clinical studies have shown that psyllium effectively treats constipation. Unlike most other herbs, psyllium has been approved by the FDA. It is referred to as a "bulk-producing laxative" because it increases in size, or bulk, when it comes in contact with water. Psyllium, probably the most popular bulk-producing laxative, is used daily in some form by approximately four million Americans.

Psyllium is a form of dietary fiber (see *Fiber* chapter). There are many health benefits of fiber, but the amount of fiber intake is often inadequate. For example, in the United States, the intake of dietary fiber is only about 50% of the recommended amount. For people with MS, this raises the possibility some "MS-associated" constipation may actually be due to inadequate fiber intake. Studies with psyllium and other sources of fiber have shown that a high fiber intake may improve many different medical conditions, including high cholesterol levels, heart disease, hypertension, stroke, diabetes, and obesity. In addition to its effects on constipation, fiber may alleviate multiple other gastrointestinal conditions, such as gastroesophageal reflux disease, duodenal ulcer, diverticulitis, and hemorrhoids.

Psyllium usually is well tolerated. However, the FDA warns that it may produce choking, especially if the intake of fluids is not adequate or an individual has swallowing difficulties. Notably, some people with MS *do* have swallowing difficulties, and they should avoid using psyllium seed or husk.

Psyllium is available in over-the-counter preparations such as Metamucil. It also may be taken in the form of the seed or husk. The FDA recommends that each dose of psyllium be taken with at least 8 ounces of water or other fluid. Oral medications should be taken 1 hour before or 4 hours after psyllium, because psyllium may alter the absorption of these drugs.

Other herbal therapies are available for constipation. One source of fiber is bran, the outer coat of grains, including wheat, oats, and rice. Bran may be consumed as a breakfast cereal, in tablet form, or as crude fiber. Other fiber-rich foods include apples, citrus fruits, and beans. Other herbs that appear to be effective for relieving constipation and are generally safe for short-term use (1 to 2 weeks) include buckthorn, cascara, castor oil, guar gum, olive oil, and senna. The long-term use of some of these herbs may lead to dependence on their use and decreased blood levels of potassium.

(?) Pycnogenol

Pycnogenol is made from the bark of the French maritime pine tree (*Pinus pinaster*), which is native to the western Mediterranean region. Pycnogenol is a mixture of chemicals known as *oligomeric proanthocyanidins* (OPCs). These chemicals, which are similar to those in grape seed extract and green tea leaves, act as antioxidants.

Pycnogenol has been touted as a treatment for many diseases, including MS. However, there are not any formal clinical studies of Pycnogenol or OPCs on MS. Also, Pycnogenol has immune-stimulating effects, which, in theory, could worsen the disease process of MS or antagonize the therapeutic effects of MS disease-modifying medications.

The safety of long-term Pycnogenol use has not been documented in the general population. Pycnogenol and other specialized antioxidant preparations generally are more expensive than are antioxidant vitamins.

Further research on the effects on MS of Pycnogenol, OPCs, and antioxidants generally is needed. Based on current evidence, Pycnogenol does not provide any beneficial effects and poses theoretical risks for people with MS.

⑦ St. John's Wort

St. John's wort (*Hypericum perforatum*) has been used for therapeutic purposes for more than 2,000 years. Its most common current use is as a treatment for depression, a condition that may occur in about one-half of people with MS.

Although St. John's wort has been studied extensively, the chemicals that produce its effects have not been clearly identified. In the past, it was thought that a chemical known as hypericin was responsible for its effects. However, more recent studies indicate that another chemical, hyperforin, may play an important role. In addition to uncertainties about its active constituents, it is not known how this herb alters brain function. Hyperforin affects multiple chemicals in the brain, including serotonin, norepinephrine, and dopamine. Effects on hormones and even the immune system have been proposed. In the end, St. John's wort (and other herbs) may be found to exert multiple biologic effects.

Many studies have investigated the antidepressant effects of St. John's wort. Most, but not all, studies indicate the St. John's wort is effective for depression that is of mild-moderate severity. St. John's wort may not be as effective as conventional medications for severe depression.

Several factors should be kept in mind when considering treatment with St. John's wort. First, depression should be discussed with a physician, because it is not a condition that people should diagnose and treat on their own. St. John's wort should not be used for severe depression (as opposed to mild or moderate depression). Although this herb is generally well tolerated, it may occasionally produce side effects, including upset stomach, sedation, dizziness, irritability, anxiety, and confusion. Rarely, St. John's wort may produce sensitivity of the skin and nerves to sun exposure (photosensitivity), especially in fair-skinned people. In those with depression or manic-depressive illness, St. John's wort may provoke conditions known as *mania* and *hypomania*, which are characterized by excessive physical and mental activity. Abrupt discontinuation of St. John's wort may cause withdrawal side effects, including headache, nausea, dizziness, insomnia, confusion, and fatigue.

Important drug interactions may occur with St. John's wort. Because of its effects on the liver, St. John's wort may decrease the blood levels of many prescription medications. These medications include oral contraceptives, which has led some to say that some "little St. Johns" may be running around now because of unexpected pregnancies that occurred with the combined use of oral contraceptives and St. John's wort. Many other drugs may be affected by St. John's wort, including medications commonly used to treat heart disease, depression, seizures, and cancer. Among these drugs of concern, several are used for MS-related symptoms: alprazolam (Xanax), carbamazepine (Tegretol), imipramine (Tofranil), phenytoin (Dilantin), phenobarbital, and primidone (Mysoline). St. John's wort may decrease blood levels of blood-thinning medication (warfarin or Coumadin). In addition, the herb should not be taken in conjunction with antidepressant medications, including those referred to as tricyclic antidepressants (such as nortriptyline [Pamelor] and amitriptyline [Elavil]); selective serotonin reuptake inhibitors (SSRIs) such as fluoxetine (Prozac), paroxetine (Paxil), and sertraline (Zoloft); and monoamine oxidase (MAO) inhibitors.

Tablets of St. John's wort are usually 300 mg. Tablets should be standardized to contain 0.3% hypericin. In most studies, 300 mg has been given three times daily.

The effectiveness and side effects of St. John's wort suggest that it may be a reasonable treatment option for depression. However, the numerous potential drug interactions with this herb raise serious concerns about its use.

ⓘ Spirulina

People have consumed Spirulina, also known as blue-green algae, for hundreds of years. It was harvested from lakes near Mexico City by the Aztecs and from Lake Chad by natives of the Sahara Desert.

Spirulina sometimes is recommended for MS. It also is claimed to be effective for many other conditions, including fatigue, cancer, obesity, arthritis, viral infections, high cholesterol levels, and hair loss. Spirulina is also known as "super seaweed" and "superfood." It is rich in vitamins, minerals, and proteins, and is available in tablets, capsules, powders, and processed foods such as snack bars. It produces a characteristic intense green color when added to drinks.

It is not entirely clear why Spirulina is recommended for MS. Vitamin B_{12} supplements are sometimes suggested for people with MS, and Spirulina contains a form of vitamin B_{12}. However, it is not clear whether vitamin B_{12} is beneficial for most people with MS. Also, it appears that much of the vitamin B_{12} in Spirulina is in a chemical form not utilized by the human body and may antagonize the effects of active forms of vitamin B_{12}.

One particular species of Spirulina contains gamma-linolenic acid (GLA), which could possibly be beneficial for MS (see the chapter on *Fats: Fish Oil and Polyunsaturated Fatty Acids*), but many other species of Spirulina do not contain GLA, and it is hard to know which species are present in any given Spirulina product.

Spirulina may be associated with MS therapy because some studies have determined that it acts on the immune system. However, these immune-system effects have been variable and of unclear significance. Some studies indicate that

Spirulina stimulates the immune system and thus, theoretically, may actually be harmful for MS. Isolated reports suggest that in individuals with other immune conditions (pemphigus vulgaris, dermatomyositis), symptoms may be provoked by Spirulina.

Finally, Spirulina may be recommended for MS because it is claimed to be effective for fatigue. No well-documented published studies support this claim.

In addition to the lack of evidence supporting its use specifically in MS, Spirulina is relatively expensive, and its safety is not known. Spirulina is at least 10 to 20 times more costly than other protein sources, such as beef and milk. Insufficient information is available about the safety of long-term Spirulina use. Although it has been consumed in some countries for hundreds of years with no apparent adverse effects, some batches of Spirulina have been found to contain mercury, lead, arsenic, radioactive metals, bird feathers, flies, and microbes. Contaminated products may cause nausea, vomiting, liver toxicity, and death.

⑦ Stinging Nettle

Stinging nettle (*Urtica dioica*) has been used traditionally in folk medicine. It is currently sometimes recommended for MS, urinary tract infections, and many other medical conditions. Nettle is notable for having stinging hairs containing chemicals that produce skin irritation.

Very little research has been conducted on nettle. There are not any clinical studies that justify the use of nettle for MS or any other medical condition. In addition, scientific studies indicate that nettle may activate the immune system cells known as T cells. These effects pose theoretical risks for people with MS. Nettle may produce sedation, and thus has the potential to worsen MS fatigue and increase the effects of sedating medications and alcohol. Because of its vitamin K content, nettle may interfere with the effects of blood-thinning medications such as warfarin or Coumadin.

✓ Valerian

Valerian (*Valeriana officinalis*) has been used as a sedating and calming herb for over 1,000 years. It is sometimes referred to as "the Valium of the nineteenth century." Valerian has a characteristic odor, which is similar to that of dirty socks—a "stink rating" is sometimes used to evaluate different valerian products.

Many studies have evaluated the pharmacological and clinical effects of Valerian. Valerian may produce its effects by an action similar to that of Valium (diazepam) and related prescription drugs (benzodiazepines), but the active chemicals and their exact biological activities have not been determined. Multiple clinical trials indicate that valerian is effective for insomnia. These studies are of variable quality.

Valerian sometimes is suggested as a treatment for anxiety, depression, and muscle stiffness (spasticity). However, due to limited clinical studies, its effects on these conditions are not known.

Sleep disorders are common in MS and may contribute to MS-associated fatigue. Sleeping difficulties may be associated with stress and anxiety. Because of the complexities of diagnosing and treating sleep disorders, this condition should be discussed with a physician.

Although valerian usually is well tolerated, the safety of long-term use has not been established. Valerian may produce excessive sedation or worsen MS fatigue, especially if it is used in combination with other sedating medications (such as lioresal [Baclofen], tizanidine [Zanaflex], and diazepam [Valium]) or alcohol. Other side effects include headache, excitability, insomnia, and possible liver toxicity.

Variable doses are given for valerian products. A typical recommendation is to take a dose of 400 to 900 mg of valerian extract 1 to 2 hours before bedtime. Valerian also may be taken as a tea (1 teaspoon of crude dried herb several times daily) or tincture (0.5 to 1 teaspoon) several times daily. The therapeutic effects of valerian may require daily use for 2 to 4 weeks (as opposed to sporadic use on an "as needed" basis).

⚠ Yohimbe and Yohimbine

Yohimbe refers to the bark obtained from a West African evergreen tree (*Pausinystalia yohimbe*), which traditionally has been used for sexual disorders and as an aphrodisiac. Yohimbine, a type of chemical known as an alkaloid, is present in yohimbe.

Limited studies have evaluated the effectiveness and safety of yohimbe for sexual disorders. Some studies indicate that yohimbe may be beneficial for erectile dysfunction in men. However, it has many serious side effects, including severe and dangerous reductions in blood pressure, abnormalities of heart rhythm (arrhythmias), heart failure, and death. Other side effects include insomnia, anxiety, tremor, high blood pressure, rapid heart rate, headache, nausea, and vomiting. The FDA has determined that yohimbe is not safe or effective and that it should not be available for over-the-counter use. Yohimbine, the active ingredient in yohimbe, is available by prescription in the United States.

People with MS may experience sexual disorders, including difficulties with erections and decreased libido. These sexual problems should be evaluated and treated by a physician or other health care professional. Yohimbine should only be used with physician supervision. For erectile dysfunction, conventional medical medications are safer and more effective than yohimbe or yohimbine.

Herbs That May Affect MS, Interact With Medications Used in MS, or Have Serious Side Effects

Many different herbs are available in the United States, especially in stores that specialize in herbal products. Their beneficial effects are sometimes described extensively, although the possible harmful effects on a specific disease such as MS are not mentioned. In this section, we consider herbs that may stimulate the immune system, worsen MS-associated symptoms, and interact with medications commonly used for MS. Potentially dangerous herbs also are discussed.

Herbs That May Interact With All MS Disease-Modifying Medications or Worsen MS: Immune-Stimulating Herbs

In scientific studies, many herbs have been shown to potentially activate the immune system (Table 3.6). These herbs have potential risks for people with MS because they could worsen the underlying disease process of MS or inhibit the therapeutic effects of MS disease-modifying medications. Some of these herbs may stimulate immune system function through the actions of specific sugar molecules, known as "polysaccharides," which are present in many herbs.

The immune system has two components, known as the *cellular* immune system and the *humoral* immune system. The immune-stimulating effects of herbs may occur on one or both of these components. Although MS research in the past has focused on abnormalities in the cellular system, both the cellular and humoral systems are involved in the disease process.

It is important to note that the effects of herbs on MS itself have never been specifically studied. Immune-stimulating effects have been observed in *scientific studies*, such as test tube experiments or animal studies. It is not known whether an herb that produces an immune effect in a scientific study will necessarily cause a harmful effect in a person with MS.

Many commonly used herbs may stimulate the immune system (see Table 3.6). Echinacea is the most well known of these herbs. Some other herbs in this category are among the most popular herbs in the United States, including alfalfa, Asian ginseng, astragalus, cat's claw, garlic, and Siberian ginseng. Additional information on Asian herbs that may have immune-stimulating effects may be found in the chapters on *Acupuncture and Traditional Chinese Medicine* and *Ayurveda*.

TABLE 3.6 HERBS THAT MAY STIMULATE THE IMMUNE SYSTEM

Alfalfa	Ginseng, American	Shiitake mushroom
Andrographis	Ginseng, Asian	South African geranium
Ashwagandha	Ginseng, Siberian	Spirulina (blue-green
Astragalus	Jiaogulan	algae)
Bupleurum	Larch arabinogalactan	Stinging nettle
Cat's claw	Maitake mushroom	Thuja
Chlorella	Mistletoe, European	Thunder god vine
Cordyceps	Neem	Tinospora cordifolia
Echinacea	Picrorhiza	Trichopus zeylanicus
Elderberry	Pycnogenol	
Garlic	Reishi mushroom	

In some herbal therapy books, MS is correctly described as an immune disorder; however, it is then assumed that MS is caused by too little immune-system activity and that immune-stimulating herbs are beneficial. Consequently, some of the herbs in Table 3.6 often are recommended for MS. MS is indeed an immune disorder, but it is caused by excessive immune-system activity. Thus, on a theoretical basis, immune-stimulating herbs may activate the disease or antagonize the effects of MS disease-modifying medications.

It is impossible to develop strict guidelines about the use of these herbs because their exact effects on MS are not known. It may be best for people with MS to simply avoid these herbs. If they are used, they probably should not be used in high doses or on a long-term basis.

Herbs That May Interact With Specific MS Disease-Modifying Medications

Herbs with immune-stimulating effects, which were previously outlined, have the potential to interfere with all of the MS disease-modifying medications. In addition, there are many other herbs that may interact with specific disease-modifying medications. Potential herb interactions for the six major categories of MS medications are outlined in the following text.

Fingolimod (Gilenya) Gilenya has several possible side effects that could be worsened by specific herbal therapies. This drug lowers the level of a specific type of white blood cell known as a "lymphocyte." This effect could be worsened by two uncommon herbs, Madagascar periwinkle and thunder god vine. Also, Gilenya may affect the liver. There are multiple herbs that might increase the risk for liver toxicity (Table 3.7). Finally, Gilenya may affect the heart by producing a slowing down of the heart rate, known as "bradycardia," or, rarely, a slowing of electrical conduction in the heart, known as "QT prolongation."

Herbs that may increase the risk of significant bradycardia include American hellebore, bacopa (brahmi), calabar bean, and huperzine A. Herbs that may provoke QT prolongation include bitter orange, country mallow, ephedra, and horny goat weed.

Glatiramer Acetate (Copaxone) There are not any known herb interactions with this drug.

Interferons (Avonex, Betaseron, Extavia, Rebif) Interferons may lower the white blood cell count. The risk for this side effect may be increased by Madagascar periwinkle and thunder god vine. Also, interferons may produce liver toxicity, an effect that may be provoked by many different herbs (Table 3.7). Of note, there are published case reports of people with MS who have developed liver toxicity while taking interferon medications and herbs with possible liver toxicity—one person was taking morinda citrifolia (noni) and the other was taking sweet clover (melilot).

Natalizumab (Tysabri) Tysabri may affect the liver. Multiple herbs may worsen this effect (Table 3.7).

Dimethylfumarate (Tecfidera) Tecfidera may rarely lower the level of a specific type of white blood cell known as a "lymphocyte." Two rarely used herbs that may provoke this effect are Madagascar periwinkle and thunder god vine.

Teriflunomide (Aubagio) Aubagio may affect the liver and multiple herbs may increase the risk for this side effect (Table 3.7).

TABLE 3.7 HERBS WITH POSSIBLE LIVER TOXICITY

Alkanna	Germander
Alpine ragwort	Golden ragwort
Bishop's weed	Gotu kola
Black cohosh	Gravel root
Boldo	Greater celandine
Borage seed oil	Groundsel
Butterbur	Hemp agrimony
Cassia cinnamon	Hound's tongue
Chaparral	Kava kava
Coltsfoot	Khella
Comfrey	Morinda citrifolia (noni)
Dusty miller	Pennyroyal oil
Echinacea	Red yeast
Eucalyptus	Sweet clover (melilot)
Fo-ti	Tansy ragwort

Herbs That May Interact With Dalfampridine (Ampyra)

Dalfampridine (Ampyra) is used to improve walking in people with MS. This drug may increase the risk of seizures. Herbs that may also increase seizure risk, and thus pose a risk to those who take Ampyra, include dendrobium, ephedra, sage, thuja, and wormwood. Also, seizure risk with Ampyra is increased in the setting of impaired kidney function. There are many herbs that may impair kidney function (Table 3.8).

Herbs That May Interact With Sedating Medications or May Cause Sedation

Many herbs may produce sedation (Table 3.9). Some of the more common herbs on this list are Asian ginseng, chamomile, goldenseal, kava kava, St. John's wort, Siberian ginseng, and valerian.

TABLE 3.8 HERBS WITH POSSIBLE KIDNEY TOXICITY

American chestnut	Hedge-hyssop
Autumn crocus	Horse chestnut
Black bryony	Larch turpentine
Bryonia	Lemon verbena
Buchu	Licorice
Bumweed	Liverwort
Calamus	Mangosteen
Castor	Marsh tea
Chaparral	Mate
Chenopodium oil	Mountain ash
Cissus quadrangularis	Myrrh
Colocynth	Oak bark
Cypress	Parsley
Goa powder	Periwinkle
Ground ivy	Peru balsam
Precatory bean	Tolu balsam
Pulsatilla	Tormentil
Rosemary	Turpentine oil
Rue	Watercress
Sarsaparilla	White sandalwood
Savin tops	Witch hazel
Sorrel	Wood sorrel
Storax	Wormseed
Tansy	Yellow dock

The sedating effects of these herbs may occur when they are taken alone or in combination with sedating medication or alcohol. This is important because fatigue is common in MS. In addition, medications with possible sedating effects are used commonly in MS, including lioresal (Baclofen), tizanidine (Zanaflex), diazepam (Valium), and clonazepam (Klonopin).

Herbs That May Interact With Steroids

Steroids sometimes are used to treat MS attacks. Some herbs (Table 3.10) probably should be avoided with steroid use because they may worsen steroid side effects (increase blood sugar or decrease blood potassium) or increase the potency of the steroids. The more commonly used herbs on this list are Asian ginseng, licorice, and senna.

TABLE 3.9 HERBS WITH POSSIBLE SEDATING EFFECTS

Ashwagandha	Hops	St. John's wort
Bitter almond	Indian snakeroot	Sassafras
Calamus	Jamaican dogwood	Sceletium
Calendula	Kava kava	Shepherd's purse
California poppy	Lavender	Skullcap
Catnip	Lemon balm	Stinging nettle
Celery	Magnolia	Sweet bay
Chamomile	Marsh tea	Valerian
Elecampane	Motherwort	Wild lettuce
Ginseng, Siberian	Passionflower	Yerba mansa
Gotu kola (hydrocotyle)	Sage	

TABLE 3.10 HERBS THAT MAY INTERACT WITH STEROIDS

Aloe	Licorice
Bayberry	Lily-of-the-valley
Buckthorn	Pheasant's eye
Cascara sagrada	Senna
Ephedra (*ma huang*)	Squill
Figwort	

Herbs That May Interact With Antidepressant Medications

There are two large classes of antidepressant medications. The newer class, known as "serotonergic" medications, includes fluoxetine (Prozac), sertraline

(Zoloft), and paroxetine (Paxil). The older class, which is known as "tricyclics," includes amitriptyline (Elavil) and nortriptyline (Pamelor). Some of these anti-depressant medications are also used to treat MS-associated pain. Multiple herbs may interact with antidepressant medications. Those that may interact with serotonergic medications include St. John's wort and a very uncommon herb known as Hawaiian baby woodrose. Herbs that may interact with tricyclic medications include angel's trumpet, belladonna, European mandrake, henbane, jimson weed, scopolia, St. John's wort, and yohimbe.

Herbs That May Interact With Amantadine

Amantadine is sometimes used to treat MS-associated fatigue. Confusion or sedation may occur if amantadine is taken along with angel's trumpet, bella-donna, European mandrake, henbane, jimson weed, or scopolia.

Herbs to Avoid With Urinary Tract Infections

Some herbs may irritate the urinary tract (Table 3.11). The most commonly used herb on this list is coffee. The herbs in this category may worsen the effects of UTIs, which occur frequently in some women with MS. In addition, frequent use or high doses of these herbs may irritate the urinary tract even when an infection does not exist (11).

Potentially Dangerous Herbs or Herbs With Unstudied Toxicity

Some herbs have been associated with significant toxic effects or have not been subjected to toxicity evaluations (Table 3.12). These herbs should be avoided. In spite of reports of toxicity, it is possible to purchase many of these herbs in the United States. For unclear reasons, some of these herbs are sometimes specifi-cally recommended for MS, including borage seed oil, chaparral, comfrey, lobelia, and yohimbe. Borage seed oil, chaparral, and comfrey may contain chemicals that are toxic to the liver. Lobelia may potentially cause a rapid heart rate, low blood pressure, seizures, coma, or death. As described previously, yohimbe may produce psychiatric problems, high blood pressure, and worsening of liver or kidney disease.

Another herb in this category, ephedra *(ma huang),* is claimed to be effective for fatigue and multiple other conditions. Ephedra use has been associated with severely increased blood pressure, abnormal heart rhythms, heart failure, and death. Also, ephedra may cause dizziness, irritability, headache, upset stomach, and heart palpitations. Due to these side effects, ephedra was banned for sale in the United States in April 2004.

TABLE 3.11 HERBS THAT MAY IRRITATE THE URINARY TRACT

American pennyroyal	Eucalyptus	Pulsatilla
Asiatic dogwood	Fragrant sumach	Red sedge
Asparagus	Grindelia	Rue
Buchu	Guarana	Sandalwood
Celery	Horseradish	Sassafras
Cinnamon	Juniper berries	Thuja
Coffee	Lovage	Thyme
Cola nut	Mate	Watercress
Copaiba oleoresin	Myrrh gum	Yerba mansa
Cubeb	Parsley	
Dill seed	Pine needles	

TABLE 3.12 HERBS WITH POTENTIAL TOXICITY OR UNINVESTIGATED TOXICITY

Blue cohosh	Foxglove	Pennyroyal
Borage	Germander	Rue
Calamus	Golden ragwort	Skullcap
Chaparral	(life root)	Tansy
Coltsfoot	Kombucha	Wormwood
Comfrey	Lobelia	Yohimbe
Dong-quai	Mistletoe	
Ephedra (*ma huang*)	Pau d'arco	

Conclusion

Herbs should be used with caution by people with MS. Many herbs with no well-documented beneficial effects may potentially worsen MS or interact with MS medications. On the other hand, some herbs may be of benefit for specific MS-related symptoms, such as cranberry for the prevention of UTIs, St. John's wort for depression, valerian for insomnia, and psyllium for constipation.

Although some information is available about herbs and MS, much more remains to be learned, even for the well-studied herbs such as echinacea and St. John's wort. In a sense, the message for herbs and MS is similar to that for unconventional medicine and MS as a whole—some of the therapies may be beneficial, some may be harmful, and nearly all are not fully understood.

Additional Readings

Books

Bauer B, ed. *Mayo Clinic Book of Alternative Medicine and Home Remedies.* New York, NY: Time Home Entertainment; 2013.

Blumenthal M, ed. *The Complete German Commission E Monographs: Therapeutic Guide to Herbal Medicines.* Austin, TX: American Botanical Council; 1998.

Bowling AC. Complementary and alternative medicine in multiple sclerosis. In: Geisser B, ed. *Primer on Multiple Sclerosis.* New York, NY: Oxford University Press; 2011:369-381.

Bowling AC. Complementary and alternative medicine: practical considerations. In: Rae-Grant A, Fox R, Bethoux F, eds. *Multiple Sclerosis and Related Disorders: Diagnosis, Medical Management, and Rehabilitation.* New York, NY: Demos; 2013:243-249.

Brinker F. *Herbal Contraindications and Drug Interactions.* OR: Eclectic Medical Publishers; 2010.

Fetrow CW, Avila JR. *Professional's Handbook of Complementary and Alternative Medicines.* Philadelphia, PA: Lippincott, Williams, & Wilkins; 2004.

Jellin JM, Batz F, Hitchens K, et al. *Natural Medicines Comprehensive Database.* Stockton, CA: Therapeutic Research Faculty; 2014.

Ulbricht CE, Basch EM, eds. *Natural Standard Herb and Supplement Reference: Evidence-Based Clinical Reviews.* St. Louis, MO: Elsevier-Mosby; 2005.

Journal Articles

Brochet B, Guinot P, Orgogozo J, et al. Double-blind, placebo controlled, multicenter study of ginkgolide B in treatment of acute exacerbations for multiple sclerosis. The Ginkgolide Study Group in multiple sclerosis. *J Neurol Neurosurg Psych.* 1995;58:360–362.

Bunchorntavakul C, Reddy KR. Review article: herbal and dietary supplement hepatotoxicity. *Aliment Pharmacol Ther.* 2013;37:3–17.

Diamond BJ, Johnson SK, Kaufman M, et al. A randomized controlled pilot trial: the effects of EGb 761 on information processing and executive function in multiple sclerosis. *Explore (NY).* 2013;9:106–107.

Etemadafir M, Sayahi F, Abtahi SH, et al. Ginseng in the treatment of fatigue in multiple sclerosis: a randomized, placebo-controlled, double-blind pilot study. *Int J Neurosci.* 2013;123:480–486.

Genuis SJ, Schwalfenberg G, Siy A-K, et al. Toxic element contamination of natural health products and pharmaceutical preparations. *PLoS One.* 2012;7: e49676.

Johnson SK, Diamond BJ, Rausch S, et al. The effect of Ginkgo biloba on functional measures in multiple sclerosis: a pilot randomized controlled trial. *Explore (NY)*. 2006;2:19–24.

Kim E, Cameron M, Lovera J, et al. American ginseng does not improve fatigue in multiple sclerosis: a single center randomized double-blind placebo-controlled crossover pilot study. *Mult Scler J*. 2011;17:1523–1526.

Korwin-Piotrowska T, Nocon D, Stankowska-Chomicz A, et al. Experience of Padma 28 in multiple sclerosis. *Phytother Res*. 1992;6:133–136.

Lovera J, Bagert B, Smoot K, et al. Ginkgo biloba for the improvement of cognitive performance in multiple sclerosis: a randomized, placebo-controlled trial. *Mult Scler*. 2007;13:376–385.

Lovera JF, Kim E, Heriza E, et al. Ginkgo biloba does not improve cognitive function in MS: a randomized placebo-controlled trial. *Neurology*. 2012;79:1278–1284.

Newmaster SG, Grguric M, Shanmughanandhan D, et al. DNA barcoding detects contamination and substitution in North American herbal products. *BMC Med*. 2013;11:222.

O'Connor K, Weinstock-Guttman, Carl E, et al. Patterns of dietary and herbal supplement use by multiple sclerosis patients. *J Neurol*. 2012;259:637–644.

⊘ Hippotherapy and Therapeutic Horseback Riding

Hippotherapy is an unusual term that refers to the use of horseback riding for therapeutic effects. The word is derived from the Greek word *hippos*, which means horse. Therapeutic horseback riding, a technique related to hippotherapy, aims to both produce therapeutic effects and teach riding skills.

Horseback riding as a therapy has been used for thousands of years. It was used in Greece in the 5th century BCE to rehabilitate injured soldiers. Hippocrates wrote of horseback riding as a "natural exercise." Similarly, wounded soldiers were treated with horseback riding in England during World War I.

More recently, Liz Hartel, a Danish woman who had polio, demonstrated the possible benefits of riding. She developed leg strength and coordination through riding, and eventually won a silver medal in dressage in the 1952 Olympic Games in Finland.

Riding therapy has been used since the 1940s in Europe, especially in Germany and Switzerland. Much of the published research in this area has been conducted in Germany. This type of therapy is a relative newcomer in the United States. The first center for therapeutic riding was established in Michigan, in 1969. More than 600 accredited therapeutic riding centers are now open in the United States.

Treatment Method

Hippotherapy and therapeutic riding often are done in conjunction with physical therapy. In riding therapy, a person is placed on a horse and monitored by a therapist, usually a trained physical therapist or occupational therapist. Typically, bareback pads are used, and straps or handholds are provided for stability. In addition to the conventional riding position, riders also may sit sideways, backwards, or even lie sideways or backwards. The person on the horse responds to the animal's movements with body movements. Unlike conventional horseback riding, in riding therapy the rider does not attempt to control the horse. Rather, the therapist, who may be on the ground or on the horse with the rider, controls the horse and adjusts the treatment as indicated.

There are newer variants of hippotherapy. *Onotherapy* utilizes methods similar to those of hippotherapy but is done on donkeys. Also, *hippotherapy simulators,* which are robotic horses that simulate horseback riding motion, are being used increasingly in research studies.

Studies in Multiple Sclerosis and Other Conditions

Hippotherapy is believed to be beneficial for people with walking difficulties because the rhythmic movements of the human pelvis while horseback riding are similar to those that occur with walking. In addition, the variations in the horse's speed, stride, and direction are thought to be beneficial for walking impairments. Some studies indicate that approximately 100 different horse movements are transmitted to the rider during each minute of riding. Some psychological benefits also may be related to developing a bond with the horse, developing relationships with the therapist and other riders, and simply being outdoors.

Several studies have evaluated hippotherapy in people with multiple sclerosis (MS) (1–5). These studies have had different designs, and some have found that different people have different responses to hippotherapy. Taken together, the most consistent benefits reported in these studies are improvement in balance and walking. Other reported beneficial effects include improvement in "emotional functioning," pain, and muscle stiffness (spasticity).

Hippotherapy and therapeutic riding have been researched extensively in children with cerebral palsy. These studies are relevant to MS because people with cerebral palsy and MS experience some of the same neurologic difficulties, including walking unsteadiness, stiffness, and weakness. Unfortunately, many of the studies on cerebral palsy have been small, poorly designed, and have not included a placebo group. In addition, inconsistent results have been obtained. In studies of once- or twice-weekly therapy, ranging from 8 to 26 weeks, therapy has been associated with improvement in walking, running, jumping, muscle strength, and muscle stiffness. In addition, one study found that children walked more efficiently and used less energy to walk after therapy. Improvement in standing and sitting postures also has been associated with hippotherapy in some studies.

Studies have been done in several other conditions. Research in the elderly and in people who have had strokes have reported improvement in walking and balance. Increased muscle strength has been reported in the elderly. A German study of people with significant arm or leg weakness found that hippotherapy improved stiffness (spasticity), urinary function, bowel function, mood, and sleep. One study of children with language disorders reported improvement in language skills and self-esteem.

Although some studies have reported positive effects in MS, cerebral palsy, and other conditions, the results of these studies are not conclusive. Clearly, better-designed studies using larger numbers of patients are needed to more fully understand the effects of this type of therapy.

Side Effects

The most obvious risk of hippotherapy and therapeutic horseback riding is falling from the horse. People with MS who are experiencing a significant exacerbation should probably avoid hippotherapy because they may be especially unstable. Also, riding may not be possible for people with difficulty sitting, decreased head control, and severe muscle stiffness or spasticity. People with severe fatigue or symptoms worsened by heat should be cautious about riding in hot weather. The American Hippotherapy Association lists a number of other conditions that should preclude hippotherapy, including severe osteoporosis, bone fractures, herniated disks, instability of the spine, severe arthritis, the use of anticoagulant medication, wounds or sores on weight-bearing surfaces, and seizures. The Association also recommends that therapy be done cautiously with some conditions, including diabetes, hip joint abnormalities, obesity, mild or moderate osteoporosis, allergies to dust or horsehair, heart disease, incontinence, and recent surgery.

Practical Information

It is best to receive hippotherapy from a qualified therapist who works at a riding center. For those with mild disability, therapeutic riding sessions provide the benefits of riding as well as riding lessons. When the riding skills are learned, riding may be done independently.

Sessions generally last 20 to 30 minutes. Fees are approximately $35 to $150 per hour. Health insurance may cover some of the cost of the therapy.

More information on hippotherapy and therapeutic horseback riding may be obtained from:

- The American Hippotherapy Association (www.americanhippotherapyassociation.org), PO Box 2014, Denver, CO 80522 (877-851-4592)
- The National Center for Equine Facilitated Therapy (www.nceft.org), 880 Runnymede Rd., Woodside, CA 94062 (650-851-2271)

Conclusion

Hippotherapy and therapeutic horseback riding are low-risk, moderate-cost therapies that offer possible benefits for multiple MS-associated symptoms, including bladder and bowel problems, depression, pain, spasticity, walking difficulties, weakness. Further studies are needed to determine the effects of this therapy more definitively.

Additional Readings
Journal Articles

Ajzenman HF, Standeven JW, Shurtleff TL. Effect of hippotherapy on motor control, adaptive behaviors, and participation in children with autism spectrum disorder: a pilot study. *Am J Occup Ther.* 2013;67:653–663.

Beinotti F, Christofoletti G, Correia N, Borges G. Effects of horseback riding therapy on quality of life in patients post stroke. *Top Stroke Rehabil.* 2013;20:226–232.

Beinotti F, Correia N, Christofoletti G, Borges G. Use of hippotherapy in gait training for hemiparetic post-stroke. *Arq Neuropsiquiatr.* 2010;68:908–913.

Bertoti DB. Effect of therapeutic horseback riding on posture in children with cerebral palsy. *Phys Ther.* 1988;68:1505–1512.

Borioni N, Marinaro P, Celestini S, et al. Effect of equestrian therapy and onotherapy in physical and psychosocial performances of adults with intellectual disability: a preliminary study of evaluation tools based on the ICF classification. *Disabil Rehabil.* 2012;34:279–287.

Bronson C, Brewerton K, Ong J, Palanca C, Sullivan SJ. Does hippotherapy improve balance in persons with multiple sclerosis: a systematic review. *Eur J Phys Rehabil Med.* 2010;46:347–353.

De Araujo TB, De Oliveira RJ, Martins WR, de Moura Pereira M, Copetti F, Safons MP. Effects of hippotherapy on mobility, strength and balance in elderly. *Arch Gerontol Geriatri.* 2013;56:478–481.

Goldmann T, Vilimek M. Kinematics of human spine during hippotherapy. *Comp Meth Biochem Biomed Eng.* 2012;15:203–205.

Hakanson M, Moller M, Lindstrom I, Mattsson B. The horse as the healer-a study of riding in patients with back pain. *J Bodyw Mov Ther.* 2009;13:43–52.

Hammer A, Nilsagard Y, Forsberg A, Pepa H, Skargren E, Oberg B. Evaluation of therapeutic riding (Sweden)/hippotherapy (United States). A single-subject experimental design study replicated in eleven patients with multiple sclerosis. *Physiother Theory Prac.* 2005;21(1):51–77.

Han JY, Kim JM, Kim SK, et al. Therapeutic effects of mechanical horseback riding on gait and balance ability in stroke patients. *Ann Rehabil Med.* 2012;36:762–769.

Homnick DN, Henning KM, Swain CV, Homnick TD. Effect of therapeutic horseback riding on balance in community-dwelling older adults with balance deficits. *J Altern Complement Med.* 2013;19:622–626.

Kim S, Yuk GC, Gak H. Effects of the horse riding simulator and ball exercises on balance of the elderly. *J Phys Ther Sci.* 2013;25:1425–1428.

MacKay-Lyons M, Conway C, Roberts W. Effects of therapeutic riding on patients with multiple sclerosis: a preliminary trial. *Proceedings of the 6th International Therapeutic Riding Congress.* 1988;8:173–178.

MacKinnon JR, Noh S, Laliberte D, et al. Therapeutic horseback riding: a review of the literature. *Phys Occup Ther Ped.* 1995;15:1–15.

MacKinnon JR, Noh S, Lariviere J, et al. A study of therapeutic effects of horse-back riding for children with cerebral palsy. *Phys Occup Ther Ped.* 1995;15:17–31.

McGibbon NH, Andrade C-K, Widener G, Cintas HL. Effect of an equine-movement therapy program on gait, energy expenditure, and motor function in children with spastic cerebral palsy: a pilot study. *Dev Med Child Neurol.* 1998;40:754–762.

Meregillano G. Hippotherapy. *Phys Med Rehabil Clin N Amer.* 2004;15:843–854.

Munoz-Lasa S, Ferriero G, Valero R, Gomez-Muñiz F, Rabini A, Varela E. Effect of therapeutic horseback riding on balance and gait of people with multiple sclerosis. *G Ital Med Lav Ergon.* 2011;33:462–467.

Pauw J. Therapeutic horseback riding studies: problems experienced by researchers. *Physiotherapy.* 2000;86:523–527.

Silkwood-Sherer D, Warmbier H. Effects of hippotherapy on postural stability in persons with multiple sclerosis: a pilot study. *J Neurol Phys Ther.* 2007;31:77–84.

Sung YH, Kim CJ, Yu BK, Kim KM. A hippotherapy simulator is effective to shift weight bearing toward the affected side during gait in patients with stroke. *NeuroRehabilitation.* 2013;33:407–412.

Sunwoo H, Chang WH, Kwon JY, Kim TW, Lee JY, Kim YH. Hippotherapy in adult patients with chronic brain disorders: a pilot study. *Ann Rehabil Med.* 2012;36:756–761.

Zadnikar M, Kastrin A. Effects of hippotherapy and therapeutic horseback riding on postural control or balance in children with cerebral palsy: a meta-analysis. *Dev Med Child Neurol.* 2011;53:684–691.

⑦ Homeopathy

Homeopathy is one of the more controversial forms of complementary and alternative medicine (CAM). Much of the controversy is due to the fact that the basic principles of homeopathy are in conflict with many of the fundamental concepts of conventional medicine as well as those of chemistry, biology, and physics. In spite of these controversial ideas, homeopathy is, on a worldwide basis, one of the most popular forms of CAM.

Homeopathy is a system of medicine that was developed in the 1800s by Samuel Hahnemann, a German physician. Homeopathy was very popular in Europe and North America in the 19th century. The use of homeopathy in the United States declined from the 1950s to the 1970s, but its popularity has rebounded since.

Homeopathy is used globally. On a worldwide basis, $1 billion to $5 billion are spent yearly on this form of treatment. Homeopathy is most popular in Europe and India. Homeopathic remedies are dispensed in pharmacies in France. In the United States, more than $150 million are spent annually on homeopathic remedies, and approximately 1% of American adults currently use homeopathy.

Treatment Method

Homeopathy is based on several principles. One is the "law of similars," which states that "like cures like." Variations of this principle have been used in other forms of medicine for thousands of years. In homeopathy, it is believed that if large doses of a substance produce specific symptoms, then very small doses of that substance will cure the same symptoms. For example, because large doses of arsenic produce stomach cramps, very low doses of arsenic may be used to treat them.

The use of very low doses of substances is another important principle of homeopathy. Natural substances, such as herbs, minerals, or animal products, are mixed with water or alcohol and then diluted 1:10 or 1:100. These dilutions are then repeated many times, so that the final solution is *extremely dilute.* In homeopathic notation, X is used for 1:10 dilutions, C is used for 1:100 dilutions, and a number is used for the number of times a specific dilution is made. For example, *12X* refers to a solution that has been diluted 12 times in a 1:10 manner, and *30C* signifies a 1:100 dilution performed 30 times.

Many homeopathic preparations are so dilute that they do not contain even a single molecule of the original substance. In this situation, it is argued that the water has a "memory" for the substance that it once contained. Also, by the laws of homeopathy, it is believed that a solution is more potent if it contains less of a substance. These ideas of water "memory" and increased potency with increased dilution generate much controversy because they defy the conventional laws of physics, chemistry, and biology. The use of these dilute solutions has raised questions about whether homeopathy is simply a way to produce a placebo response.

Homeopathy is focused on identifying both symptoms and the personal features of the patient. In addition, homeopathic treatment aims to use the body's natural healing processes. This is in contrast to conventional medicine, in which symptoms are used primarily to diagnose an underlying disease—the personal characteristics of an individual are not a critical component of the diagnostic process or choice of therapy, and treatment involves the use of drugs and other therapies that improve the disease process but do not necessarily alter the body's natural healing abilities.

Because of the detailed evaluation process, homeopaths probably become more familiar with their patients and spend more time with them than do physicians who practice conventional medicine. One study found that physicians in the United States who practice homeopathy spend more than twice as much time with their patients than do physicians who do not practice homeopathy. The in-depth relationship that develops in homeopathy may be important for the healing process and may certainly augment any type of placebo effect.

A variety of homeopathic remedies has been suggested for multiple sclerosis (MS). The treatment regimen depends on the individual and the specific symptoms. Homeopathic remedies sometimes recommended for MS include *Argentum nitricum, Aurum muriaticum,* and *Plumbum metallicum.* Much of the beneficial effect of homeopathy may be a placebo response because the approach of homeopaths may be conducive to producing placebo effects and homeopathic remedies may not actually contain any active compounds. Even if it is a placebo response, it may be helpful in certain situations. It is known that placebos are generally 30% to 40% effective. For situations in which conventional medicine has no particularly effective therapy, homeopathy may be a way to provide at least a placebo response. Jeremy Swayne, an English homeopath, writes: "If homeopathy is placebo, it presents us with a rich and systematic study of the working of the placebo response, which fully deserves to be taken seriously and investigated. If it is not, then the implications are even more startling" (1). Homeopathy includes both classic and nonclassic approaches. The classic approach involves a detailed evaluation of the patient by a practitioner who develops a personalized treatment plan on the basis of the clinical evaluation. In contrast, the nonclassic approach does not involve a homeopath. Instead, a certain condition is identified, and treatment for that condition is then given. In the nonclassic approach, the condition may be identified by the affected individual or by a nonhomeopath practitioner who uses homeopathic therapy.

Studies in MS and Other Conditions

Whether homeopathic therapy produces effects that are greater than those produced by placebos is subject to controversy. Many clinical studies have evaluated homeopathic treatment for a variety of conditions. Unfortunately, many of these studies have been poorly conducted and the results often are not conclusive.

To attempt to clarify this area, several studies have analyzed the results from multiple homeopathic clinical trials. The Cochrane Collaboration, an authoritative scientific review committee, found that homeopathic medicines did not have effects beyond placebo for multiple conditions, including cancer, attention-deficit hyperactivity disorder, asthma, dementia, influenza, and induction of labor (2). A 2005 study evaluated multiple homeopathic and conventional medicine clinical trials (3). Overall, the quality of the homeopathy trials was higher than that of the conventional medicine trials. When large trials of high quality were examined, it was found that homeopathy generally produced a much weaker treatment effect than did conventional medicine. The authors of the study concluded that these results were consistent with the concept that the clinical effects of homeopathy are placebo effects.

Homeopathy is not one of the more commonly used forms of CAM among people with MS in the United States. In contrast, homeopathy appears to be used frequently by people with MS in Europe. Studies have shown that, among people with MS, homeopathy is the most popular form of CAM in Holland and one of the most popular CAM therapies in Germany.

Specific homeopathic remedies sometimes are recommended for MS. The medical literature contains isolated reports (anecdotes) of individuals with

MS treated with homeopathy. However, no well-documented large studies have investigated the effect of homeopathic treatment on MS.

Homeopathy has produced mixed results for neurologic diseases other than MS. Variable results or limited evidence for a therapeutic effect have been observed in studies of migraine, pain, and vertigo.

Viral infections, such as the common cold and flu, may lead to MS attacks. As a result, it may be helpful for people with MS to try to prevent viral infections or to shorten the time that they are affected by a viral infection. Limited options are available for the treatment or prevention of viral infections. These include simple preventive measures (such as hand-washing and avoiding exposure to infected people), the flu vaccination, and prescription medications that decrease the duration and severity of the flu. Supplements of unproven effectiveness for the common cold (echinacea, garlic, zinc, vitamin C) pose a theoretical risk for people with MS because of possible immune-stimulating activity.

Given the limited options, some people consider the use of homeopathy for preventing or treating viral infections. Studies of homeopathic therapies for viral syndromes have produced mixed results. Although homeopathy does not appear to be effective for flu prevention, positive results have been obtained in some studies of flu treatment—the significance of these results is not clear. For people with an interest in homeopathic remedies, this approach may be a reasonable possibility for the treatment of viral infections. If homeopathy is used, available conventional therapies, especially those for the flu, should be discussed with a physician, and it must be kept in mind that the homeopathic therapies are not proven to be effective.

Side Effects

Overall, homeopathy is generally well tolerated. Homeopathy should not be used in lieu of conventional medical therapy since this could lead to delay in the diagnosis and treatment of potentially serious medical conditions. There are very rare cases of severe allergies and serious toxicity with homeopathic preparations. Toxicity has been associated with preparations that contain metals (arsenic, cadmium, mercury, iron), aconitum, kerosene, and thallium.

Homeopaths note several precautions that should be taken. One is that treatment should be discontinued when a symptom resolves. Otherwise, the treatment may produce recurrence of the symptom. Also, *antidotes* may interfere with treatment. Antidotes include coffee, acupuncture, x-rays, and dental drilling. Finally, a person should notify his or her homeopath of any conventional medical treatment that is being used because this information may affect the homeopathic interpretation of symptoms.

Practical Information

Initial visits with a homeopath are typically 60 minutes in length and cost between $100 and $140. Follow-up visits are 20 to 30 minutes and cost about $60.

More information on homeopathy can be obtained from:

- The National Center for Homeopathy (NCH) (www.nationalcenterforhomeopathy.org), 1760 Old Meadow Rd., McLean, VA 22102 (703-506-7667)

Conclusion

Homeopathy is a low-risk, low- to moderate-cost therapy with unproven effectiveness. No rigorous studies have specifically evaluated the effect of homeopathy on MS. Limited studies suggest that it may be beneficial for pain and vertigo. For people with MS who are interested in this approach, it may be worth considering for mild conditions (such as viral infections or mild MS-related symptoms) or for conditions for which conventional medical therapy is ineffective or only partially effective. Homeopathy should not be used in place of conventional medicine. Specifically, homeopathic treatment should not be used for controlling MS disease activity in place of conventional Food and Drug Administration (FDA)-approved MS medications.

Additional Readings

Books

Bauer B, ed. *Mayo Clinic Book of Alternative Medicine and Home Remedies.* New York, NY: Time Home Entertainment; 2013:144.

Ernst E, ed. *The Desktop Guide to Complementary and Alternative Medicine: An Evidence-Based Approach.* Edinburgh, UK: Mosby; 2001:53–55.

Jellin JM, Gregory PJ, Batz F, et al. *Pharmacist's Letter/ Prescriber's Letter Natural Medicines Comprehensive Database.* Stockton, CA: Therapeutic Research Faculty; 2014.

Micozzi MS, ed. *Fundamentals of Complementary and Alternative Medicine.* Philadelphia, PA: Saunders Elsevier; 2011:343–354.

Swayne J. *Homeopathic Method: Implications for Clinical Practice and Medical Science.* New York, NY: Churchill Livingstone; 1998.

Synovitz LB, Larson KL. *Complementary and Alternative Medicine for Health Professionals: A Holistic Approach to Consumer Health.* Burlington, MA: Jones and Bartlett Learning; 2013:128–134.

Journal Articles

Davidson JR, Crawford C, Ives JA, Jonas WB. Homeopathic treatments in psychiatry: a systematic review of randomized placebo-controlled studies. *J Clin Psych.* 2011;72:795–805.

Ernst E. Homeopathy: what does the "best" evidence tell us? *Med J Aust.* 2010;192:458–460.

Haresnape C. An exploration of the relationship between placebo and homeopathy and the implications for clinical trial design. *JSRM Short Rep.* 2013;4:2042533313490927.

Jonas WB, Kaptchuk TJ, Linde K. A critical overview of homeopathy. *Annals Int Med.* 2003;138:393–399.

Kleijnen J, Knipschild P, ter Riet G. Clinical trials of homoeopathy. *Br Med J.* 1991;302:316–326.

Linde K, Clausius N, Ramirez G, et al. Are the clinical effects of homoeopathy placebo effects? A meta-analysis of placebo-controlled trials. *Lancet.* 1997;350: 834–843.

Linde K, Scholz M, Ramirez G, Clausius N, Melchart D, Jonas WB. Impact of study quality on outcome in placebo-controlled trials of homeopathy. *J Clin Epidemiol.* 1999;52:631–636.

Mathie RT, Frye J, Fisher P. Homeopathic Oscillococcinum for preventing and treating influenza and influenza-like illness. *Cochrane Database Syst Rev.* 2012;12:CD001957.

Posadzki P, Alotaibi A, Ernst E. Adverse effects of homeopathy: a systematic review of published case reports and case series. *Int J Clin Pract.* 2012;66: 1178–1188.

Shang A, Huwiler-Muntener K, Nartey L, et al. Are the clinical effects of homeopathy placebo effects? Comparative study of placebo-controlled trials of homeopathy and allopathy. *Lancet.* 2005;366:726–732.

Weiser M, Strosser W, Klein P. Homeopathic vs conventional treatment of vertigo: a randomized double-blind clinical study. *Arch Otolaryngol Head Neck Surg.* 1998;124:879–885.

Whitmarsh TE. Homeopathy in multiple sclerosis. *Complement Ther Nurs Midwifery.* 2003;9:5–9.

⚠ Hyperbaric Oxygen

Hyperbaric oxygen treatment is a form of oxygen therapy. It is claimed to be an effective treatment for a large number of diseases, including multiple sclerosis (MS). Unfortunately, many of the claims about this therapy are not supported by research evidence.

Treatment Method

In this type of treatment, a person breathes oxygen under increased pressure in a specially designed chamber. The procedure increases the oxygen content of the blood and thereby increases the amount of oxygen in different body tissues. The increased oxygen level in the blood and tissues is believed to be helpful for a variety of medical conditions.

Studies in MS and Other Conditions

The original study that generated interest in hyperbaric oxygen and MS was published in the prestigious *New England Journal of Medicine* in 1983 (1). In this study of 17 people with MS, 12 showed improvement and 5 had long-lasting improvement. In addition to this clinical study, animal studies have produced positive results. In animals, hyperbaric oxygen protects against experimental allergic encephalomyelitis (EAE), an experimental form of MS.

Advocates of hyperbaric oxygen therapy for MS cite the positive clinical study from 1983. However, seven studies performed after the 1983 study did *not* demonstrate any consistent therapeutic effect for hyperbaric oxygen. In a few studies, a mild improvement in bladder problems was noted. A 1995 review of hyperbaric oxygen treatment trials in MS concluded that hyperbaric oxygen did not produce significant benefits in MS and that this therapy should not be used for MS (2). Another analysis of hyperbaric oxygen trials in MS, published in 2004, concluded that this therapy did not produce consistent evidence for a therapeutic effect, should not be used on a routine basis, and should not be investigated further in MS (3). The methodology and the interpretation of the results of past trials of hyperbaric oxygen in MS have been criticized (4). A 2010 reanalysis of past trials and publications noted that it was conceivable that hyperbaric oxygen might produce improvement with prolonged treatment or in a subgroup of people with MS (5). However, the overall assessment of this review was that there was "no plausible benefit" of hyperbaric oxygen on the clinical course of MS, that the routine treatment of MS with hyperbaric oxygen "is not recommended," and that further research in this area is "difficult to justify."

Hyperbaric oxygen is an accepted therapy for a limited number of specific medical conditions. For example, it is an effective treatment for burns and severe infections. Other rare uses included decompression sickness (as a result of deep-sea diving), carbon monoxide poisoning, air bubbles in the bloodstream caused by medical procedures, and tissue injury caused by radiation exposure.

Side Effects

In general, hyperbaric oxygen is well tolerated. Mild and reversible visual changes may sometimes occur. Rarely, more serious side effects may occur, including seizures, pressure injury to the ear, cataracts, and collapsed lungs.

Practical Information

Hyperbaric oxygen therapy is time-consuming and expensive. Each session lasts for 1 to 5 hours, and a course of therapy may require 20 sessions. Individual sessions cost between $75 and $300. A course of treatment may cost several thousand dollars. Hyperbaric oxygen therapy is costly because the equipment is expensive, technicians monitor the equipment during therapy, and many treatment sessions usually are involved.

Conclusion

No consistent evidence supports the use of hyperbaric oxygen therapy in MS. Multiple clinical trials and reviews of these trials have concluded that it is not an effective treatment for MS. In addition, it may be very expensive, requires much time and effort, and occasionally produces serious side effects.

Additional Readings

Journal Articles

Bennett M, Heard R. Hyperbaric oxygen therapy for multiple sclerosis. *Cochrane Database Syst Rev.* 2004;(1):CD003057.

Bennett M, Heard R. Hyperbaric oxygen therapy for multiple sclerosis. *CNS Neurosci Ther.* 2010;16:115–124.

Kleijnen J, Knipschild P. Hyperbaric oxygen for multiple sclerosis: review of controlled trials. *Acta Neurol Scand.* 1995;91:330–334.

Neubauer RA, Neubauer V, Gottlieb SF. The controversy over hyperbaric oxygenation therapy for multiple sclerosis. *J Amer Phys Surgeons.* 2005;10:112–115.

Tibbles PM, Edelsberg JS. Hyperbaric oxygen therapy. *N Engl J Med.* 1996;334:1642–1648.

⊘ Hypnosis

Hypnosis uses mental processes to alter physical processes. In this way, hypnosis, like biofeedback and meditation, is a type of mind–body therapy.

Medical interest in hypnosis has existed for hundreds of years. In the late 1700s, Franz Mesmer, an Austrian physician, used calming gestures and words to relax patients and, presumably, balance their magnetic energy. A commission appointed by the French Academy criticized this technique, known as *mesmerism,* and Mesmer was claimed to be a fraud. More recently, a magical, evil, mind-controlling view of hypnosis was promoted by vaudeville performers and magicians.

Hypnosis has gained some acceptance by conventional medicine despite these negative representations of the technique. It was deemed a valid medical treatment in England in 1955 and in the United States in 1958. Research studies support the use of hypnosis for some conditions. However, many physicians and other mainstream health care professionals do not readily incorporate hypnosis into their medical practices.

Treatment Method

In hypnosis, an individual enters a trancelike state. In this state of focused concentration, which is generally produced by a hypnotherapist, an individual is particularly vulnerable to suggestion. As a result, during hypnosis, a therapist makes suggestions of therapeutic value. For example, anxiety may be improved with suggestions for relaxation, and pain may be relieved with suggestions for numbness. In self-hypnosis, individuals make specific suggestions themselves. Self-hypnosis usually is most effective when it is taught by a trained therapist.

There is great variability in the success of hypnosis. Some of this variability is due to the fact that different people have different degrees of susceptibility to hypnotic suggestion. Approximately two-thirds of the population is moderately susceptible to suggestion, and 5% to 10% are extremely susceptible. Children and young adults are especially responsive to hypnosis.

Studies in Multiple Sclerosis and Other Conditions

Several studies have specifically evaluated the possible benefits of hypnosis for multiple sclerosis (MS). There are two clinical trials from the University of Washington that evaluated the effects of self-hypnosis on MS-associated pain. One of these trials, which included 22 people with MS, found that self-hypnosis was superior to a technique known as progressive muscle relaxation (1). The other study, conducted on 15 people, found that self-hypnosis was most effective for pain when combined with *cognitive restructuring,* a psychotherapeutic approach that aims to identify and modify dysfunctional thought processes (2). There is also a study of the effects of *autogenic training,* a technique similar to hypnosis, on 22 people with MS (3). Autogenic training involves mental exercises using relaxation and suggestion. It is aimed at teaching people to recognize the origin of certain physical and mental disorders and use that awareness for self-treatment. In the study of MS, autogenic training was associated with increased energy and less limitation in roles due to physical and emotional difficulties. Finally, there are published *case reports* of individual people with MS who experienced improvement in multiple MS-related symptoms with hypnosis (4,5).

Symptoms that may occur with MS have been investigated in people with other conditions. Anxiety, which occurs frequently in MS, may be reduced through hypnosis-induced relaxation. Also, hypnosis appears to relieve different types of pain, including headache and pain associated with surgery, cancer, and fibromyalgia, a rheumatologic condition. Hypnosis may be used during surgery to reduce the amount of anesthesia or to completely eliminate the need for anesthesia in some cases. Hypnosis also has produced beneficial effects in some studies of insomnia as well as fatigue.

The effects of hypnosis on immune-system function have been investigated in limited studies. Hypnotic suggestions may be made to attempt to specifically alter immune function. Mixed results have been obtained in these studies. Further research is needed to determine if hypnosis produces immunologic changes that are significant enough to affect disease processes.

Side Effects

Hypnosis usually is safe. Although some movies and television shows portray hypnotized individuals performing evil tasks, this is not an accurate view. People cannot be forced into hypnosis, and hypnotized people cannot be unwittingly instructed to commit undesirable acts. Rarely, relaxation induced by hypnosis (and other mind–body methods) may paradoxically *increase* anxiety and cause disturbing thoughts and fear of losing control. People with psychiatric disorders may experience adverse effects and should discuss their situation with a psychiatrist before considering hypnosis.

Practical Information

Hypnotherapy sessions are generally 30 to 90 minutes in length and cost between $60 and $150. An average course of treatment involves 6 to 12 weekly sessions. Several organizations provide information about hypnosis:

- The American Society of Clinical Hypnosis (www.asch.net), 140 North Bloomingdale Rd., Bloomingdale, IL 60108 (630-980-4740)

- Society for Clinical and Experimental Hypnosis (www.sceh.us), PO Box 252, Southborough, MA 01772 (508-598-5553)

- Some health insurance companies reimburse for hypnosis.

Conclusion

Hypnosis is a well-tolerated, low- to moderate-cost therapy. Hypnosis may relieve some MS-associated symptoms, including anxiety, fatigue, pain, and insomnia.

Additional Readings
Books

Bauer B, ed. *Mayo Clinic Book of Alternative Medicine and Home Remedies.* New York, NY: Time Home Entertainment; 2013:102.

Benham G, Nash MR. Hypnosis. In: Oken BS, ed. *Complementary Therapies in Neurology.* London, UK: Parthenon Publishing; 2004:169–187.

Cassileth BR. *The Alternative Medicine Handbook.* New York, NY: W.W. Norton; 1998:122–130.

Ernst E, ed. *The Desktop Guide to Complementary and Alternative Medicine: An Evidence-Based Approach.* Edinburgh, UK: Mosby; 2001:56–58.

Micozzi MS, ed. *Fundamentals of Complementary and Alternative Medicine.* Philadelphia, PA: Saunders Elsevier; 2011:120,121.

Synovitz LB, Larson KL. *Complementary and Alternative Medicine for Health Professionals: A Holistic Approach to Consumer Health.* Burlington, MA: Jones and Bartlett Learning; 2013:206,207.

Journal Articles

Dane JR. Hypnosis for pain and neuromuscular rehabilitation with multiple sclerosis: case summary, literature review, and analysis of outcomes. *Int J Clin Exp Hypn.* 1996;44:208–231.

Dhanani NM, Caruso TJ, Carinci AJ. Complementary and alternative medicine for pain: an evidence-based review. *Curr Pain Headache Rep.* 2011;15:39–46.

Finnegan-John J, Molassiotis A, Richardson A, Ream E. A systematic review of complementary and alternative medicine interventions for the management of cancer-related fatigue. *Integr Cancer Ther.* 2013;12:276–290.

Hall H, Minnes L, Olness K. The psychophysiology of voluntary immunomodulation. *Int J Neurosci.* 1993;69:221–234.

Hammond DC. Hypnosis in the treatment of anxiety- and stress-related disorders. *Expert Rev Neurother.* 2010;10:263–273.

Jensen MP, Barber J, Romano JM, et al. A comparison of self-hypnosis versus progressive muscle relaxation in patients with multiple sclerosis and chronic pain. *Int J Clin Exp Hypn.* 2009;57:198–221.

Jensen MP, Ehde DM, Gertz KJ, et al. Effects of self-hypnosis training and cognitive restructuring on daily pain intensity and catastrophizing in individuals with multiple sclerosis and chronic pain. *Int J Clin Exp Hypn.* 2011;59:45–63.

Landolt AS, Milling LS. The efficacy of hypnosis as an intervention for labor and delivery pain: a comprehensive methodological review. *Clin Psychol Rev.* 2011;31:1022–1031.

Lazarus AA, Mayne TJ. Relaxation: some limitations, side effects, and proposed solutions. *Psychotherapy.* 1990;27:261–266.

Miller GE, Cohen S. Psychological interventions and the immune system: a meta-analytic review and critique. *Health Psychol.* 2001;20:47–63.

Smith GR, McKenzie JM, Marmer DJ, Steele RW. Psychologic modulation of the human immune response to *Varicella zoster. Arch Intern Med.* 1985;145:221–235.

Sutcher H. Hypnosis as adjunctive therapy for multiple sclerosis: a progress report. *Am J Clin Hypn.* 1997;39:283–290.

Sutherland G, Andersen MB, Morris T. Relaxation and health-related quality of life in multiple sclerosis: the example of autogenic training. *J Behav Med.* 2005;28:249–256.

Torem MS. Mind-body hypnotic imagery in the treatment of auto-immune disorders. *Am J Clin Hypn.* 2007;50:157–170.

Wahbeh H, Haywood A, Kaufman K, Zwickey H. Mind-body medicine and immune system outcomes: a systematic review. *Open Complem Med J.* 2009;1:25–34.

⑦ Low-Dose Naltrexone

Naltrexone is an oral medication approved by the U.S. Food and Drug Administration (FDA) for the treatment of opiate and alcohol addiction. It has been proposed that low-dose naltrexone (LDN) is effective in preventing multiple sclerosis (MS) attacks, slowing the progression of MS, and treating MS symptoms. LDN is claimed to be effective for multiple other diseases, including cancer, AIDS, rheumatoid arthritis, and Crohn's disease. Dr. Bernard Bihari, a physician in New York City, was the first to propose that LDN may be an effective treatment for MS and other diseases. A patent for the use of naltrexone in MS has been awarded by the U.S. Patent Office.

Treatment Method

Naltrexone typically is used in oral doses of 50 mg daily. LDN treatment uses much lower oral daily doses of 1.5 to 4.5 mg.

Studies in MS and Other Conditions

Multiple theories have been proposed about how LDN might produce therapeutic effects in MS. For slowing down the disease process, it has been claimed that LDN may produce immune changes that would be beneficial for MS. It has also been proposed that LDN decreases the formation of harmful chemicals known as free radicals, which then decreases *excitotoxicity*, a biochemical process that injures nerve cells (1). In terms of possibly relieving MS symptoms, it has been hypothesized that LDN enhances opiate effects by increasing the body's production of its own opiate chemicals, known as *endorphins,* and by increasing the body's sensitivity to endorphins. Through this process, LDN could conceivably produce an *endorphin high* (without exercise) and thereby relieve multiple symptoms.

Limited animal studies have been conducted with LDN in experimental auto-immune encephalomyelitis (EAE), the animal model of MS. Two studies in this animal model show that LDN decreases the amount of brain inflammation and also decreases the severity of the disease (2,3).

Three clinical trials of LDN in MS have produced variable results. An Italian study in primary progressive MS found improvement in spasticity, worsening of pain, and no effect on multiple other symptoms, including fatigue, depression, and quality of life (4). In two other trials, very similar research protocols were used in people with relapsing and progressive MS. One of these studies reported improvement in pain and mental health (5), while the other did not find any beneficial effects (6).

LDN has undergone limited testing in a wide range of other medical conditions. Promising, but not definitive, results have been obtained in clinical trials of fibromyalgia-associated pain, irritable bowel syndrome, and Crohn's disease.

Side Effects

Based on available evidence, LDN appears to be generally well-tolerated. In one of the MS clinical trials, there was neurological worsening in one patient with progressive MS. In people who are treated with opiate medications, LDN could provoke withdrawal. The safety of LDN use, especially on a long-term basis, is not known. Anecdotally, it has been reported that LDN may increase muscle stiffness and increase wakefulness (1).

Practical Information

Due to limited information about LDN, its use should be discussed with a health professional. It is not known if LDN affects the disease course in MS. As a result, LDN should not be used *instead* of FDA-approved disease-modifying medications.

Conclusion

LDN is generally well-tolerated, but the safety of long-term LDN use is not known. LDN should be avoided in those who take opiate medications. Limited clinical trial testing of LDN in people with MS has produced inconsistent results. Further work is needed in this area.

Additional Readings

Journal Articles

Agrawal YP. Low dose naltrexone therapy in multiple sclerosis. *Med Hypotheses.* 2005;64:721–724.

Bowling AC. The 411 on low dose naltrexone. *Momentum.* Spring 2009:44–46.

Cree BA, Kornyeyeva E, Goodin DS. Pilot trial of low-dose naltrexone and quality of life in multiple sclerosis. *Ann Neurol.* 2010;68:145–150.

Gironi M, Martinelli-Boneschi F, Sacerdote P, et al. A pilot trial of low-dose naltrexone in primary progressive multiple sclerosis. *Mult Scler.* 2008;14:1076–1083.

Kariv R, Tiomny E, Grenshpon R, et al. Low-dose naltrexone for the treatment of irritable bowel syndrome: a pilot study. *Dig Dis Sci.* 2006;51:2128–2133.

Sharafaddinzadeh N, Moghtaderi A, Kashipazha D, Majdinasab N, Shalbafan B. The effect of low-dose naltrexone on quality of life of patients with multiple sclerosis: a randomized placebo-controlled trial. *Mult Scler.* 2010;16:964–969.

Smith JP, Field D, Bingaman SI, Evans R, Mauger DT. Safety and tolerability of low-dose naltrexone therapy in children with moderate to severe Crohn's disease: a pilot study. *J Clin Gastroenterol.* 2013;47:339–345.

Smith JP, Stock H, Bingaman S, Mauger D, Rogosnitzky M, Zagon IS. Low-dose naltrexone therapy improves active Crohn's disease. *Am J Gastroenterol.* 2007;102:820–828.

Younger Y, Noor N, McCue R, Mackey S. Low-dose naltrexone for the treatment of fibromyalgia: findings of a small, randomized, double-blind, placebo-controlled, counterbalanced, crossover trial assessing pain levels. *Arth Rheum.* 2013;65:529–538.

Magnets and Electromagnetic Therapy

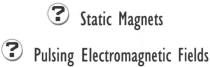

? Static Magnets

? Pulsing Electromagnetic Fields

The use of magnets and electromagnetic fields is a type of *energy medicine*. Magnets and electricity have been used for medicinal purposes for thousands of years. They were used in ancient China to stimulate acupuncture sites. In the 11th and 12th centuries, it was claimed that lodestones, minerals with natural magnetic qualities, relieved a variety of medical conditions. Paracelsus, a 16th-century Swiss physician and alchemist, used magnets to treat seizures. In the 18th century, Franz Mesmer, an Austrian physician, proposed a theory of *animal magnetism* and wrote a book on the subject, *On the Medicinal Uses of the Magnet*. It was later found that his therapy was based on hypnotism (see the chapter on *Hypnosis*), not on any therapeutic effects of magnets. A large number of magnetic and electrical devices were promoted during the 19th century, which is sometimes referred to as the *golden age of medical electricity*. These devices included magnetic insoles, belts, girdles, and caps. The manufacture and sale of magnetic devices in the United States is now limited by the Food, Drug, and Cosmetic Act and the Medical Devices Amendment of 1976. Several recent research studies on magnets have increased interest in this type of therapy.

Treatment Method

Magnets and electricity are used in both conventional and unconventional medicine. In conventional medicine, small amounts of electrical energy produced by the body are measured for diagnostic reasons. For example, an electroencephalogram (EEG) records the electrical energy produced by the brain, whereas an electrocardiogram (ECG or EKG) detects electrical currents produced by the heart. MRI machines use very powerful magnets to produce images of different parts of the body.

A unique therapeutic use of electrical energy has been employed recently to treat tremors in people with multiple sclerosis (MS), Parkinson's disease, and other neurologic disorders. In this treatment, an electrode is implanted in a brain region that controls body movements. Electrical stimulation of the electrode may significantly improve the tremor.

Magnets and electricity have many unconventional uses. Two types of electro-magnetic therapy usually are considered for MS. One type of therapy, known as static magnetic therapy, uses magnets that are available as bracelets, belts, and even large mats that may be placed on a bed. The other form of therapy, known as pulsed electromagnetic field therapy, uses devices that produce pulsing magnetic fields at a specific frequency. The pulsing magnetic fields usually are weak, but some studies have used strong fields.

Multiple hypotheses exist about how magnets could produce therapeutic effects. For strong magnets placed on the spine, it has been proposed that the magnetic field alters nerve activity in the spinal cord in such a way that it decreases muscle stiffness. For weaker magnetic devices, it is often claimed that they correct disease-causing electrical imbalances in the body. For devices placed on acupuncture points, it is proposed that acupuncture-like effects occur, such as increases in the release of pain-relieving chemicals (opioids) in the body. Multiple other mechanisms have been proposed, including an alteration of the flow of electrically charged atoms (such as calcium) and changes in hormone levels and immune-system function.

Studies in MS and Other Conditions

There are several placebo-controlled clinical studies of pulsed electromagnetic therapy in MS. One of these used strong fields applied to the spine—the others used weak electromagnetic fields.

One study using strong fields was reported by a Danish group in 1996 (1). In 38 people with MS, it was found that the electromagnetic treatment was associated with a decrease in spasticity, compared with those who received sham therapy.

For studies using weak electromagnetic fields, variable results have been reported:

- A promising two-part study of electromagnetic therapy in people with MS was reported from Hungary in 1987 (2). In the first part of this study, which included the use of a placebo therapy, 70% to 80% of the 20 treated participants benefited from pulsed electromagnetic therapy applied to the spine and legs. Spasticity, pain, and bladder function improved. In the second part of the investigation, electromagnetic treatment was used in 104 people in a less rigorous manner. Once again, symptoms improved in approximately 80% of people.

- In 1997, a placebo-controlled study from the University of Washington examined the effects of a pulsing device applied to three acupuncture points on 30 people with MS (3). Benefits were noted with spasticity, bladder function, cognitive problems, fatigue, mobility, and vision.

- In 2003, another placebo-controlled study treated 117 people with MS with a pulsing device placed on an acupuncture point near the shoulder (4). Beneficial effects were noted for fatigue and overall quality of life. No therapeutic effect for bladder function was noted. Variable results were obtained with spasticity.

- A two-part study, reported in 2009 (5) and 2011 (6), investigated the effects of a magnetic mattress on fatigue in 37 people with MS. This study was placebo-controlled for 12 weeks, and then *open-label* (not placebo-controlled) for 3 years. Improvement in fatigue was reported for both portions of the study.

- A 2012 placebo-controlled study evaluated the effects of a magnetic mattress on fatigue in 50 people with MS (7). This study found that the magnetic mattress did not produce statistically significant beneficial effects on fatigue.

Due to the inconsistent findings and the lack of rigor in some of these clinical trials, further research is needed to determine whether this therapy has any definite therapeutic effects in MS.

In addition to these studies of large groups of people with MS, reports exist of individuals with MS who experienced improvement in multiple symptoms using electromagnetic therapy. These reports are difficult to interpret because each study involved only a single person with MS.

Magnets have been investigated in other conditions. Among neurologic disorders, small studies have found that magnet therapy may be beneficial for people with nerve pain associated with diabetes and other conditions. Variable results have been obtained in studies of magnet therapy for low back pain, neck pain, and arthritis pain.

Pulsing electromagnetic therapy stimulates the healing of bone fractures; it also may decrease swelling resulting from ankle sprains, promote healing of bedsores, and improve joint mobility and pain in people with arthritis. Pulsing devices are approved by the Food and Drug Administration (FDA) for the treatment of bone fractures that do not heal.

A fascinating area of research involves applying pulsing high-intensity magnetic fields to the scalp. This technique, known as *transcranial magnetic stimulation*, takes advantage of the ability of magnetic fields to pass through bone.

In this procedure, a very strong magnetic field applied to the scalp passes through the skull and stimulates the underlying brain tissue. For example, magnetic stimulation to the brain region that controls movement results in movement of the corresponding part of the body. Some studies indicate that this therapy may be effective for a wide range of conditions, including depression, schizophrenia, and pain. The FDA has approved transcranial magnetic stimulation devices for some types of depression and migraine headaches.

Side Effects

The use of magnets and pulsing electromagnetic fields is generally well tolerated, but the long-term safety of these therapies is not known. Women who are pregnant and people with pacemakers and other implanted electronic medical devices should consult a physician before using this type of therapy. When using one of the pulsing devices with a weak field, warnings are given that it should not be used by those with epilepsy, cancer, diabetes, or heart or kidney disease. High-intensity magnetic fields, such as those used in transcranial magnetic stimulation, may have significant side effects (headaches, hearing loss, seizures, and other possible unknown effects) and should only be used under the direction of qualified clinicians. There is a case report of a person with MS who experienced a seizure while receiving transcranial magnetic stimulation.

Practical Information

A large number of magnets and pulsing electromagnetic devices are available. These vary greatly in terms of strength, size, shape, composition, and cost. Although some companies claim that their products are better because they produce a stronger electromagnetic field, it is not clear that a stronger field necessarily provides more benefit.

Conclusion

Low-intensity magnets and pulsing electromagnetic fields are usually well tolerated. Several studies suggest that pulsing electromagnetic fields may improve multiple MS symptoms, including spasticity and fatigue. However, these studies have produced inconsistent results. Further studies are required to determine definitively whether electromagnetic therapy in MS is effective.

Transcranial magnetic stimulation is a very specific type of magnetic therapy that is FDA-approved for some forms of depression and migraine. Transcranial magnetic stimulation and other approaches that use high-intensity magnetic stimulation may cause serious side effects—their use must be monitored by trained clinicians.

Additional Readings

Books

Bauer B, ed. *Mayo Clinic Book of Alternative Medicine and Home Remedies.* NewYork, NY: Time Home Entertainment; 2013:125,126.

Cassileth BR. *The Alternative Medicine Handbook.* NewYork, NY: W.W. Norton; 1998:299–304.

Jellin JM, Gregory PJ, Batz F, et al. *Pharmacist's Letter/ Prescriber's Letter Natural Medicines Comprehensive Database.* Stockton, CA: Therapeutic Research Faculty; 2014.

Micozzi MS, ed. *Fundamentals of Complementary and Alternative Medicine.* Philadelphia, PA: Saunders Elsevier; 2011:144–152.

Polman CH, Thompson AJ, Murray TJ, Bowling AC, Noseworthy JH. *Multiple Sclerosis: The Guide to Treatment and Management.* NewYork, NY: Demos Medical Publishing; 2006:157–159.

Synovitz LB, Larson KL. *Complementary and Alternative Medicine for Health Professionals: A Holistic Approach to Consumer Health.* Burlington, MA: Jones and Bartlett Learning; 2013:227–229.

Weintraub MI. Magnetic biostimulation in neurologic illness. In: Weintraub MI, Micozzi MS, eds. *Alternative and Complementary Treatments in Neurologic Iillness.* NewYork, NY: Churchill Livingstone; 2001:278–286.

Journal Articles

Aleman A. Use of repetitive transcranial magnetic stimulation for treatment in psychiatry. *Clin Psychopharmacol Neurosci.* 2013;11:53–59.

Colbert AP, Cleaver J, Brown KA, et al. Magnets applied to acupuncture points as therapy—a literature review. *Acupunct Med.* 2008;26:160–170.

deCarvalho ML, Motta R, Konrad G, Battaglia MA, Brichetto G. A randomized placebo-controlled cross-over study using a low frequency magnetic field in the treatment of fatigue in multiple sclerosis. *Mult Scler J.* 2012;18:82–89.

Fregni F, Pascual-Leone A. Transcranial magnetic stimulation for the treatment of depression in neurologic disorders. *Curr Psych Rep.* 2005;7:381–390.

George MS, Lisanby SAH, Sackeim HA. Transcranial magnetic stimulation: applications in neuropsychiatry. *Arch Gen Psych.* 1999;56:300–311.

Guseo A. Pulsing electromagnetic field therapy of multiple sclerosis by the Gyuling-Bordas device: double-blind, cross-over and open studies. *J Bioelec.* 1987;6:23–35.

Haupts MR, Daum S, Ahle G, Holinka B, Gehlen W. Transcranial magnetic stimulation as a provocation for epileptic seizures in multiple sclerosis. *Mult Scler.* 2004;10:475,476.

Hovington CL, McGirr A, Lepage M, Berlim MT. Repetitive transcranial magnetic stimulation (rTMS) for treating depression and schizophrenia: a systematic review of recent meta-analyses. *Ann Med.* 2013;45:308–321.

Hug K, Roosli M. Therapeutic effects of whole-body devices applying pulsed electromagnetic fields (PEMF): a systematic literature review. *Bioelectromagnetics.* 2011. [Epub ahead of print]. doi: 10.1002/bem.20703.

Lappin MS, Lawrie FW, Richards TL, Kramer ED. Effects of a pulsed electromagnetic therapy on multiple sclerosis fatigue and quality of life: a double-blind, placebo controlled trial. *Altern Ther Health Med.* 2003;9:38–48.

Macfarlane GJ, Paudyal P, Doherty M, et al. A systematic review of evidence for the effectiveness of practitioner-based complementary and alternative therapies in the management of rheumatic diseases: osteoarthritis. *Rheumatology.* 2012;51:2224–2233.

Markov MS. Magnetic field therapy: a review. *Electromagn Biol Med.* 2007; 26:1–23.

Nielsen JF, Sinkjaer T, Jakobsen J. Treatment of spasticity with repetitive magnetic stimulation: a double-blind placebo-controlled study. *Mult Scler.* 1996;2: 227–232.

Piatkowski J, Haase R, Ziemssen T. Long-term effects of bio-electromagnetic-energy-regulation therapy on fatigue in patients with multiple sclerosis. *Altern Ther Health Med.* 2011;17:22–28.

Piatkowski J, Kern S, Ziemssen T. Effect of BEMER magnetic field therapy on the level of fatigue in patients with multiple sclerosis: a randomized, double-blind controlled trial. *J Altern Complement Med.* 2009;15:507–511.

Pittler MH, Brown EM, Ernst E. Static magnets for reducing pain: systematic review and meta-analysis of randomized trials. *CMAJ.* 2007;177:736–742.

Richards TL, Lappin MS, Acosta-Urquidi J, et al. Double-blind study of pulsing magnetic field effects on multiple sclerosis. *J Alt Complement Med.* 1997;3:21–29.

Vallbona C, Hazlewood CF, Jurida G. Response of pain to static magnetic fields in postpolio patients: a double-blind pilot study. *Arch Phys Med Rehabil.* 1997;78:1200–1203.

⑦ Marijuana

Marijuana is derived from the plant known as *Cannabis,* one of the oldest cultivated plants. It was grown in China nearly 5,000 years ago and has been used medicinally in many different cultures for thousands of years. There are two major types, or "subspecies," of *Cannabis*—one of these is a tall, angular plant known as *Cannabis sativa,* while the other, which is shorter and bushier, is known as *Cannabis indica.*

Marijuana contains many different chemical compounds, of which about 60 are pharmacologically active chemicals known as "cannabinoids." One of the main cannabinoids is known as delta-9-tetrahydrocannabinol or THC, which produces much of the euphoria of marijuana. Another cannabinoid, known as cannabidiol or CBD, appears to produce other effects. The *Cannabis sativa* subspecies contains mainly THC while *Cannabis indica* contains both THC and CBD. Many different types of cannabis hybrid plants have been developed by cross-breeding *Cannabis sativa* and *Cannabis indica.*

There is a growing trend for legalization of marijuana for medical and recreational use. In the United States, 20 states and the District of Columbia have legalized marijuana for medical use—two states, Colorado and Washington, have legalized recreational use. In spite of these state laws, marijuana remains illegal at the federal level in the United States. In Canada, the use of marijuana for medical purposes is considered a constitutional right. In Europe, The Netherlands has a long history of tolerance for marijuana use and several other countries have decriminalized its use. In South America, Uruguay has legalized recreational use.

In the United States, the state laws generally allow for medical marijuana use by those with MS and other "approved conditions." The exact wording of these laws varies from state to state but, with regard to multiple sclerosis (MS), usually refers in some way to "spasticity" or "pain" due to MS or simply to "multiple sclerosis."

Treatment Method

Marijuana is available in several forms. Most simply, the leaf may be smoked or eaten in the form of "edible" products, such as candy or baked goods. To avoid exposure to smoke, vaporizers may be used. The resin of the plant, hashish, also may be smoked or eaten.

Marijuana-derived chemicals may also be used medically. THC, the main active constituent, is available by prescription as a pill, known as dronabinol or Marinol. A synthetic form of THC, known as nabilone or Cesamet, also is available in pill form. Both dronabinol and nabilone are available by prescription in the United States.

Oils may be used to make "extracts" of marijuana that contain many of the active chemicals. One of these extracts, known as Sativex or nabiximols, is an oral spray that is derived from a patented cannabis hybrid plant that is grown in a secret location in the United Kingdom. Sativex is standardized to contain approximately equal amounts of THC and CBD. Sativex is not available in the United States but is available by prescription in several other countries. Another standardized extract that is used in research studies is known as "Cannador," which contains a THC:CBD ratio of about 2:1 and is available for research purposes from the Society for Clinical Research in Germany.

Studies in MS and Other Conditions

The biologic effects of cannabinoids have been extensively investigated. These chemicals bind to proteins in the central nervous system (CNS) that decrease nerve cell activity. These proteins are known as *CB1 receptors.* Theoretically, binding to CB1 receptors could decrease some MS-associated symptoms, such as pain and spasticity. Also, cannabinoids bind to another type of protein known as *CB2 receptors.* Binding to these proteins, which are present on immune cells, may mildly suppress the immune system and could thus potentially slow down the disease course in MS. Other effects of cannabinoids, including antioxidant properties and inhibitory effects on a harmful process known as *excitotoxicity,* could also theoretically be beneficial for MS.

The effects of marijuana, THC, and nabilone have been studied in many diseases, including MS. Some of the recent interest in medical marijuana was generated by a 1999 report by the National Academy of Sciences/Institute of Medicine (NAS/IOM) that analyzed the scientific and clinical literature on the potential therapeutic effects of marijuana. The NAS/IOM report indicated that marijuana and THC may relieve the spasticity or muscle stiffness associated with MS and also may be effective in the treatment of pain, nausea associated with chemotherapy, and weight loss associated with AIDS and cancer. The report also cautioned against the long-term use of smoked marijuana, indicated that effective prescription medications are available for many conditions treated with marijuana, and suggested that methods of taking the drug, other than smoking, should be developed.

There is a long history of MS-related studies of marijuana. Various studies have evaluated the effects of marijuana on the animal model of MS, known as experimental autoimmune encephalomyelitis (EAE). In one study, mice with EAE exhibited spasticity and tremor—THC and two other marijuana-derived chemicals reduced both spasticity and tremor in these animals. Other studies in EAE have shown that high doses of cannabinoids decrease the overall severity of disease.

There are many clinical trials that have evaluated the effects of marijuana on MS symptoms. Many people, including health professionals, may not know the results of these studies or may not even be aware that the studies have been conducted. The first published article, reported in 1979 in the prestigious *Journal of the American Medical Association,* indicated that marijuana may relieve MS-associated spasticity (1). Since that initial publication, there have been nearly 20 additional MS clinical trials of low, moderate, and high quality—these trials, which are technically classified as "Class I, II, or III," have had 10 or more participants and have included a placebo-treated group.

It is important to recognize that a wide range of marijuana products has been used in these studies. The majority of the studies have used marijuana extracts in the form of Sativex or the standardized research preparation known as "Cannador." Six studies have used THC or Marinol, while only two have used smoked marijuana.

Many different MS symptoms have been evaluated in these studies (2–13). The symptoms that have most consistently shown improvement are pain and "subjective spasticity," which refers to an individual's sense of how much spasticity, or muscle stiffness, he or she is experiencing. It is interesting to note that "objective spasticity," a formal measure of muscle stiffness that is determined by a clinician, has generally *not* shown improvement in these studies. Several trials in MS (and other conditions) have reported improvement in sleep with marijuana. Positive as well as negative results have been reported with bladder function—the strongest evidence for benefit has been seen with Sativex for increased frequency of urination. No benefit has been found for tremor.

As noted, limited MS studies have focused on smoked marijuana, which may be the most common form of marijuana used by those with MS. Two relatively small clinical trials on people with MS have been conducted. The largest study, which included 30 people with MS, reported improvement in objectively measured spasticity but worsening of cognitive function (3). The other study found that participants felt that their ability to balance improved but objective measures showed that balance actually worsened (4). Several survey-based studies using questionnaires have evaluated the effects of smoked marijuana in people with MS (14). In these surveys, symptoms that are commonly reported to be improved include pain, spasticity, and sleeping difficulties. Surveys such as these are generally less reliable than formal clinical trials. However, they may provide important information because, as noted, clinical trial information on smoked marijuana is limited and also these survey studies may in some ways be more representative of the "real world" situation than a clinical trial.

An independent review panel, commissioned by the American Academy of Neurology, used rigorous standards to formally evaluate the studies of marijuana (and other forms of CAM) and MS symptoms (13). With these standards, the panel, of which I was a member, was not able to make any conclusions about smoked marijuana due to the limited number of studies. For THC and extracts, the following conclusions were made:

- Likely Effective
  - Pain: THC, extracts (Sativex and Cannador)
  - Subjective spasticity: THC, extracts (Sativex and Cannador)
  - Frequency of urination: Sativex
- Likely or Possibly *Not* Effective
  - Objective spasticity: THC, Sativex
  - Tremor: THC
  - Urinary incontinence: Sativex

There are very limited human studies of the potential effects of marijuana on the immune system and the overall disease course in people with MS. As noted, marijuana has biological effects that could, in theory, slow down the disease course, and studies in the animal model indicate that marijuana may have a "disease-modifying" effect. However, contrary to what might be expected, one human study found that marijuana-derived chemicals actually produced immune-stimulating effects. Another study of blood samples from people in a large MS study known as the CAMS study found that oral THC and marijuana extract did not produce any effects on multiple immune markers. Finally, a large and rigorous study of nearly 500 people with progressive MS in the United Kingdom, known as the CUPID Study, did not find any effect of THC on slowing down the progression of disability (15).

Side Effects

Smoked marijuana and marijuana-derived products may have adverse effects. Some of the safety information is limited because it is challenging to methodically study standardized marijuana use in large numbers of people over an extended period of time.

In MS studies, marijuana products have generally been well tolerated (13). Some studies have shown neurological side effects, including dizziness, impaired balance, sedation, lightheadedness, memory difficulties, and difficulty concentrating. About 10% of participants have experienced gastrointestinal side effects, such as increased appetite, nausea, vomiting, constipation, and dry or sore mouth. Less common side effects have included muscle pain, increased spasticity, seizures, leg weakness, dehydration, temporary psychosis, and hallucinations. Oral "ulcers," which are similar to canker sores, have been reported with Sativex.

Additional possible side effects have been reported in studies in the general population. Long-term use has been associated with depression, psychosis, and addiction. Other adverse effects that have been reported include impaired driving, incoordination, and visual difficulties. Chronic use may impair lung function, cause heart attacks, cause dependence and apathy, and increase the risk of cancer of the lung, head, and neck. Marijuana products may increase the sedating effects of medications and alcohol. They may also increase the activating effects of stimulating medications. Marijuana may interfere with blood-thinning medications such as warfarin (Coumadin). Some of the side effects that may be specifically associated with marijuana smoke, such as cancer and lung conditions, may be avoided by using vaporizers or oral preparations such as edible marijuana products, extracts, and pills that contain THC or nabilone.

In the United States, there may be safety issues related to the quality of marijuana products. States that have medical or recreational marijuana laws generally do not monitor the quality of the products that are sold. For example, in Colorado, which has legalized marijuana for medical and recreational use, one independent laboratory analyzed the THC content of 13 edible products and found that none of the products contained the amount of THC that was listed on the label (16). Most products contained significantly less than what was listed on the label—three products had only 0.2% to 0.4% of the claimed amount of THC. One product contained nearly 50% more THC than was listed on the label. Also in Colorado, marijuana products have labels that warn users about uncertainties with purity and potency as well as overall safety and effectiveness:

Warning: There may be health risks associated with the consumption of this product…. The product was produced without regulatory oversight for health, safety, or efficacy…. The marijuana product contained within this package has not been tested for potency, consume with caution. The marijuana product contained within this package has not been tested for contaminants.

Unresolved Issues, Unanswered Questions

Although a large amount of research has been done on marijuana and MS, there are significant challenges with "translating" this research into clinical practice. First, the majority of the MS studies have been done with extracts of marijuana (Sativex and Cannador) that are standardized to contain very specific amounts of cannabinoids. However, these extracts are not generally available for medical (or recreational) use in the United States and many other countries. The extracts or edible products that are available may not be standardized and may be of uncertain quality. Also, there are not any guidelines on how to apply research results on extracts to smoked forms of marijuana.

There are many other unanswered questions about marijuana use in MS:

- For medical use, products are available from many different cannabis hybrid plants and each of these plants has its own unique composition of cannabinoids—when smoked, eaten, or used as an extract, are some hybrids more effective or safe than others?

- What dose, how often, and in what form (smoked, eaten, extract) should marijuana products be used to optimize effectiveness and safety?

- For treating MS symptoms, should marijuana products be used on their own or in combination with medications?

- In terms of overall safety and effectiveness for symptoms such as pain or spasticity, how do marijuana products compare with conventional medications?

- Are marijuana products safe and effective when used in combination with MS disease-modifying medications or medications that are commonly used to treat MS symptoms?

Conclusion

Marijuana is legal for use in MS in some states and countries. As a result, it is sometimes assumed that marijuana has been proven to be safe and effective in MS. Indeed, some marijuana products may relieve some MS symptoms. However, information about marijuana's effectiveness in MS is limited, marijuana may produce side effects, and there are many unanswered questions about how to use marijuana in MS.

Studies in MS have primarily used extracts and THC. Studies of extracts and THC indicate that some, but not all, of these products decrease pain and "subjective spasticity" and improve bladder function and sleep. These products do not appear to improve tremors or objectively measured spasticity. Smoked marijuana has undergone very limited investigation in MS. There are potential serious side effects with all forms of marijuana. Also, there may be safety issues due to the lack of standard-ized preparations and quality control. Marijuana use should be discussed with a physician. Users should be aware that marijuana use may be illegal.

Further research and improved quality control is needed in this area. Future research should include studies that are rigorous and are specifically designed to address the multiple unresolved issues. Also, for marijuana products that are sold for medical (or recreational) use, there should be quality standards and monitoring procedures for purity and potency.

Additional Readings

Books

Bowling AC. Complementary and alternative medicine: practical considerations. In: Rae-Grant A, Fox R, Bethoux F, eds. *Multiple Sclerosis and Related Disorders: Diagnosis, Medical Management, and Rehabilitation.* New York, NY: Demos; 2013:243–249.

Iversen LL. *The Science of Marijuana.* New York, NY: Oxford University Press; 2008.

Jellin JM, Gregory PJ, Batz F, et al. *Pharmacist's Letter/ Prescriber's Letter Natural Medicines Comprehensive Database.* Stockton, CA: Therapeutic Research Faculty; 2014.

Journal Articles

Anon. Adverse effects of marijuana. *Prescrire Int.* 2011;20:18–23.

Baca R. Labels fudge THC levels: with no standard for testing, buyers can't trust items' potency. *Denver Post.* March 9, 2014:1A, 17A.

Baker D, Pryce G, Croxford J, et al. Cannabinoids control spasticity and tremor in a multiple sclerosis model. *Nature.* 2000;404:84–87.

Baker D, Pryce G, Giovannoni G, Thompson AJ. The therapeutic potential of cannabis. *Lancet Neurol.* 2003;2:291–298.

Borgelt LM, Franson KL, Nussbaum AM, Wang GS. The pharmacologic and clinical effects of medical cannabis. *Pharmacotherapy.* 2013;33:195–209.

Bowling AC. Cannabinoids in MS—are we any closer to knowing how best to use them. *Mult Scler.* 2006;12:523–525.

Bowling AC. Marijuana and MS—an unfinished story. *Momentum.* Fall 2010:33–35.

Bowling AC. Worthless weed or pot of gold. *Int J MS Care.* 2004;5:138,166.

Clark AJ, Ware MA, Yazer E, Murray TJ, Lynch ME. Patterns of cannabis use among patients with multiple sclerosis. *Neurology.* 2004;62:2098–2100.

Corey-Bloom J, Wolfson T, Gamst A, et al. Smoked cannabis for spasticity in multiple sclerosis: a randomized, placebo-controlled trial. *CMAJ.* 2012;184: 1143–1150.

Fox P, Bain PG, Glickman S, Carroll C, Zajicek J. The effect of cannabis on tremor in patients with multiple sclerosis. *Neurology.* 2004;62:1105–1109.

Greenberg HS, Werness SA, Puch JE, Andrus RO, Anderson DJ, Domino EF. Short-term effects of smoking marijuana on balance in patients with multiple sclerosis and normal volunteers. *Clin Pharmacol Ther.* 1994;55:324–328.

Katona S, Kaminski E, Sanders H, Zajicek J. Cannabinoid influence on cytokine profile in multiple sclerosis. *Clin Exp Immunol.* 2005;140:580–585.

Killestein J, Hoogervorst ELJ, Reif M, et al. Immunomodulatory effects of orally administered cannabinoids in multiple sclerosis. *J Neuroimmunol.* 2003;137: 140–143.

Koppel BS, Brust JCM, Fife T, et al. Systematic review: efficacy and safety of medical marijuana in selected neurologic disorders: report of the Guideline Development Subcommittee of the American Academy of Neurology. *Neurology.* 2014;82:1556–1563.

Petro DJ, Ellenberger C. Treatment of human spasticity with tetrahydrocannabinol. *J Clin Pharmacol.* 1981;21:413S–416S.

Pryce G, Cabranes A, Fernandez-Ruiz J, et al. Control of experimental spasticity by targeting the degradation of endocannabinoids using selective fatty acid amide hydrolase inhibitors. *Mult Scler J.* 2013;19:1896–1904.

Thomas G, Kloner RA, Rezkalla S. Adverse cardiovascular, cerebrovascular, and peripheral vascular effects of marijuana inhalation: what cardiologists need to know. *Am J Cardiol.* 2014;113:187–190.

Ungerleider JT. Therapeutic issues of marijuana and THC. *Int J Addict.* 1985;20:691–699.

Ungerleider JT, Andrysiak T, Fairbanks L, Ellison GW, Myers LW. Delta-9-THC in the treatment of spasticity associated with multiple sclerosis. *Pharmacol Issues Alc Subst Abuse.* 1988;7:39–50.

Vaney C, Heinzel-Gutenbrunner M, Jobin P, et al. Efficacy, safety and tolerability of an orally administered cannabis extract in the treatment of spasticity in patients with multiple sclerosis: a randomized, double-blind, placebo-controlled, crossover study. *Mult Scler.* 2004;10:417–424.

Wade DT, Makela PM, House H, Bateman C, Robson P. Long-term use of a cannabis-based medicine in the treatment of spasticity and other symptoms in multiple sclerosis. *Mult Scler.* 2006;12:639–645.

Wade DT, Makela P, Robson P, House H, Bateman C. Do cannabis-based medicinal extracts have general or specific effects on symptoms in multiple sclerosis: a double-blind, randomized, placebo-controlled study on 160 patients. *Mult Scler.* 2004;10:434–441.

Yadav V, Bever C, Bowen J, et al. Summary of evidence-based guideline: complementary and alternative medicine in multiple sclerosis: report of the Guideline Development Subcommittee of the American Academy of Neurology. *Neurology.* 2014;82:1–10.

Zajicek J, Ball S, Wright D, et al. Effect of dronabinol on progression in progressive multiple sclerosis (CUPID): a randomized, placebo-controlled trial. *Lancet Neurol.* 2013;12:857–865.

Zajicek J, Fox P, Sanders H, et al. Cannabinoids for treatment of spasticity and other symptoms related to multiple sclerosis (CAMS study): multicentre randomised placebo-controlled trial. *Lancet.* 2003;362:1517–1526.

Zajicek J, Sanders HP, Wright DE, et al. Cannabinoids in multiple sclerosis (CAMS) study: safety and efficacy data for 12 months follow up. *J Neurol Neursurg Psych.* 2005;76:1664–1669.

Zajicek JP, Apostu VI. Role of cannabinoids in multiple sclerosis. *CNS Drugs.* 2011;25:187–201.

⊘ Massage

Massage is a healing method that has been used for thousands of years. It was a recommended therapy in ancient China and Egypt. Many common forms of massage now used in the United States are derived from Swedish massage, which was developed by a Swedish physician in the 19th century. Massage may be provided on its own, or it may be a component of other forms of alternative healing, including Ayurveda, traditional Chinese medicine, and aromatherapy. Reflexology is a specific type of foot massage (see chapter on *Reflexology*).

Treatment Method

Massage usually is done on a specially designed table in a warm, quiet room with soft lighting and relaxing music. The individual receiving the massage is partially or completely undressed; a sheet or towel is used to cover parts of the body that are not being massaged. The therapist uses a variety of techniques, including pressing, stroking, rubbing, slapping, and tapping. Oil or lotion usually is used to make the movements smoother.

Massage may be effective through several possible mechanisms. First, massage appears to relax muscles (although only limited studies have formally evaluated this effect). This effect may be helpful for conditions that are worsened by muscle stiffness, such as headaches, neck pain, and low back pain. Also, massage may release chemicals known as *endorphins,* which reduce pain. Through a theoretical process known as *gate control,* which presumes that only a certain number of impulses may reach the brain from a specific body part, stimulation by massage in a painful area may decrease the number of pain impulses received by the brain from that area. Finally, the simple act of touching that occurs with massage may convey positive feelings that are difficult to evaluate rigorously, such as caring, comfort, and acceptance. Touching is a simple and possibly beneficial act that often is missing from interactions between patients and physicians and other mainstream health care providers.

Studies in MS and Other Conditions

Several studies have specifically evaluated massage therapy in people with multiple sclerosis (MS). In one of the earliest studies, reported in 1998, 24 people with MS who received massage therapy were compared with those who did not (1). In this small study, massage therapy was associated with multiple benefits, including increased self-esteem, improved social functioning, and reduced anxiety and depression. In addition, those who received massage had better self-perception of their bodies and the progression of their disease.

There are two studies that show that massage therapy improves *self-efficacy*, which refers to the strength of belief in one's own ability to complete tasks and reach goals (2,3). In general, higher self-efficacy is associated with higher levels of optimism and lower levels of hopelessness. The MS studies, which used weekly massage for 8 to 16 weeks, found that the self-efficacy effect of massage persisted for 4 weeks, but not 8 weeks, after discontinuation of massage therapy. This indicates that ongoing massage may be needed for the self-efficacy effect.

Another study evaluated the effects of massage and exercise on multiple MS symptoms (4). This 5-week study of 48 people with MS used four different approaches—massage, exercise, massage in combination with exercise, and no treatment. Massage or massage combined with exercise were most effective and improved multiple symptoms, including pain, balance, and walking speed. The effects on walking and balance are interesting and not necessarily what one would expect with massage—of note, possible beneficial effects of massage on walking have also been noted in limited studies in those with Parkinson's disease, cerebral palsy, and spinal cord injury. Further research in this area is needed.

There are several other small studies of massage in MS. One found improvement in constipation with 4 weeks of abdominal massage that was administered by people with MS or their caregivers (5). Another small trial found that slow, stroking massage movements over the spine were associated with improvement in anxiety and in the electrophysiological measures of muscle stiffness (6). A small preliminary study of two people with MS found that massage along with aromatherapy was associated with improvements in mobility, personal hygiene, and dressing ability (7).

Conditions that may occur with MS have been studied in medical conditions other than MS. Nearly all these studies have serious limitations, and, consequently, the results must not be taken as definitive. Some studies have shown a reduction in stress, anxiety, and depression. It is often stated that spasticity or stiffness in the arms or legs may improve with massage—studies in this area are surprisingly limited. Some studies in conditions other than MS indicate that abdominal massage may improve constipation. Several forms of pain, including low back pain and cancer-related pain, may improve with massage. The National Cancer Institute recognizes massage as a nonmedication therapy for pain. In terms of general health effects, several studies have found that massage modestly reduces blood pressure.

In addition to its effects on specific symptoms, massage also may have a beneficial effect on self-esteem and overall quality of life through its "healing touch" properties. Dr. Elizabeth Forsythe, an English physician with MS, wrote about her experiences with massage in the book *Multiple Sclerosis: Exploring Sickness and Health*: "Her patience, acceptance, and her remarkable hands began to lessen my loathing for my body. The massage also relieved much of the muscle spasm and tension in my body. Being massaged by somebody known and trusted is a good start to the building or rebuilding of a personal world of trust" (8).

The effects of massage on the immune system are not well understood. Various effects of massage on immune function have been reported, but the significance of these effects is not known.

Side Effects

Massage usually is well tolerated. Minor adverse effects that have been reported include headache, muscle pain, and lethargy. There are also rare, isolated reports of more serious complications, such as bleeding into the liver with deep abdominal massage.

To prevent complications, there are certain conditions for which massage should be avoided or practiced with caution. The following guidelines should be followed:

- Recent injuries, such as fractures and open skin lesions, should not be massaged.

- Abdominal massage should be avoided by people with ulcers or enlargement of the liver or spleen.

- People with fever, infection, clotted blood vessels (thrombosis), and jaundice should avoid massage.

- Those with cancer, arthritis, and heart disease should consult a physician before receiving massage therapy.

- Women who are pregnant should only receive massage from therapists who are experienced in pregnancy massage.

Practical Information

Massage often is performed by a therapist, but it also may be done on one's own without a therapist. Massage therapy sessions typically last from 30 to 90 minutes and cost $30 to $60 per hour. The expense of massage therapy is covered by some insurance plans. You can locate a massage therapist in the yellow pages of the telephone book.

More information about massage and qualified massage therapists is available from:

- The American Massage Therapy Association (www.amtamassage.org), 500 Davis Street, Evanston, IL 60201 (877-905-0577)

- National Certification Board for Therapeutic Massage and Bodywork (www.ncbtmb.com), 1901 South Meyers Rd., Suite 240, Oakbrook Terrace, IL 60181 (800-296-0664)

Conclusion

Massage is a relatively safe, low- to moderate-cost therapy that may have several benefits. Although it has not been extensively studied in MS, limited studies in other conditions suggest that it may be helpful for some MS-associated symptoms, including anxiety, depression, constipation, muscle stiffness (spasticity), pain, and walking. Also, massage may mildly reduce blood pressure.

Additional Readings

Books

Bauer B, ed. *Mayo Clinic Book of Alternative Medicine and Home Remedies*. New York, NY: Time Home Entertainment; 2013:131–135.

Micozzi MS, ed. *Fundamentals of Complementary and Alternative Medicine*. Philadelphia, PA: Saunders Elsevier; 2011:211–231.

Oken BS, ed. *Complementary Therapies in Neurology*. London, UK: Parthenon Publishing; 2004.

Synovitz LB, Larson KL. *Complementary and Alternative Medicine for Health Professionals: A Holistic Approach to Consumer Health*. Burlington, MA: Jones and Bartlett Learning; 2013:184–188.

Vickers A. *Massage and Aromatherapy: A Guide for Health Professionals*. London, UK: Chapman & Hall; 1996.

Weintraub MI, Micozzi MS, eds. *Alternative and Complementary Treatments in Neurologic Illness*. New York, NY: Churchill Livingstone; 2001.

Journal Articles

Billhult A, Lindholm C, Gunnarsson R, Stener-Victorin E. The effect of massage on immune function and stress in women with breast cancer—a randomized controlled trial. *Auton Neurosci.* 2009;150:111–115.

Braun LA, Stanguts C, Casanelia L, et al. Massage therapy for cardiac surgery patients—a randomized trial. *J Thor Cardiovasc Surg.* 1012;144:1453–1459.

Brouwer B, de Andrade VS. The effects of slow stroking on spasticity in patients with multiple sclerosis: a pilot study. *Physiother Theory Pract.* 1995;11:13–21.

Donoyama N, Ohkoshi N. Effects of traditional Japanese massage therapy on various symptoms in patients with Parkinson's disease: a case-series study. *J Alt Complement Ther.* 2012;18:294–299.

Finch P, Becker P. Changes in the self-efficacy of multiple sclerosis patients following massage therapy. *J Bodywork Movement Ther.* 2007;11:267–272.

Finch P, Bessonnette S. A pragmatic investigation into the effects of massage therapy on the self efficacy of multiple sclerosis clients. *J Bodywork Movement Ther.* 2014;18:11–16.

Givi M. Durability of effect of massage therapy on blood pressure. *Int J Prev Med.* 2013;4:511–516.

Hernandez-Reif M, Field T, Field T, et al. Multiple sclerosis patients benefit from massage therapy. *J Bodywork Movement Ther.* 1998;2:168–174.

Hou WH, Chiang PT, Hsu TY, Chiu SY, Yen YC. Treatment effects of massage therapy in depressed people: a meta-analysis. *J Clin Psychiatry.* 2010;71:894–901.

Krohn M, Listing M, Tjahjono G, et al. Depression, mood, stress, and Th1/Th2 immune balance in primary breast cancer patients undergoing classical massage therapy. *Support Care Cancer.* 2011;19:1303–1311.

McClurg D, Hagen S, Hawkins S, Lowe-Strong A. Abdominal massage for the alleviation of constipation symptoms in people with multiple sclerosis: a randomized controlled feasibility study. *Mult Scler J.* 2011;17:223–233.

Negahban H, Rezaie S, Goharpey S. Massage therapy and exercise therapy in patients with multiple sclerosis: a randomized controlled pilot study. *Clin Rehabil.* 2013;27:1126–1136.

Pan YQ, Yang KH, Wang YL, Zhang LP, Liang HQ. Massage interventions and treatment-related side effects of breast cancer: a systematic review and meta-analysis [published online ahead of print November 26 2013]. *Int J Clin Oncol.* 2013.

Rapaport MH, Schettler P, Bresee C. A preliminary study of the effects of repeated massage on hypothalamic-pituitary-adrenal and immune function in healthy individuals: a study of mechanisms of action and dosage. *J Altern Complement Med.* 2012;18:789–797.

Rosen J, Lawrence R, Bouchard M, Doros G, Gardiner P, Saper R. Massage for perioperative pain and anxiety in placement of vascular access devices. *Adv Mind Body Med.* 2013;27:12–23.

Sinclair M. The use of abdominal massage to treat chronic constipation. *Jo Bodywork Movement Ther.* 2011;15:436–445.

Supa'at I, Zakaria Z, Maskon O, Aminuddin A, Nordin NA. Effects of Swedish massage therapy on blood pressure, heart rate, and inflammatory markers in hypertensive women. *Evid Based Complement Altern Med.* 2013;2013:171852.

Vanderbilt S. Searching for comfort: alternative therapies and multiple sclerosis. *Massage and Bodywork.* 2004;Aug/Sept:50–59.

Walsh E, Wilson C. Complementary therapies in long-stay neurology in-patient settings. *Nurs Stand.* 1999;13:32–35.

✅ Meditation

Meditation is a type of mind–body therapy, a class of therapies that also includes biofeedback, hypnosis, and guided imagery. For thousands of years, meditation has been practiced in some form, especially in the context of religious practice. Also, meditation is one of several components of some complementary and alternative medicine (CAM) therapies, including Ayurveda (which uses transcendental meditation or TM) and traditional Chinese medicine.

Meditation is a way of producing the *relaxation response*, which has been described extensively by Dr. Herbert Benson at the Harvard Medical School and The Mind/Body Medical Institute. The relaxation response is a state of relaxation associated with decreased anxiety, muscle relaxation, and lowering of blood pressure. It is believed to be the opposite of the physiologic response known as the *fight-or-flight response*, characterized by the activation or stimulation of multiple body processes, such as increases in heart rate, blood pressure, and breathing rate.

Treatment Method

Many different meditation methods are used. All these techniques elicit relaxation by focusing concentration, relaxing the body, and diverting attention from stressful thoughts and feelings. One of the simplest strategies, outlined years ago by Dr. Herbert Benson in *The Relaxation Response*, is as follows:

1. Sit in a comfortable position in a quiet room and close your eyes.

2. Relax your muscles by starting with the feet and slowly working up the body to the face.

3. Each time you exhale, say a word silently.

4. Try to avoid distracting thoughts.

5. Continue this process for 10 to 20 minutes.

Other, more formal meditation methods include TM, mindfulness meditation (or *vipassana),* and meditation techniques associated with Zen (the Chinese word for meditation) and yoga. Mindfulness meditation and mindfulness-based stress reduction have been extensively researched by Dr. Jon Kabat-Zinn and others—these approaches are discussed in the *Mindfulness* chapter of this book. The relaxation response may be evoked by hypnosis, guided imagery, biofeedback, and prayer, all of which are discussed in detail elsewhere in this book.

Studies in Multiple Sclerosis and Other Conditions

Studies of meditation and multiple sclerosis (MS) are surprisingly limited. One study evaluated the effects of a meditation class on 22 people—10 had MS and 12 had a different condition known as peripheral neuropathy (1). The class was provided weekly for 2 months and those in the meditation group were compared to a control group who received standard medical care. Relative to the controls, the meditation group showed improvement in pain and overall quality of life—there was also improvement in fatigue. Another meditation study evaluated 40 people, nine of whom had MS, and found that meditation along with imagery decreased both anxiety and physical complaints during the physical rehabilitation process (2).

Other research studies have examined meditation effects on symptoms and conditions that may occur with MS but have involved people with conditions other than MS. In studies of variable quality, it has been found that meditation may improve stress, anxiety, depression, fatigue, various types of pain, and sleeping difficulties. Although difficult to study formally, feelings of control, empowerment, and self-esteem may develop through meditation.

Limited studies indicate that meditation may improve thinking problems such as memory and attention. Also, MRI studies have found that meditation is associated with thickening of the outer surface of the brain, known as the *cerebral cortex* or *grey matter*, which is important for cognitive function.

Interestingly, meditation and other relaxation methods may produce changes in immune function. Various immune-system changes have been described. However, the precise effects and their impact on MS are not fully understood at this time.

Meditation has been investigated in a number of other medical conditions. In terms of general health, meditation, especially TM, may reduce blood pressure. Also, limited studies indicate that meditation may improve blood sugar control, which could be helpful for people with diabetes.

Side Effects

Meditation does not usually involve any serious risks. Rarely, the state of relaxation elicited by meditation may produce fear of losing control, disturbing thoughts, and anxiety. Meditation may produce difficulties in people with serious psychiatric diseases, such as severe depression and schizophrenia. Meditation should not be used in place of conventional therapy to treat MS or serious MS-associated symptoms.

Practical Information

Meditation may be done independently by following techniques described in books such as *The Relaxation Response.* Classes in meditation techniques often are available through hospitals, health clubs, and community centers. Individual classes are typically 30 to 90 minutes in length and cost $60 to $150 per session. Group sessions are 60 minutes and cost $15 to $35. If meditation is pursued, it is important to keep in mind that it often does not have immediate effects. It may take several weeks or months of practice to achieve significant relaxation. More information about meditation may be obtained from:

- The American Meditation Society (www.americanmeditationsociety.org), 750 Dogwood Terrace, Boiling Springs, PA 17001 (717-240-0392)
- The World Wide Online Meditation Center (www.meditationcenter.com)

Conclusion

Meditation is a well-tolerated, low-cost therapy that may provide medical benefits without the use of medication. Limited studies indicate that meditation may be helpful for relieving stress, anxiety, depression, fatigue, insomnia, pain, and cognitive problems. It also may improve self-esteem and feelings of control. For general health, meditation may reduce blood pressure and improve blood glucose control.

Additional Readings

Books

Bauer B, ed. *Mayo Clinic Book of Alternative Medicine and Home Remedies.* New York, NY: Time Home Entertainment; 2013:104–107.

Benson H. *The Relaxation Response.* New York, NY: HarperTorch; 2000.

Jellin JM, Gregory PJ, Batz F, et al. *Pharmacist's Letter/ Prescriber's Letter Natural Medicines Comprehensive Database.* Stockton, CA: Therapeutic Research Faculty; 2014.

Kabat-Zinn J. *Wherever You Go, There You Are: Mindfulness Meditation in Everyday Life.* New York, NY: Hyperion; 2005.

Micozzi MS, ed. *Fundamentals of Complementary and Alternative Medicine.* Philadelphia, PA: Saunders Elsevier; 2011:117–120.

Rakel D. Recommending meditation. In: Rakel D, Faass N. *Complementary Medicine in Clinical Practice.* Boston, MA: Jones and Bartlett; 2006.

Synovitz LB, Larson KL. *Complementary and Alternative Medicine for Health Professionals: A Holistic Approach to Consumer Health.* Burlington, MA: Jones and Bartlett Learning; 2013:196–204.

Journal Articles

Brook RD, Appel, LF, Rubenfire M, et al. Beyond medications and diet: alternative approaches to lowering blood pressure: a scientific statement from the American Heart Association. *Hypertension.* 2013;61:1360–1383.

Chaipanont S. Hypoglycemic effect of sitting breathing meditation exercise on type 2 diabetes at Wat Khee Nok Primary Health Center in Nonthatburi province. *J Med Assoc Thai.* 2008;91:93–98.

Chen KW, Berger CC, Manheimer E, et al. Meditative therapies for reducing anxiety: a systematic review and meta-analysis of randomized controlled trials. *Depress Anx.* 2012;29:545–562.

Fan Y, Tang YY, Ma Y, Posner MI. Mucosal immunity modulated by integrative meditation in a dose-dependent fashion. *J Altern Complem Med.* 2010;16:151–155.

Fang CY, Reibel DK, Longacre ML, Rosenzweig S, Campbell DE, Douglas SD. Enhanced psychosocial well-being following participation in a mindfulness-based stress reduction program is associated with increased natural killer cell activity. *J Altern Complem Med.* 2010;16:531–538.

Hurley RV, Patterson TG, Cooley SJ. Meditation-based interventions for family caregivers of people with dementia: a review of the empirical literature. *Aging Ment Health.* 2013;18:281–288.

Kang DH, Jo HJ, Jung WH, et al. The effect of meditation on brain structure: cortical thickness mapping and diffusion tensor imaging. *Soc Cogn Affect Neurosci.* 2013;8:27–33.

Kim YH, Kim HJ, Ahn SD, Seo YJ, Kim SH. Effects of meditation on anxiety, depression, fatigue, and quality of life of women undergoing radiation therapy for breast cancer. *Complem Ther Med.* 2013;21:379–387.

Kwekkeboom KL, Dherwin CH, Lee JW, Wanta B. Mind-body treatments for the pain-fatigue-sleep disturbance symptom cluster in persons with cancer. *J Pain Symptom Man.* 2010;39:126–138.

Lavretsky H, Epel ES, Siddarth P, et al. A pilot study of yogic meditation for family dementia caregivers with depressive symptoms: effects on mental health, cognition, and telomerase activity. *Int J Geriatric Psych.* 2013;28:57–65.

Lazar SW, Kerr CE, Wasserman RH, et al. Meditation experience is associated with increased cortical thickness. *Neuroreport.* 2005;16:1893–1897.

Lazarus AA, Mayne TJ. Relaxation: some limitations, side effects, and proposed solutions. *Psychotherapy.* 1990;27:261–266.

Luders E, Thompson PM, Kurth F, et al. Global and regional alterations of hippocampal anatomy in long-term meditation practitioners. *Hum Brain Map.* 2013;34:3369–3375.

Mandel AR, Keller SM. Stress management in rehabilitation. *Arch Phys Med Rehabil.* 1986;67:375–379.

Marciniak R, Sheardova K, Cermakova P, Hude ek D, Sumec R, Hort J. Effect of meditation on cognitive functions in context of aging and neurodegenerative diseases. *Front Behav Neurosci.* 2014;8:17.

Newberg AB, Serruya M, Wintering N, Moss AS, Reibel D, Monti DA. Meditation and neurodegenerative diseases. *Ann N Y Acad Sci.* 2014;1307:112–123.

Paul-Labrador M, Polk D, Dwyer JH, et al. Effects of a randomized controlled trial of transcendental meditation on components of the metabolic syndrome in subjects with coronary heart disease. *Arch Intern Med.* 2006;166:1218–1224.

Reiner K, Tibi L, Lipsitz JD. Do mindfulness-based interventions reduce pain intensity? A critical review of the literature. *Pain Med.* 2013;14:230–242.

Smith GR, McKenzie JM, Marmer DJ, Steele RW. Psychologic modulation of the human immune response to *Varicella zoster. Arch Int Med.* 1985;145:2110–2112.

Tavee J, Rensel M, Planchon SM, Butler RS, Stone L. Effects of meditation on pain and quality of life in multiple sclerosis and peripheral neuropathy. *Int J MS Care.* 2011;13:163–168.

Wahbeh H, Elsas S-M, Oken BS. Mind-body interventions: applications in neurology. *Neurology.* 2008;70:2321–2328.

Zachariae R, Kristensen JS, Hokland P, Ellegaard J, Metze E, Hokland M. Effect of psychological intervention in the form of relaxation and guided imagery on cellular immune function in normal healthy subjects: an overview. *Psychother Psychosom.* 1990;54:32–39.

⊘ Mindfulness

Mindfulness is a mind–body therapy that has the potential to provide multiple health benefits to those with multiple sclerosis (MS) and many other medical conditions. Mindfulness may elicit deep states of relaxation and alleviate some physical symptoms. In addition, it may help people lead fuller and deeper lives.

Mindfulness is quite different from other relaxation approaches. In mindfulness, one actually focuses on day-to-day distractions that are minimized in guided imagery and many forms of meditation. Mindfulness, which is derived from Buddhist tradition, dates back about 2500 years. In the United States, Dr. Jon Kabat-Zinn began research on mindfulness in the 1980s and has applied it to a wide range of medical conditions.

Treatment Method

In mindfulness, attention is used to develop calmness and stability. When feelings or thoughts arise, they are not ignored or suppressed. Instead, they are observed nonjudgmentally in a moment-to-moment manner. This approach can lead to a different frame of reference and a deeper perspective on the stresses of life. A key element of mindfulness is the quality of awareness in each moment, not the topic or subject upon which one is focused. Mindfulness training aims to make people more aware in their lives and with what is occurring in the moment.

Studies in MS and Other Conditions

Limited studies have evaluated mindfulness in people with MS. The largest study, which included 150 people with MS, evaluated the effects of 8 weeks of mindfulness training. Those who received the training had improvement in anxiety as well as depression, fatigue, and overall quality of life (1). In a different type of study of mindfulness, which included 119 people with MS, training in mindfulness was not provided. Rather, people were administered tests to determine their degree of mindfulness, and the results of that test were correlated with other psychological measures (2). This study found that higher levels of mindfulness were associated with lower levels of stress, better coping skills, increased resilience, and higher quality of life. A smaller study that used multiple forms of mindfulness meditation in a group of people who had MS or another neurological condition known as *peripheral neuropathy* found that mindfulness improved pain and overall quality of life in those with MS (3). Another form of mindfulness known as *mindfulness of movement* is a component of tai chi and has produced beneficial effects in MS (see the *Tai Chi and Qigong* chapter).

Mindfulness has been extensively studied in other medical conditions and in the general population. These studies demonstrate that mindfulness is effective for stress and anxiety. Mindfulness also appears to be beneficial for depression and fatigue. More limited studies indicate that mindfulness-based approaches improve pain and sleeping difficulties.

Side Effects

Mindfulness is usually well tolerated. Relaxation approaches may rarely produce anxiety, fear of losing control, and disturbing thoughts. In people with psychiatric conditions, these approaches may produce difficulties and should be used with caution.

Practical Information

Information about mindfulness and a listing of mindfulness teachers may be found through the mindfulness center at the University of Massachusetts, which was started by Dr. Kabat-Zinn:

- The Center for Mindfulness (Univ. of Massachusetts): www.umassmed .edu/cfm/home/index.aspx

Dr. Kabat-Zinn has also written a classic book on the topic of mindfulness:

- *Wherever You Go There You Are* (New York: Hyperion, 2005).

Conclusion

Mindfulness is a low-risk approach that may alleviate multiple MS-related symptoms, including anxiety, depression, fatigue, pain, and sleeping difficulties.

Mindfulness has been extensively studied in several medical conditions, but studies in MS are extremely limited. Further MS studies in this area are needed.

Additional Readings

Books

Bauer B, ed. *Mayo Clinic Book of Alternative Medicine and Home Remedies.* New York, NY: Time Home Entertainment; 2013.

Kabat-Zinn J. *Wherever You Go There You Are.* New York, NY: Hyperion; 2005.

Micozzi MS, ed. *Fundamentals of Complementary and Alternative Medicine.* Philadelphia, PA: Saunders Elsevier; 2011.

Journal Articles

Garland EL, Howard MO. Mindfulness-oriented recovery enhancement reduces pain attentional bias in chronic pain patients. *Psychother Psychosom.* 2013;82: 311–318.

Gross CR, Kreitzer MJ, Reilly-Spong M, et al. Mindfulness-based stress reduction versus pharmacotherapy for chronic primary insomnia: a randomized controlled clinical trial. *Explore (NY).* 2011;7:76–87.

Grossman R, Kappos L, Gensicke H, et al. MS quality of life, depression, and fatigue improve after mindfulness training: a randomized trial. *Neurology.* 2010;75:1141–1149.

Johansson B, Bjuhr H, Ronback L. Mindfulness-based stress reduction (MBSR) improves long-term mental fatigue after stroke or traumatic brain injury. *Brain Inj.* 2012;26:1621–1628.

Lazarus AA, Mayne TJ. Relaxation: some limitations, side effects, and proposed solutions. *Psychotherapy.* 1990;27:261–266.

Pakenham KI, Samios C. Couples coping with multiple sclerosis: a dyadic perspective on the roles of mindfulness and acceptance. *J Behav Med.* 2013;36: 389–400.

Reiner K, Tibi L, Lipsitz JD. Do mindfulness-based interventions reduce pain intensity: A critical review of the literature. *Pain Med.* 2013;14:230–242.

Senders A, Bourdette D, Hanes D, Yadav V, Shinto L. Perceived stress in multiple sclerosis: the potential role of mindfulness in health and well-being. *J Evid Based Complement Altern Med.* 2014;19:104–111.

Simpson R, Booth J, Lawrence M, Byrne S, Mair F, Mercer S. Mindfulness based interventions in multiple sclerosis: a systematic review. *BMC Neurol.* 2014;14:15.

Tavee J, Rensel M, Planchon SM, Butler RS, Stone L. Effects of meditation on pain and quality of life in multiple sclerosis and peripheral neuropathy. *Int J MS Care*. 2011;13:163–168.

Van der Lee ML, Garssen B. Mindfulness-based cognitive therapy reduces chronic cancer-related fatigue: a treatment study. *Psychooncology*. 2012;21:264–272.

Winbush NY, Gross CR, Kreitzer MJ. The effects of mindfulness-based stress reduction on sleep disturbance: a systematic review. *Pain Med*. 2013;14:230–242.

⊘ Music Therapy

As its name implies, music therapy uses music to facilitate healing. This type of therapy has been practiced for thousands of years. It was used in some form in ancient Egypt and ancient Greece. Singing and drumming are also components of shamanic and Native American healing.

In the United States, music therapy degrees were first granted in the 1940s. The National Association for Music Therapy established music therapy as an official discipline in 1950. Conventional medicine has increasingly recognized music therapy. About 5,000 professional and student music therapists practice in the United States.

The exact mechanism by which music therapy may be therapeutic for MS and other neurological conditions is not known. Listening to music involves two major neurological processes—perception and emotional processing. Perception allows one to recognize the physical characteristics of music, such as tone, harmony, and rhythm. Emotional processing evokes a wide range of feeling states, including happiness, sadness, and relaxation. Perceiving and feeling music activates a remarkable number of interconnected brain regions. Dancing or creating music activates an even larger number of brain regions.

The widespread activation of the brain that occurs with music suggests that music may play a critical role in human existence. It has been proposed that music preceded language in human evolution, thus making it a core human characteristic. Music appears to be involved in sexual attraction, and, more generally, music may promote social bonding.

There are many theories about music's potential neurological and psychological effects. Because the brain pathways for music-associated emotional responses are different from those for verbal communication, music may be a novel way to stimulate emotions, facilitate emotional processing, and produce emotional change. Some of music's benefits may be related to music-induced relaxation. In addition, for people with movement difficulties such as incoordination or walking disorders, music therapy may elicit *entrainment*, which essentially means that moving to the music makes movements more rhythmic, regular, and efficient.

Treatment Method

Importantly, pursuing music therapy does not require musical talent. There are many people, including those who are tone-deaf, who are passionate about music and could potentially benefit from music therapy.

Music may be pursued on one's own or by working with a professional music therapist. In formal music therapy, the appropriate form of therapy for a specific person is determined by a trained music therapist. Music therapy may be practiced on an individual or group basis. *Rhythmic auditory stimulation* is a specific type of music therapy that uses the rhythm and timing of music to improve the intrinsic rhythmic movements of walking. Music is also sometimes used to facilitate imagery (see the *Guided Imagery* and *Hypnosis* chapters).

There are many ways that music may be pursued on one's own:

- Listening to Music

Many people listen to music casually. It may be helpful to be more attentive to music and more mindful about the types of music one chooses.

- Creating Music

There are many options for creating music, including joining a chorus or choir, playing an instrument, or simply making rhythmic sounds with an object, such as a drumstick, along with music.

- Moving to Music

Options in this category range from formal dancing lessons to just moving parts of the body in time with music.

Studies in Multiple Sclerosis and Other Conditions

Music therapy has undergone limited investigation in multiple sclerosis (MS). One study of 20 people with MS found that music therapy improved self-esteem, depression, and anxiety (1). Another study of 225 people with MS reported that group music therapy may provide psychological support, improve depression and anxiety, and assist in coping with the disease (2). In a small investigational study of people with advanced MS, music therapy improved respiratory muscle weakness (3). In one small MS study, rhythmic auditory stimulation, the method that uses the rhythm of music to improve walking, has been shown to improve walking in people with MS (4). One study of music therapy for 38 people with MS-associated cognitive difficulties did not find benefit for the whole group but did find possible benefit in those with less cognitive impairment (5).

In people with other conditions, music therapy has produced beneficial effects. Music therapy has been shown to decrease anxiety and depression in some studies. Limited clinical testing suggests that rhythmic auditory stimulation improves balance and walking in several neurological conditions, including Parkinson's disease, cerebral palsy, stroke, traumatic brain injury, and Huntington's disease. In studies of a wide range of medical conditions, music therapy has improved coordination, cognitive function, pain, and sleep. Studies of music therapy and fatigue have produced inconsistent results. In the area of general health, music therapy may mildly decrease blood pressure.

Side Effects

Music therapy is essentially risk-free, although excessive noise (greater than 90 decibels) may impair hearing and increase blood pressure.

Practical Information

More information about music therapy and qualified music therapists may be obtained from:

- The American Music Therapy Association (www.musictherapy.org), 8455 Colesville Road, Suite 1000, Silver Spring, MD 20910 (301-589-3300)

Conclusion

Music therapy is a safe and inexpensive approach that may be beneficial for some MS symptoms. Although no large definitive studies in people with MS have been undertaken, limited studies in MS and studies in other groups of people suggest that music therapy may be helpful for anxiety, depression, self-esteem, coping, cognitive problems, coordination, pain, sleep, and walking difficulties. Also, music therapy may mildly reduce blood pressure. Further research of music therapy in MS and other conditions is needed.

Additional Readings

Books

Bauer B, ed. *Mayo Clinic Book of Alternative Medicine and Home Remedies.* New York, NY: Time Home Entertainment; 2013:109.

Levitin DJ. *This Is Your Brain on Music.* New York, NY: Penguin Group; 2006.

Sacks O. *Musicophilia: Tales of Music and the Brain.* New York, NY: Alfred A. Knopf; 2007.

Spencer JW, Jacobs JJ. *Complementary and Alternative Medicine: An Evidence-Based Approach.* St. Louis, MO: Mosby; 2003.

Storr A. *Music and the Mind.* New York, NY: Ballantine Books; 1992.

Journal Articles

Bernatzky G, Bernatzky P, Hesse HP, Staffen W, Ladurner G. Stimulating music increases motor coordination in patients afflicted with Morbus Parkinson. *Neurosci Lett.* 2004;361:4–8.

Bernatzky G, Presch M, Anderson M, et al. Emotional foundations of music as a non-pharmacologic pain management tool in modern medicine. *Neurosci Biobehav Rev.* 2011;35:1989–1999.

Bowling AC. Music and the brain may be a therapeutic duet. *Momentum.* Fall 2009;2:43–45.

Bradt J, Dileo C, Grocke D, et al. Music interventions for improving psychological and physical outcomes in cancer patients. *Cochrane Database Syst Rev.* 2011;8:CD006911.

Chanda ML, Levitin DJ. The neurochemistry of music. *Trends Cogn Sci.* 2013;17:179–193.

Conklyn D, Stough D, Novak E, Paczak S, Chemali K, Bethoux F. A home-based walking program using rhythmic auditory stimulation improves gait performance in patients with multiple sclerosis: a pilot study. *Neurorehabil Neural Rep.* 2010;24:835–842.

deDreu MJ, van der Wilk AS, Poppe E, Paczak S, Chemali K, Bethoux F. Rehabilitation, exercise therapy and music in patients with Parkinson's disease: a meta-analysis of the effects of music-based movement therapy on walking ability, balance and quality of life. *Parkinson Relat Disord. Suppl.* 2012;18:S114–S119.

de Niet G, Tiemens B, Lendemeijer B, et al. Music-assisted relaxation to improve sleep quality: meta-analysis. *J Adv Nurs.* 2009;65:1356–1364.

Hars M, Herrmann FR, Gold G, Rizzoli R, Trombetti A. Effect of music-based multitask training on cognition and mood in older adults. *Age Ageing.* 2014;43: 196–200.

Kim SJ, Kwak EE, Park ES, et al. Changes in gait patterns with rhythmic auditory stimulation in adults with cerebral palsy. *NeuroRehabilitation*. 2011;29:233–241.

Kim SJ, Kwak EE, Park ES, Cho SR. Differential effects of rhythmic auditory stimulation and neurodevelopmental treatment/Bobath on gait patterns in adults with cerebral palsy: a randomized controlled trial. *Clin Rehabil*. 2012;26:904–914.

Kozasa EH, Hachul H, Monson C, et al. Mind-body interventions for the treatment of insomnia: a review. *Rev Bras Psiquiatr*. 2010;32:437–443.

Kwekkeboom KL, Cherwin CH, Lee JW, et al. Mind-body treatments for the pain-fatigue-sleep disturbance symptom cluster in persons with cancer. *J Pain Symptom Man*. 2010;39:126–138.

Lengdobler H, Kiessling WR. Group music therapy in multiple sclerosis: initial report of experience. *Psychother Psychosom Med Psychol*. 1989;39:369–373 [in German].

Lim HA, Miller K, Fabian C. The effects of therapeutic instrumental music performance on endurance, self-perceived fatigue level, and self-perceived exertion of inpatients in physical rehabilitation. *J Music Ther*. 2011;48:124–148.

Marwick C. Music therapists chime in with data on medical results. *JAMA*. 2000;283:731-733.

Moore KS, Peterson DA, O'Shea G, et al. The effectiveness of music as a mnemonic device on recognition memory for people with multiple sclerosis. *J Music Ther*. 2008;XLV:307–329.

Moreira SV, Franca DD, Moreira MA, et al. Musical identity of patients with multiple sclerosis. *Arq Neuropsiquiatr*. 2009;67:46–49.

Ostermann T, Schmid W. Music therapy in the treatment of multiple sclerosis: a comprehensive literature review. *Expert Rev Neurother*. 2006;6:469–477.

Sarkamo T, Soto D. Music listening after stroke: beneficial effects and potential neural mechanisms. *Ann N Y Acad Sci*. 2012;1252:266–281.

Schmid W, Aldridge D. Active music therapy in the treatment of multiple sclerosis patients: a matched control study. *J Music Ther*. 2004;61:225–240.

Suh JH, Han SJ, Jeon SY, et al. Effect of rhythmic auditory stimulation on gait and balance in hemiplegic stroke patients. *NeuroRehabilitation*. 2014;34:193–199.

Wiens ME, Reimer MA, Guyn HL. Music therapy as a treatment method for improving respiratory muscle strength in patients with advanced multiple sclerosis: a pilot study. *Rehabil Nurs*. 1999;24:74–80.

Wittwer Je, Webster KE, Hill K. Rhythmic auditory cueing to improve walking in patients with neurological conditions other than Parkinson's disease—what is the evidence? *Disabil Rehabil*. 2013;35:164–176.

Zhang JM, Wang P, Yao JX, et al. Music interventions for psychological and physical outcomes in cancer: a systematic review and meta-analysis. *Support Care Cancer*. 2012;20:3043–3053.

⊛ Obesity and Weight Management

Obesity is a common and serious condition. It may increase the risk for many diseases, including multiple sclerosis (MS). Also, in those with MS, obesity may impair neurological function and overall quality of life. Unlike many other medical conditions, obesity is preventable or treatable with lifestyle modifications.

Obesity is common. In the United States, about one-third of adults are obese. In addition, many American children and adolescents are obese and the rate of obesity in these younger age groups is rising.

Obesity increases the risk for a wide range of medical conditions, some of which may ultimately be life-threatening. For example, the risk of diabetes is increased 10 to 20 times in those who are obese. Other conditions whose risk is increased with obesity include heart disease, stroke, high blood pressure, high blood cholesterol, and some forms of cancer.

Several approaches may be used to determine if one is obese. One of these is the *body mass index (BMI)*. The BMI is used as an approximate guideline since age, gender, ethnicity, and body type may impact how BMI actually relates to body fat. To calculate the BMI, weight (W), in pounds, and height (H), in inches, are used:

$$BMI = W/H^2 \times 705$$

The reference ranges for BMIs are as follows:

- Underweight: less than 18.5
- Normal: 18.5 to 24.9

- Overweight: 25.0 to 29.9
- Obese: greater than 30.0

Treatment Method

There are many approaches to weight management, some of which are dangerous and expensive. The safest and most effective strategy for losing weight is to consume a healthy diet, exercise, and change unhealthy lifestyle habits. This strategy must be ongoing and lifelong. Basic aspects of this strategy are as follows:

- Healthy Diet: If calories are consumed but not used, they are stored as fat. Thus, taking in fewer calories is a critical aspect of effective weight management. The appropriate number of calories that should be taken in on a daily basis depends on several factors, including age and activity level. Calorie goals that are needed for weight loss may be obtained from primary care doctors, dietitians, or reputable weight-loss programs.

- Exercise: Exercise is essential for using up the calories that are consumed. Aerobic activities may be used to decrease body fat, while resistance training may increase lean muscle tissue. Moderate amounts of exercise may be challenging for many people with MS due to a variety of factors, including disability, fatigue, and heat-induced worsening of symptoms. Physical therapists and physiatrists (rehabilitation physicians) are best-suited for developing appropriate and doable exercise programs for those with MS.

- Changing Unhealthy Behavior: Unhealthy approaches to eating and physical activity may be deeply entrenched. Identifying and changing these approaches is required for a weight management program to be successful over the long term. This aspect of weight management may be done on one's own or through consultation with health professionals, including primary care physicians, dietitians, and weight-loss specialists.

More aggressive weight-loss methods are sometimes needed. Medications that may be used include sibutramine (Meridia) and orlistat (Xenical). Also, weight-loss surgery may be very effective in appropriate situations.

Many dietary supplements are claimed to be effective for weight loss. However, most of these have not been adequately tested for effectiveness. In addition, some have serious and potentially fatal side effects, including ephedra, bitter orange, and country mallow.

Studies in MS and Other Conditions

Studies of obesity specifically in those with MS are limited. One study found that 50–55% of people with MS were overweight or obese (1). With regard to obesity and the immune system, it is known that obesity produces a chronic, low grade level of inflammation that could increase the risk for immune conditions such as MS. Indeed, obesity before age 20 has been associated with increased risk for MS. Also, obesity and other common features of the "Western lifestyle," such as diets that are high in fat and salt, are increasingly recognized as risk factors for a wide range of autoimmune conditions, including psoriasis, diabetes, inflammatory bowel disease, and rheumatoid arthritis.

There are multiple ways in which obesity could adversely affect those with MS. First, obesity increases the risk for other medical conditions, such as diabetes, heart disease, high blood pressure, high cholesterol, and arthritis. In people with MS, the presence of some of these other "nonneurological" conditions may actually decrease neurological function and lower overall quality of life. Also, obesity is known to provoke some symptoms that are common in MS, including fatigue, sleeping problems (sleep apnea), urinary difficulties, and depression. As a result, obesity in people with MS may increase the risk or severity of these symptoms. Finally, the risk of vitamin D deficiency, which may adversely affect MS, is higher in those who are obese.

Practical Information

Additional information about obesity and weight management may be obtained from several websites:

- Academy of Nutrition and Dietetics: www.eatright.org/Public/content .aspx?id=6843
- International Food Information Council Foundation: www.foodinsight .org/Resources/Weight-Management
- Steps to a Healthier Weight, U.S. Dept. of Agriculture: www.Choose MyPlate.gov
- My Food-a-Pedia, U.S. Dept. of Agriculture: www.myfoodapedia.gov
- Weight-Control Information Network: www.niddk.nih.gov/index.htm

Conclusion

Obesity in childhood and adolescence is associated with an increased risk of developing MS. In those who have MS, obesity may provoke MS symptoms and increase the risk for other diseases, such as diabetes, heart disease, and arthritis, which may worsen neurological function and overall quality of life. Likewise, weight management may be a valuable and underutilized "nondrug" approach to prevent or manage symptoms and also to optimize neurological function and quality of life in those with MS.

Additional Readings

Books

Bauer B, ed. *Mayo Clinic Book of Alternative Medicine and Home Remedies.* New York, NY: Time Home Entertainment; 2013:186–187.

Duyff RL. *American Dietetic Association Complete Food and Nutrition Guide.* Boston, MA: Houghton Mifflin Harcourt; 2012:21–52.

Jellin JM, Batz F, Hitchens K. *Natural Medicines Comprehensive Database.* Stockton, CA: Therapeutic Research Faculty; 2014.

Rinzler CA. *Nutrition for Dummies.* Hoboken, NJ: Wiley; 2011:39–52.

Journal Articles

Burgio KL, Newman DK, Rosenberg MT, Sampselle C. Impact of behavior and lifestyle on bladder health. *Int J Clin Pract.* 2013;67:494–504.

Hedstrom AK, Bomfim IL, Barcellos L, et al. Interaction between adolescent obesity and HLA risk genes in the etiology of multiple sclerosis. *Neurology.* 2014;82:865–872.

Hedstrom AK, Olsson T, Alfredsson L. High body mass index before age 20 is associated with increased risk for multiple sclerosis in both men and women. *Mult Scler.* 2012;18:1334–1336.

Langer-Gould A, Brara SM, Beaber BE, Koebnick C. Childhood obesity and risk of pediatric multiple sclerosis and clinically isolated syndrome. *Neurology.* 2013;80:548–552.

Manzel A, Muller DN, Hafler DA, Erdman SE, Linker RA, Kleinewietfeld M. Role of "Western diet" in inflammatory autoimmune diseases. *Curr Allergy Asthma Rep.* 2014;14:404.

Marrie RA, Beck CA. Obesity and HLA in multiple sclerosis: weighty matters. *Neurology.* 2014;82:826–827.

Munger K, Chitnis T, Ascherio A. Body size and risk of MS in two cohorts of US women. *Neurology.* 2009;73:1543–1550.

Pilutti LA, Dlugonski D, Pula JH, Motl RW. Weight status in persons with multiple sclerosis: implications for mobility outcomes. *J Obes.* 2012;868256.

Ponsonby AL, Lucas RM, Dear K, et al. The physical anthropometry, lifestyle habits and blood pressure of people presenting with a first clinical demyelinating event compared to controls: the Ausimmune study. *Mult Scler.* 2013;19:1717–1725.

Salem R, Bamer AM, Alschuler KN, et al. Obesity and symptoms and quality of life indicators of individuals with disabilities. *Disabil Health J.* 2014;7:124–130.

⑦ Paleolithic Diets

For the past few decades, Paleolithic diets, also known as the *Hunter-Gatherer Diets* or *Caveman Diets*, have been proposed for the prevention and management of multiple sclerosis (MS) as well as many other diseases. A major article that raised mainstream medical interest in the Paleolithic diet was published in 1985 in the prestigious *New England Journal of Medicine* by Drs. Melvin Konner and S. Boyd Eaton.

Paleolithic diets are controversial. Proponents of these diets, which are based on the presumed diet of Paleolithic humans, state that the current Western diet is the cause for many "diseases of civilization," such as heart disease, high blood pressure, obesity, and diabetes. It is claimed that a return to "caveman" diets may prevent and treat these diseases. Paleolithic diet advocates point out that some medical conditions, such as high blood pressure and diabetes, are less common in modern foraging humans who live in more "primitive" ways and do not eat typical Western diets. Also, proponents claim that dietary changes in Western nations have been too rapid for human evolution. Thus, it is thought that Western diseases are caused by an unhealthy mismatch between modern diets and Paleolithic genetics.

Critics challenge many of the underlying assumptions and beliefs regarding Paleolithic diets. They claim that it is difficult to determine what constitutes a Paleolithic diet because "Paleolithic" refers to very different human ancestors (such as *Australopithecus* and *Homo erectus*) who lived in very diverse geographic areas (such as coastal and inland areas on different continents) and had different forms of hunting, foraging, and agriculture. Due to all of these variables, critics state that the diets of Paleolithic people were very diverse and cannot be condensed into a single dietary approach. Also, critics note that, in spite of extensive anthropological studies, the food intake of different Paleolithic humans has not been established and some of the foods that were known to be consumed thousands of years ago are not currently available. Critics also believe that evolution of the human body has occurred since Paleolithic times and that, even over the course of a single lifetime, the human body has the ability to adapt to dietary changes.

Treatment Method

Paleolithic diets generally encourage the intake of fish, grass-fed meats, eggs, fruits, vegetables, nuts, seeds, and "healthy" oils (such as olive, walnut, and flaxseed). Foods that are excluded or minimized include grains, beans, dairy products, potatoes, processed oils, salt, and refined vegetable oils. There are many variants of this dietary approach. One variant, the "Wahls Diet," has been proposed by Dr. Terry Wahls, a physician who has MS. The "Wahls Protocol" is a broad-based strategy that uses the Wahls Diet along with other therapies, which may include 10 to 30 different dietary supplements, toxin elimination, exercise, electrical stimulation of muscles, and stress management (1,2).

Studies in MS and Other Conditions

Since the publication of the article on Paleolithic nutrition in the *New England Journal of Medicine* in 1985, many studies of this dietary approach have been conducted.

In the area of MS, there has been minimal research on the Paleolithic diet. There are no studies that have specifically evaluated the effects of this diet on MS. One small preliminary study of the Wahls Protocol, which included Paleolithic dietary changes as well as other therapies, found improvement in fatigue (3). Dr. Wahls' personal, beneficial experience with protocol has been described (4). Based on current research, it is not possible to make any conclusions about the effectiveness of the Paleolithic diet in MS.

The Paleolithic diet has been much more extensively studied in common "Western" diseases, such as heart disease and diabetes. Some of these studies have produced encouraging results. However, there are still uncertainties about the effectiveness of the Paleolithic diet, especially relative to other "healthful" diets that utilize current nutrition guidelines to decrease the intake of unhealthy foods and increase the intake of healthy foods. Drs. Konner and Boyd, the authors of the Paleolithic diet publication in 1985, recently wrote a follow-up article and stated that, in spite of some positive research results related to the diet, "much more research needs to be done" and that "the ultimate validity" of the Paleolithic approach has not been proven (5).

Side Effects

The Paleolithic diet is generally well tolerated. However, it is difficult for some people to adhere to the diet. Also, there is concern that people who follow Paleolithic diets may not obtain the health benefits of grains, dairy products, and other dietary approaches that have more definitive evidence of beneficial health effects.

In 2014, *U.S. News and World Report* commissioned a 22-member panel of nationally recognized nutrition experts to independently score 32 diets, including the Paleolithic diet, on the basis of seven different criteria, including nutritional completeness, ease of use, ability to produce short- and long-term weight loss, and safety and effectiveness in managing and preventing heart disease and diabetes. In this review, the Paleolithic diet tied for "last place" in overall score and was among the three lowest ranked diets in all of the seven criteria.

Conclusion

The Paleolithic diet is generally safe. However, its effectiveness in MS, as well as other medical conditions, has not been established. Further studies of the potential benefits of this diet, especially relative to other "healthful diets," are needed.

Additional Readings

Books

Wahls T. *The Wahls Protocol*. New York, NY: Penguin Group; 2014.

Zuk M. *Paleofantasy: What Evolution Really Tells Us About Sex, Diet, and How We Live*. New York, NY: WW Norton & Co; 2014.

Journal Articles

Anon. Best diets 2014. *U.S. News and World Report*; 2014. http://health.usnews.com/best-diet

Bisht B, Darling WG, Grossmann RE, et al. A multimodal intervention for patients with secondary progressive multiple sclerosis: feasibility and effect on fatigue. *J Altern Complement Med*. 2014;20:347–355.

Jonsson T, Granfeldt Y, Ahren B, et al. Beneficial effects of a Paleolithic diet on cardiovascular risk factors in type 2 diabetes: a randomized cross-over pilot study. *Cardiovasc Diabetol*. 2009;8:35.

Jonsson T, Granfeldt Y, Lindeberg S, et al. Subjective satiety and other experiences of a Paleolithic diet compared to a diabetes diet in patients with type 2 diabetes. *Nutr J*. 2013;12:105.

Konner M, Eaton SB. Paleolithic nutrition: twenty-five years later. *Nutr Clin Pract.* 2010;25:594–601.

Lindeberg S. Paleolithic diets as a model for prevention and treatment of Western disease. *Am J Human Biol.* 2012;24:110–115.

O'Keefe JH, Cordain L. Cardiovascular disease resulting from a diet and life-style at odds with our Paleolithic genome: how to become a 21st-century hunter-gatherer. *Mayo Clin Proc.* 2004;79:101–108.

Osterdayl M, Kocturk T, Koochek A, et al. Effects of a short-term intervention with a Paleolithic diet in healthy volunteers. *Eur J Clin Nutr.* 2008;62:682–685.

Schardt D. Pondering paleo: channeling your inner caveperson. *Nutr Action Healthletter.* 2013;40:9–11.

Turner BL, Thompson AL. Beyond the Paleolithic prescription: incorporating diversity and flexibility in the study of human diet evolution. *Nutr Rev.* 2013;71:501–510.

✓ Pets

Pets are a part of everyday life for many people, but they may provide special benefits for people with medical conditions. The concept that pets may be therapeutic is not new. In the 19th century, the nurse Florence Nightingale, who loved pets and had exotic pets of her own, wrote: "A small pet animal is often an excellent companion for the sick ... " (1).

Recently, pets have been used increasingly in medical settings, and studies indicate that they may provide health benefits. The potential therapeutic effects of pets relate to the more general concepts of *biophilia* and *ecotherapy*. Biophilia is a term that was proposed by Dr. Edward O. Wilson to explain a connection that humans subconsciously need and seek out with other forms of life. According to this concept, human health depends on one's relations with the natural environment. Ecotherapy aims to provide connection, balance, guidance, and healing to people by deepening their relationships with the natural environment. The term *Vitamin G* has been coined to refer to the potential therapeutic effects of natural or *green* settings.

There are many ways in which people may interact with animals for possible medical benefits:

- *Pet Ownership* Most simply, one may own a pet by purchasing, adopting, or rescuing an animal.
- *Service Animals* Trained pets may be helpful to those with physical disabilities. Dogs are the most commonly used service animals—in rare cases, monkeys and miniature horses are used for this purpose. Service animals

may assist by performing physical tasks, such as retrieving items, or by stabilizing people who have walking difficulties.

■ *Animal-Assisted Therapy* Animals are sometimes used to assist people with physical rehabilitation, which may involve physical, occupational, or speech therapy.

Emotionally, it has been claimed that pets provide "unconditional love"—they are accepting and noncritical companions. Pet ownership has been associated with relaxation. Pets also may improve self-esteem and increase independence, responsibility, and companionship. Pets sometimes are brought into the hospital to provide possible psychological benefits for children.

Studies in Multiple Sclerosis and Other Conditions

There are many clinical studies of the potential therapeutic effects of pet ownership. Unfortunately, studies that are relevant to those with multiple sclerosis (MS) are limited. No large, well-designed studies have been conducted in people with MS. In other conditions, some studies indicate that pets may alleviate symptoms that occur with MS, including anxiety, depression, and pain. Also, pets may produce a sense of community and enhance socializing. However, the studies in these various areas are generally of low quality and have not produced consistent results.

In the area of heart disease, there are many studies of pet ownership. Some of these studies have associated pet ownership with improved survival after heart attacks and also improvement in risk factors for heart disease, such as higher levels of physical activity, lower blood pressure, and improved levels of cholesterol and other *lipids*. The most consistent finding in these studies has been increased physical activity in those who own pets, especially dogs. In 2013, the American Heart Association published a formal review of pet ownership and concluded that pet ownership, particularly dog ownership, is "probably associated" with decreased risk of heart disease (2).

Side Effects

Pets generally are well tolerated. However, some considerations should be kept in mind. Obviously, people with allergies should avoid pets that provoke allergies, and people who feel uncomfortable or stressed around pets probably would not benefit from their presence. Adequate care and an appropriate amount of space should be provided. Finally, pets should not substitute for the basic emotional needs that should be obtained from humans. They may be used for a certain level of companionship, but this should not lead to social isolation.

Practical Information

More information on service animals can be obtained from:

- Canine Companions for Independence (www.cci.org.), PO Box 446, Santa Rosa, CA 95402 (866-224-3647)

- Pet Partners (www.petpartners.org), 875 124th Avenue Northeast, Ste. 101, Bellevue, WA 98055 (425-679-5530)

- Service Dogs for Independence (www.servicedogsforindependence.com), 520-909-0531

Conclusion

Caring for a pet is a low-risk, low- to moderate-cost activity that may provide some medical benefits. However, many of the clinical studies of pet ownership are of limited quality and have produced variable results. In the general population, pet ownership may be associated with higher levels of physical activity and reduced risks of heart disease. Trained pets may be helpful to those with weakness, incoordination, or walking difficulties.

Additional Readings

Books

Selhub EM, Logan AC. *Your Brain on Nature*. Mississauga, Ontario, Canada: John Wiley & Sons Canada; 2012:127–149.

Journal Articles

Allen K, Shykoff BE, Izzo JL. Pet ownership, but on ACE inhibitor therapy, blunts home blood pressure responses to mental stress. *Hypertension*. 2001;38:815–820.

Barak Y, Savorai O, Mavashev S, Beni A. Animal-assisted therapy for elderly schizophrenic patients: a one-year controlled trial. *Am J Ger Psychiatr*. 2001;9: 439–442.

Christian HE, Westgarth C, Bauman A, et al. Dog ownership and physical activity: a review of the evidence. *J Phys Activ Health*. 2013;10:750–759.

Cline KM. Psychological effects of dog ownership: role strain, role enhancement, and depression. *J Soc Psychol*. 2010;150:117–131.

Dossey L. The healing power of pets: a look at animal-assisted therapy. *Altern Ther Health Med*. 1997;3:8–16.

Friedmann E, Thomas SA, Son H. Pets, depression and long term survival in community living patients following myocardial infarction. *Anthrozoos*. 2011;24: 273–285.

Giaquinto S, Valentini F. Is there a scientific basis for pet therapy? *Disabil Rehabil*. 2009;31:595–598.

Gillum RG, Obisesan TO. Living with companion animals, physical activity and mortality in a US national cohort. *Int J Environ Res Public Health*. 2010;7: 2452–2459.

Gretebeck KA, Radius K, Black DR, et al. Dog ownership, functional ability, and walking in community-dwelling older adults. *J Phys Activ Health*. 2013;10: 646–655.

Hall PL, Malpus Z. Pets as therapy: effects on social interaction in long-stay psychiatry. *Br J Nurs*. 2000;9:2220–2225.

Levine GN, Allen K, Braun LT, et al. Pet ownership and cardiovascular risk: a scientific statement from the American Heart Association. *Circulation*. 2013;127:2353–2363.

Marcus DA, Bernstein CD, Constantin JM, et al. Impact of animal-assisted therapy for outpatients with fibromyalgia. *Pain Med*. 2013;14:43–51.

Mayon-White R. Pets—pleasures and problems. *Br Med J*. 2005;331:1254–1255.

McNicholas J, Gilbey A, Rennie A, et al. Pet ownership and human health: a brief review of evidence and issues. *Br Med J*. 2005;331:1252–1254.

Palley LS, O'Rourke PP, Niemi SM. Mainstreaming animal-assisted therapy. *Inst Lab Animal Res J*. 2010;51:199–207.

Qureshi AI, Memon MZ, Vazquez G, et al. Cat ownership and the risk of fatal cardiovascular diseases. Results from the second National Health and Nutrition Examination Study mortality follow-up study. *J Vasc Interv Neurol*. 2009;2: 132–135.

Ruzic A, Miletic B, Ruzic T, Persić V, Laskarin G . Regular dog-walking improves physical capacity in elderly patients after myocardial infarction. *Coll Antropol. Suppl*. 2011;35:73–75.

Terra VC, Sakamoto AC, Machado HR, et al. Do pets reduce the likelihood of sudden unexplained death in epilepsy? *Seizure*. 2012;21:649–651.

Toohey AM, McCormack GR, Doyle-Baker PK, et al. Dog-walking and sense of community in neighborhoods: implications for promoting regular physical activity in adults 50 years and older. *Health Place*. 2013;22:75–81.

Wells DL. Associations between pet ownership and self-reported health status in people suffering from chronic fatigue syndrome. *J Altern Complement Med*. 2009;15:407–413.

Yabroff KR, Troiano RP, Berrigan D. Walking the dog: is pet ownership associated with physical activity in California? *J Phys Activ Health*. 2008;5:216–228.

⊘ The Pilates Method and PhysicalMind Method

The Pilates method and a variant of Pilates, the PhysicalMind method, are two types of bodywork that are intended to increase flexibility and strength. The Pilates method was created during World War I by Joseph H. Pilates, a German inventor, boxer, and dancer. He developed the technique to help soldiers recover from war injuries. In the United States, Pilates has been practiced since the 1920s. Its popularity has grown significantly during the past decade in the United States. In parallel with this increased use of Pilates, there has been a dramatic rise in Pilates-related research and medical publications over the past several years.

In several ways, Pilates is significantly different from many conventional exercise programs. In Pilates, individuals concentrate on specific body movements. This approach, unlike many conventional exercise programs, focuses much more on the quality, rather than the quantity, of movement. With Pilates, which includes more than 500 specific movements, attention is focused on which muscles are used and how they are controlled. Also in contrast to many conventional exercise programs, Pilates is designed specifically to strengthen the body's core muscles by developing abdominal control and pelvic stability. With Pilates, an emphasis also is placed on posture and on deep, coordinated breathing.

The unique aspects of Pilates, especially the focus on the quality of movement and the core muscles, may provide a unique form of exercise and *physical education*, especially for those who do not have a strong sense of the physicality of their bodies generally or their abdominal muscles specifically. Other unconventional therapies that focus on awareness of movement include Feldenkrais, tai chi, yoga, and Tragerwork.

The PhysicalMind method was developed in response to a lawsuit regarding the Pilates name. In this spin-off of the original technique, more focus is placed on the position of the body.

Both Pilates and the PhysicalMind method may use specialized exercise equipment. The earliest equipment developed for Pilates was the *Reformer*, a wooden device with cables, pulleys, springs, and sliding boards. This device allows individuals to perform specific range-of-motion exercises with the muscles of the abdomen, upper legs, back, and buttocks. Current Pilates programs use similar equipment or may simply use floor-based exercises.

Pilates and the PhysicalMind method are claimed to have several beneficial effects. They are supposed to improve strength and flexibility without increasing the size of muscles. Consequently, these methods are particularly popular among dancers.

Studies in Multiple Sclerosis and Other Conditions

Pilates research is burgeoning. At this time, there are actually several limited multiple sclerosis (MS) studies of Pilates. One of these studies, which was conducted in Turkey, evaluated the effects of Pilates in 26 people with MS. Relative to people who did not receive treatment, those who were treated with Pilates had improvement in balance, arm and leg strength, and overall mobility (1). Another study of 57 people with MS found that Pilates produced improvement in the *Timed Up and Go Test,* an established assessment of balance and functional ability that measures how quickly one can rise from a chair, walk 10 feet, turn around, walk back to the chair, and sit back down in the chair (2). A Pilates study specifically of people with MS who require the use of a wheelchair reported improvement in sitting posture, shoulder and back pain, and confidence in day-to-day activities (3). A large study of Pilates is currently being conducted at several MS centers in the United Kingdom—this study is primarily evaluating the effects of Pilates on walking and balance (4).

In limited studies of other conditions, Pilates has produced several other possible therapeutic effects. Pilates may improve low back and neck pain. In the elderly, multiple studies indicate that Pilates may increase muscle strength, improve walking ability, and decrease the risk of falling. Limited studies indicate improvement in sleep and overall quality of life with Pilates. The stretching movements of Pilates have the potential to improve muscle stiffness (spasticity), but this has not been researched. Finally, Pilates may be helpful for weight loss.

There are claims that Pilates improves sexual function and heightens sexual experience in women as well as men. However, there are not any formal studies in this area in MS or in the general population. There are similar claims about sex and yoga (see *Yoga* chapter). It is plausible that Pilates and yoga improve awareness, coordination, and strength of the pelvis in a way that leads to improved sexual function and heightened sexual experience. Research is needed in this area.

Side Effects

It is generally assumed that the Pilates and the PhysicalMind method are well tolerated.

Practical Information

Pilates and the PhysicalMind method are taught either individually or in small groups. The techniques should be learned from a trained and certified instructor. These methods may be adapted for those with disabilities. The exercises may be done individually after receiving training. Adequate training usually requires a total of 20 to 30 sessions—each session generally costs $30 to $70. More information may be obtained from:

- United States Pilates Association (www.unitedstatesPilatesassociation.com), 1500 E. Broward Blvd., Ste. 250, Ft. Lauderdale, FL 33301 (888-484-8772)

- Balanced Body (www.Pilates.com), 8220 Ferguson Ave., Sacramento, CA 95828 (800-745-2837)

Conclusion

Pilates is a low-risk, moderate-cost form of bodywork. Limited studies indicate that it may improve low back and neck pain, sleep, walking, weakness, posture, and overall quality of life. Pilates may also promote weight loss. There are not any studies of Pilates and sexual function. Pilates may be a very effective method to increase awareness and education about appropriate body movements and abdominal and pelvic muscles, especially for those who do not have a strong sense of the physicality of their bodies. Additional studies of Pilates are needed and are currently being conducted in those with MS and a wide range of other medical conditions.

Additional Readings

Books

Bauer B, ed. *Mayo Clinic Book of Alternative Medicine and Home Remedies.* New York, NY: Time Home Entertainment; 2013:110.

Journal Articles

Bird ML, Fell J. Pilates exercise has positive long term effects on the aged-related decline in balance and strength in older, community dwelling men and women. *J Aging Phys Act.* 2014;22(3):342–347.

Borges J, Baptista AF, Santana N, et al. Pilates exercises improve low back pain and quality of life in patients with HTLV-1 virus: a randomized crossover clinical trial. *J Bodywork Mov Ther.* 2014;18:68–74.

Cakmakci O. The effect of 8 week Pilates exercise on body composition in obese women. *Coll Anthropol.* 2011;35:1045–1050.

Freeman J, Fox E, Gear M, Hough A. Pilates based core stability training in ambulant individuals with multiple sclerosis: protocol for a multi-centre randomized controlled trial. *BCM Neurol.* 2012;12:19.

Granacher U, Golhofer A, Hortobagyi T, Kressig RW, Muehlbauer T. The importance of trunk muscle strength for balance, functional performance, and fall prevention in seniors: a systematic review. *Sports Med.* 2013;43:627–641.

Guclu-Gunduz A, Citaker S, Irkec C, Nazliel B, Batur-Caglayan HZ. The effects of Pilates on balance, mobility, and strength in patients with multiple sclerosis. *NeuroRehabilitation.* 2013;33:293–298.

Irez GB, Ozdemir RA, Evin R, Irez SG, Korkusuz F. Integrating Pilates exercise into an exercise program for 65+ year-old women to reduce falls. *J Sports Sci Med.* 2011;10:105–111.

Leopoldino AA, Avelar NC, Passos GB, et al. Effect of Pilates on sleep quality and quality of life of sedentary population. *J Bodywork Mov Ther.* 2013;17:5–10.

Mallin G, Murphy S. The effectiveness of a 6-week Pilates programme on outcome measures in a population of chronic neck pain patients: a pilot study. *J Bodywork Mov Ther.* 2013;17:376–384.

Marandi SM, Nejad VS, Shanazari S, Zolaktaf V A comparison of 12 weeks of Pilates and aquatic training on the dynamic balance of women with multiple sclerosis. *Int J Prev Med. Suppl.* 2013;4:S110–S117.

Medonca TM, Terreri MT, Silva CH, et al. Effects of Pilates exercises on health-related quality of life in individuals with juvenile idiopathic arthritis. *Arch Phys Med Rehabil.* 2013;94:2093–2102.

Miyamoto GC, Costa LO, Cabral CM. Efficacy of the Pilates method for pain and disability in patients with chronic low back pain: a systematic review with meta-analysis. *Braz J Phys Ther.* 2013;17:517–532.

Newell D, Shead V, Sloane L. Changes in gait and balance parameters in elderly subjects attending an 8-week supervised Pilates programme. *J Bodywork Mov Ther.* 2012;16:549–554.

Notamicola A, Fischetti F, Maccagnanao G, Comes R, Tafuri S, Moretti B. Daily Pilates exercise or inactivity for patient with low back pain: a clinical prospective observational study. *Eur J Phys Rehabil Med.* 2014;50:59–66.

Ruiz-Montero PJ, Castillo-Rodriguez A, Micalacki M, Nebojsa C, Korovljev D. 24-weeks Pilates-aerobic and educative training to improve body fat mass in elderly Serbian women. *Clin Interv Aging.* 2013;9:243–248.

Segal NA, Hein J, Basford JR. The effects of Pilates training on flexibility and body com position: an observational study. *Arch Phys Med Rehabil.* 2004;85:1977–1981.

van der Linden M, Bulley C, Geneen LJ, Hooper JE, Cowan P, Mercer TH. Pilates for people with multiple sclerosis who use a wheelchair: feasibility, efficacy, and participant experiences. *Disabil Rehabil.* 2014;36:932–939.

Vieira FT, Faria LM, Wittmann JI, Teixeira W, Nogueira LA. The influence of Pilates method in quality of life of practitioners. *J Bodywork Mov Ther.* 2013;17:483–487.

✅ Prayer and Spirituality

Religion has been a fundamental aspect of human culture for tens of thousands of years. The term *religion* generally refers to beliefs, practices, and rituals related to the sacred, which may be God or, in Eastern religious traditions, the Ultimate Truth or Reality. Religion is often organized and practiced within a community. Surveys in the United States indicate that about 75% of the general population believes that there is a God.

Spirituality, which is related to religion, has many definitions. Spirituality is not necessarily associated with religious worship or a specific belief system. Rather, spirituality refers to a connection with self and others, development of a personal value system, and a search for meaning in life. Spirituality takes many forms—for some it may involve belief in a higher power, prayer, religious observance, or meditation, while for others it may be found in art, music, or nature.

Prayer is a component of religious practice that may be used to give thanks to, or obtain help from, a higher power. Prayer is used to attempt to influence processes and events that are beyond human control, including health and disease. Prayer generally is practiced in conjunction with conventional medical care, but followers of some religions, such as the Christian Science Church, pray in lieu of using conventional medicine. *Intercessory prayer*, which has been studied in medical settings, involves one person praying for another individual who may be in a different geographic location.

There has been a growth in interest about the possible therapeutic effects of prayer and spirituality. Important issues that have been raised are whether spirituality improves health and whether prayer can improve the course of a disease or lessen the severity of a specific symptom.

Methods

Most religions involve some type of prayer. Praying may be done individually or in groups. It may be a type of meditation, or may involve recitations of words silently or aloud. As noted, intercessory prayer involves one person praying for another. It is important to recognize that prayer is one of many components of religious practice and that it may not be effective if done independently of the other aspects of religious belief.

In addition to prayer, spirituality is an active area of research. Whether spiritual belief produces effects beyond those of the placebo response has not been established. It has been claimed that spirituality may be an especially potent means of producing the placebo effect because placebo effects require belief and religious belief may be the most profound form of belief.

There are several common features to being spiritual (1):

- *Identify and focus on personal goals*: Identifying what is most meaningful in life may build and strengthen one's spirituality.

- *Release control:* Feeling that one is part of a greater whole may relieve the stress and burden of day-to-day life and improve one's ability to share the positives and negatives of life with others.

- *Increase one's social network:* Sharing of spiritual expression with others—through organized religion or other means—may lead to strong and meaningful relationships.

- *Connect to the world:* Feeling that one has a place and a purpose in the world may provide inner peace and alleviate feelings of being alone.

There are specific strategies that may be used to strengthen one's spirituality. Prayer, meditation, and relaxation approaches may be used. Keeping a journal, confiding in a friend or family member, or reading inspirational stories may help to identify and nurture what is meaningful in life. Finally, new experiences within organized religion or in the arts or nature may help build/or expand one's spirituality.

Studies of Multiple Sclerosis and Other Conditions

One frequently described case of multiple sclerosis (MS) that appears to have responded dramatically to prayer and faith involves Rita Klaus (2). She was diagnosed with MS in 1960, at the age of 20—she was a nun at the time. Because of the effects of her illness, she was given dispensation of her vows and left the convent. She eventually married and had three children. Over the years, her disease progressed to the point of significant disability. Also, her religious faith dwindled and she became skeptical of God and religion in general. At the urging of her husband, she became more committed religiously and prayed regularly. One evening in 1986, 26 years after her diagnosis of MS, she prayed for healing of her disease. The following morning, she had unusual warm and itching sensations in her legs. She was able to move her legs, get out of her wheelchair, and walk. She returned to her job as a schoolteacher and now gives public lectures on her experience.

Studies in several countries have formally evaluated religion and spirituality in those with MS. A U.S. study of more than 1,000 people with MS in the Midwest reported that nearly two-thirds used religious services to improve their health or well-being (3). A study of people with MS in Lebanon found that religious involvement was associated with a higher overall quality of life (4). However, in another study, conducted in Greece, religious involvement was associated with a *lower* quality of life among caregivers of those with MS (5). A German study evaluated religion and spirituality in people with MS and other chronic medical conditions, such as cancer and chronic pain (6). It was found that 16% of people with MS categorized themselves as both religious and spiritual, while about one-third described themselves as neither religious nor spiritual. Relative to people with other chronic conditions, those with MS were less likely to be both religious and spiritual. Another German study found that religious faith was not associated with disability, fatigue, depression, or overall life satisfaction (7).

Studies of religious involvement and spirituality in other conditions have produced mixed, but generally positive, results with regard to mental health. Religious involvement and spirituality have been associated with improved ability to cope with stress and less depression and anxiety. However, these studies have limitations. Also, some studies have associated religious involvement with *increased* anxiety and depression. These findings indicate that religious involvement and spirituality are individualized and that there may be healthy as well as unhealthy ways to be religious or spiritual.

As with studies of religious involvement, research on prayer has produced some positive findings with anxiety and depression. However, many of these studies have limitations and therefore it is difficult to draw firm conclusions.

There are several ways in which prayer could have therapeutic effects. Prayer may promote relaxation and well-being since it, like meditation, elicits the relaxation response (see the chapter on *Meditation*). Prayer may also provide a way for people to cope, especially with threatening or stressful medical situations that are felt to be uncontrollable. Finally, prayer may lead to more positive and proactive approaches that include other health-promoting behaviors, such as healthy eating habits, exercise, and avoidance of tobacco.

There have been many studies of intercessory prayer. Much of the medical interest in this form of prayer was generated by a 1988 study that reported that intercessory prayer decreased the risk of medical complications after heart attacks. However, multiple subsequent studies did not find any consistent medical benefits of intercessory prayer and a review of the various studies of intercessory prayer concluded: "We are not convinced that further trials of this intervention should be undertaken and would prefer to see any resources available for such a trial used to investigate other questions in health care" (8).

Side Effects

Prayer, religious involvement, and spirituality are generally safe. Some people have expressed concern that negative thoughts about an individual could lead to negative health outcomes. Prayer and spirituality should not be used in place of conventional medical care and should not be used to avoid making necessary life changes.

Conclusion

Prayer, religious involvement, and spirituality are low risk and inexpensive. The health effects of these approaches have not been established. Some studies indicate that prayer, religious involvement, and spirituality may improve coping and be beneficial for anxiety and depression.

Additional Readings

Books

Bauer B, ed. *Mayo Clinic Book of Alternative Medicine and Home Remedies.* New York, NY: Time Home Entertainment; 2013:112,113.

Benson H. *Timeless Healing: The Power and Biology of Belief.* New York, NY: Simon & Schuster; 1996.

Dossey L. *Reinventing Medicine: Beyond Mind-Body to a New Era of Healing.* San Francisco, CA: HarperCollins; 1999.

Hirshberg C, Barasch MI. *Remarkable Recovery: What Extraordinary Healings Tell Us About Getting Well and Staying Well.* New York, NY: Berkley; 1996.

Kiresuk TJ, Trachtenburg AI, Boucher TA. Psychiatric disorders. In: Oken BS, ed. *Complementary Therapies in Neurology.* London, UK: Parthenon Publishing; 2004:417–419.

Klaus R. *Rita's Story.* Cape Cod, MA: Paraclete Press; 1995.

Mueller P. Religious involvement, spirituality and medicine: subject review and implications for clinical practice. In: Oken BS, ed. *Complementary Therapies in Neurology.* London, UK: Parthenon Publishing; 2004:189–207.

Spencer JW, Jacobs JJ. *Complementary and Alternative Medicine: An Evidence-Based Approach.* St Louis, MO: Mosby; 2003.

Journal Articles

Argyriou AA, Iconomou G, Ifanti AA, et al. Religiosity and its relation to quality of life in primary caregivers of patient with multiple sclerosis: a case study in Greece. *J Neurol.* 2011;258:1114–1119.

Benjamins MR, Finlayson M. Using religious services to improve health: findings from a sample of middle-aged and older adults with multiple sclerosis. *J Aging Health.* 2007;19:537–553.

Bonelli RM, Koenig HG. Mental disorders, religion and spirituality 1990-2010: a systematic review. *J Relig Health.* 2013;52:657–673.

Bussing A, Ostermann T, Koenig HG. Relevance of religion and spirituality in German patients with chronic diseases. *Int J Psych Med.* 2007;37:39–57.

Bussing A, Wirth A-G, Humbroich K, et al. Faith as a resource in patients with multiple sclerosis. *Evid Based Complement Alternat Med.* 2013;2013:128575.

Garrusi B, Nakhaee N. Religion and smoking: a review of recent literature. *Int J Psychiatr Med.* 2012;43:279–292.

Koenig HG. Research on religion, spirituality, and mental health: a review. *Can J Psych.* 2009;54:283–291.

Kohls N, Sauer S, Offenbacher M, Giordano J. Spirituality: an overlooked predictor of placebo responses. *Philos Trans Roy Soc Long B Biol Sci.* 2011;366: 1838–1848.

Masters KS, Spielmans GI. Prayer and health: review, meta-analysis, and research agenda. *J Behav Med.* 2007;30:329–338.

Powell-Wiley TM, Banks-Richard K, Williams-King E, et al. Churches as targets for cardiovascular disease prevention: comparison of genes, nutrition, exercise, wellness and spiritual growth (GoodNEWS) and Dallas County populations. *J Public Health (Oxf).* 2013;35:99–106.

Roberts L, Ahmed I, Hall S, Davison A. Intercessory prayer for the alleviation of ill health. *Cochrane Database Syst Rev.* 2009;2:CD000368.

Salmoirago-Blotcher E, Fitchett G, Hovey KM, et al. Frequency of private spiritual activity and cardiovascular risk in postmenopausal women: the Women's Health Initiative. *Ann Epid.* 2013;23:239–245.

Tan MM, Chan CK, Reidpath DD. Religiosity and spirituality and the intake of fruit, vegetable, and fat: a systematic review. *Evid Based Complement Alternat Med*. 2013;2013:146214.

Visser A, Garssen B, Vingerhoets A. Spirituality and well-being in cancer patients: a review. *Psychooncology*. 2010;19:565–572.

Wachholtz AB, Pearce MJ. Does spirituality as a coping mechanism help or hinder coping with chronic pain? *Curr Pain Headache Rep*. 2009;13:127–132.

Yamout B, Issa Z, Herlopian A, et al. Predictors of quality of life among multiple sclerosis patients: a comprehensive analysis. *Eur J Neurol*. 2013;20:756–764.

⑦ Probiotics and the Gut Microbiome

There is much interest, as well as confusion, regarding the use of probiotics in multiple sclerosis (MS) and other medical conditions. Probiotics represent a novel approach with great potential for treating a wide range of diseases, including MS. However, there are many different types of probiotics and unanswered questions about the effectiveness and safety of specific probiotics in specific medical conditions.

There are common misunderstandings about what constitutes a probiotic. Probiotics are defined as bacteria and other microorganisms, which, when given to humans, provide health benefits. Contrary to some popular belief, there are hundreds of potential probiotics. Probiotics are typically administered orally and designed to colonize the gut with beneficial organisms. Since the gut is able to support hundreds of species of organisms, many of which have not been identified, many different organisms could be used as probiotics.

Probiotics are a fascinating approach to alter immune function. It is known that organisms that colonize the gut, referred to collectively as the *gut microbiome*, have a significant impact on immune system function in the gut but also throughout the body. Thus, in MS, the use of probiotics to alter the organisms in the gut could produce beneficial immune changes that ultimately decrease the severity of nervous system injury. This "gut-brain connection" provides a novel strategy to control the disease process of MS through the use of microorganisms.

There are several positive features of probiotics. They are generally inexpensive. Also, since taken orally, they are easy to administer. Finally, if the organisms do colonize the gut, probiotics may be administered over a short time period yet provide long-lasting health benefits.

Treatment Method

There are many different sources of probiotics. They may be obtained from foods such as yogurt, kefir, cheese, tempeh, miso, and some juices and soy drinks. Probiotics are also available as tablets, capsules, powders, and suppositories. Many probiotics are in the investigational stage and are not currently commercially available.

Probiotic products contain specific subtypes of bacteria, known as *species* or *strains*. Types of bacteria that are commonly used in commercially available probiotics are known as *Lactobacillus* and *Bifidobacteria*. Two popular products contain specific species and strains of these bacteria:

- Activia: contains bacteria known as *Bifidobacterium animalis* DN 173,010 strain

- Yakult: contains two bacteria known as *Lactobacillus casei* Shirota strain and *Bifidobacterium breve* Yakult strain

Consuming specific organisms through probiotics is the most direct approach to alter the gut microbiome. Some "non-probiotic" components of the diet, such as salt, may affect the gut microbiome indirectly by producing an environment that is better suited to some organisms than others (see *Salt* chapter).

Studies in MS and Other Conditions

There are limited MS-specific studies of probiotics at this time. The MS-relevant studies have focused on two types of organisms, bacteria and parasites such as whipworms (*Trichuris suis*). Most studies have been in experimental autoimmune encephalomyelitis (EAE), the animal model of MS.

In the bacteria research, several studies indicate that bacterial probiotics produce beneficial effects in EAE. However, other studies have shown no effect or worsening of EAE.

Whipworms and other parasites have been studied in EAE and, to a limited extent, in people with MS. Several studies indicate that parasitic infections are beneficial for animals with EAE. Also, limited studies in South America indicate that MS is less severe in people with MS who happen to get infected with parasites. Based on these observations, one small clinical study was done to evaluate the effects of deliberately producing whipworm infections in the intestines of people with MS. This study found that this approach was well tolerated and that there was a trend for beneficial MRI and immune effects (1). Further studies of this unique treatment approach in MS are underway (2).

Side Effects

In general, probiotics are well tolerated. Gas and bloating may occur. In children with suppressed immune function, there are rare cases of probiotics causing severe, life-threatening infections, known as *sepsis*.

In the specific situation of MS and other autoimmune conditions, there is concern that some probiotics may activate the immune system and thereby worsen the disease or inhibit the therapeutic effects of MS disease-modifying medications.

Conclusion

Probiotics are a promising treatment for MS. However, studies of the safety and effectiveness of probiotics in MS are extremely limited at this time. Some probiotics may have immune-stimulating effects and thus pose theoretical risks to those with MS. Further research of probiotics in MS is needed.

Additional Readings

Books

Bauer B, ed. *Mayo Clinic Book of Alternative Medicine and Home Remedies.* New York, NY: Time Home Entertainment; 2013:92.

Duyff RL. *American Dietetic Association Complete Food and Nutrition Guide.* Boston, MA: Houghton Mifflin Harcourt; 2012:144.

Jellin JM, Batz F, Hitchens K. *Natural Medicines Comprehensive Database.* Stockton, CA: Therapeutic Research Faculty; 2014.

Journal Articles

Ezendam J, van Loveren H. *Lactobacillus casei* Shirota administered during lactation increases the duration of autoimmunity in rats and enhances lung inflammation in mice. *Br J Nutr.* 2008;99:83–90.

Fleming JO, Isaak A, Lee JE, et al. Probiotic helminth administration in relapsing-remitting multiple sclerosis: a phase I study. *Mult Scler J.* 2011;17: 743–754.

Kobayashi T, Kato I, Nanno M, et al. Oral administration of probiotic bacteria, *Lactobacillus casei* and *Bifidobacterium breve,* does not exacerbate neurological symptoms in experimental autoimmune encephalomyelitis. *Immunopharmacol Immunotoxicol.* 2010;32:116–124.

Kwon H-K, Kim G-C, Kim Y, et al. Amelioration of experimental autoimmune encephalomyelitis by probiotic mixture is mediated by a shift in T helper cell immune response. *Clin Immunol.* 2013;146:217–227.

Lavasani S, Dzhambazov B, Nouri M, et al. A novel probiotic mixture exerts a therapeutic effect on experimental autoimmune encephalomyelitis mediated by IL-10 producing regulatory T cells. *PLoS One.* 2010;5:e9009.

Maasen CBM, Claassen E. Strain-dependent effects of probiotic lactobacilli on EAE autoimmunity. *Vaccine.* 2008;26:2056,2057.

Manzel A, Muller DN, Hafler D, Erdman SE, Linker RA, Kleinewietfeld M. Role of "Western diet" in inflammatory autoimmune diseases. *Curr Allergy Asthma Rep.* 2014;14:404.

Ozdemir O. Any role for probiotics in the therapy or prevention of autoimmune diseases? Up-to-date review. *Complem Integr Med.* 2013;10:229–250.

Wang Y, Kasper LH. The role of microbiome in central nervous system disorders. *Brain Behav Immun.* 2014;38:1–12.

⟨?⟩ Prokarin

The preparation known as Prokarin was developed by Elaine DeLack, a nurse with multiple sclerosis (MS), who lives in Washington. It is claimed that Prokarin, which was originally named Procarin, improves many MS-related symptoms.

Treatment Method

Prokarin contains histamine and caffeine. It was originally administered by a skin patch applied to the thigh for 8 hours with two patches used daily. It is now available as a once daily disc that is applied to the skin. Prokarin is administered through the skin because histamine is not absorbed if it is taken by mouth.

Prokarin was developed on the basis of a theory about histamine developed by Dr. Bayard Horton and Dr. Hinton Jonez in the 1940s and 1950s. Histamine treatment presumably decreases allergic reactions and enlarges blood vessels. Caffeine acts as a stimulant.

Studies in MS and Other Conditions

Information about the effectiveness of Prokarin itself is limited. Elaine DeLack claims that her MS was dramatically improved by using Prokarin. There is a preliminary report of Prokarin use in 10 people with MS in Washington State (1). It is claimed that 7 of the 10 people in this study experienced improvement in one or more MS symptoms, including bladder and bowel difficulties, incoordination, weakness, speech problems, walking unsteadiness, and fatigue (1).

One published study evaluated the effects of Prokarin use in 55 people with MS (2). It was found that 67% of people experienced improvement in MS symptoms after 6 weeks of treatment. Improvement was noted in a wide range of symptoms, including weakness, numbness, walking difficulties, pain, fatigue, and depression. This study is limited by the fact that neither caffeine alone nor a placebo treatment was used. Also, the effectiveness of the therapy was determined by self-assessment, an approach that is subject to inaccuracy.

A placebo-controlled study of Prokarin was reported in 2002 (3). This was a 12-week study of 29 people with MS. Prokarin was reported to improve fatigue. A question raised in the study was whether the fatigue-relieving effect was due to the caffeine in Prokarin. Blood caffeine levels were similar for the Prokarin- and placebo-treated groups. This suggests that caffeine was not the critical factor in decreasing fatigue, but the results of this relatively small study are not conclusive. Prokarin did not produce changes in brain chemistry (as measured by a technique known as *magnetic resonance* spectroscopy) and did not improve thinking abilities, walking, or arm coordination.

There have not been any clinical studies of Prokarin in people with MS since 2002.

Older reports of histamine treatment for MS, published in the late 1940s and the early 1950s, used intravenous histamine along with another medication (tubocurarine), physical therapy, and allergy testing. Beneficial effects of this multimodality treatment were noted. However, the significance of these findings for histamine treatment alone is not clear because several different therapies were used simultaneously, and strict clinical trial guidelines (such as the use of placebo-treated groups) were not followed.

Histamine has effects on the animal model of MS, known as EAE (experimental allergic encephalomyelitis). However, these effects are complex and their relevance to the treatment of MS is not clear.

In response to information about Prokarin's reported benefits, the Clinical Advisory Committee of the Greater Washington Chapter of the National Multiple Sclerosis Society released a statement in 1999. In this statement, physicians and nurses expressed the opinion that they did not believe that Prokarin was beneficial for their MS patients. They also had concerns that Prokarin was being used instead of prescription medications with established effectiveness for treating MS.

Side Effects

Limited information is available on the safety of Prokarin. The histamine in Prokarin may potentially worsen asthma, and there have been reports that Prokarin has caused severe asthmatic attacks. One person taking baclofen

(Lioresal) experienced irritability and loss of appetite while taking Prokarin. Rashes have occurred at the site where the patch is applied.

Prokarin should not be used *instead* of conventional Food and Drug Administration (FDA)-approved MS medications. Also, information from the company that manufactures Prokarin states that specific drugs and herbs may decrease the effectiveness of Prokarin:

- Antihistamines that block the histamine-2 receptors, such as ranitidine (Zantac), famotidine (Pepcid), and cimetidine (Tagamet).

- Anti-spasticity medications, including baclofen (Lioresal) and tizanidine (Zanaflex).

- Licorice root.

Practical Information

Prokarin is available only by prescription and costs approximately $200 per month.

Conclusion

Prokarin is expensive, and limited information exists about its safety and effectiveness. One small study suggests that it may improve fatigue. Prokarin should not be used by people with asthma because it contains histamine, which may provoke asthma.

Additional Readings

Books

EDMS, LLC. *Off-Label Drug Booklet for Prokarin.* Stanwood, WA: EDMS, LLC; [no date].

Journal Articles

Alonso A, Jick SS, Hernan MA. Allergy, histamine 1 receptor blockers, and the risk of multiple sclerosis. *Neurology.* 2006;66:572–575.

Gillson G, Richards TL, Wright JV, Smith RB, Wright, JV A double-blind pilot study of the effect of Prokarin on fatigue in multiple sclerosis. *Mult Scler.* 2002;8:30–35.

Gillson G, Wright JV, Ballasiotes G. Transdermal histamine in multiple sclerosis. Part 1: clinical experience. *Alt Med Rev.* 1999;4:424–428.

Horton BT, Wagener HP, Aita JA, et al. Treatment of multiple sclerosis by the intra venous administration of histamine. *JAMA.* 1944;124:800,801.

Jonez HD. Management of multiple sclerosis. *Postgrad Med.* 1952;2:415–422.

Panula P, Nuutinen S. The histaminergic network in the brain: basic organization and role in disease. *Nat Rev Neurosci.* 2013;14:472–487.

Passani MB, Ballerini C. Histamine and neuroinflammation: insights from murine experimental autoimmune encephalomyelitis. *Front Syst Neurosci.* 2012;6:32.

Saligrama N, Case LK, del Rio R, Noubade R, Teuscher C. Systemic lack of canonical histamine receptor signaling results in increased resistance to autoimmune encephalomyelitis. *J Immunol.* 2013;191:614–622.

⑦ Reflexology

Reflexology is a therapy based on applying pressure to specific parts of the foot. It is similar to acupressure and shiatsu. In the United States, reflexology was initially developed in the early 1900s by Dr. William Fitzgerald, an ear, nose, and throat specialist in Connecticut. He named the treatment *zone therapy*. Subsequently, in the 1930s, Eunice Ingham, an American nurse and physical therapist, modified the method and named it *reflexology*. Her nephew, Dwight Byers, is one of the current authorities in this area and is president of the International Institute of Reflexology.

Treatment Method

In reflexology, specific parts of the foot are believed to correspond to different body parts. The application of pressure to reflex points (referred to as *cutaneo-organ reflex points*) on the foot is claimed to affect specific parts of the body. The left foot is associated with the left half of the body, while the right foot is associated with the right half.

Reflexology is intended to improve health by increasing energy flow to specific parts of the body. In this way, it is similar to other healing systems that believe in a life force, such as traditional Chinese medicine and Ayurvedic medicine.

Reflexology usually is provided by a trained reflexologist. It also may be done individually. Sessions usually start with a foot massage and are followed by application of pressure to reflex points.

Studies in Multiple Sclerosis and Other Conditions

Clinical studies of reflexology are limited. There are several clinical studies of reflexology in multiple sclerosis (MS). The largest study included 73 people with MS (1). Participants were treated weekly for 10 weeks with reflexology or with a placebo, or *sham,* treatment. The sham treatment resembled reflexology but was actually a *nonspecific foot massage* that was designed to avoid stimulation of reflexology points. The focus of this study was pain—multiple other MS symptoms were monitored as well. It was found that after 10 weeks of reflexology, there was improvement in pain as well as fatigue, depression, disability, spasms, and quality of life. However, similar therapeutic effects were seen in those who received the placebo treatment. This indicates that the beneficial effects may have been due to a placebo response or possibly *nonspecific* stimulation of the foot. Similarly, another study evaluated the effects of reflexology on 20 people with MS who had moderate to severe disability and found that, over the course of 8 weeks, there was improvement in multiple MS symptoms with reflexology or sham massage of the foot and calf (2). Another study of 71 people with MS evaluated the effects of reflexology or sham massage over 11 weeks (3). This study found that reflexology was more effective than sham massage in producing improvement in muscle stiffness and sensory and bladder symptoms. Interestingly, the sham massage in this study, unlike the two other studies, only involved the calf. These various MS studies have produced inconsistent results. Taken together, they raise important questions about whether reflexology simply evokes a placebo response and also whether reflexology actually has specific beneficial effects or if these same effects may be produced simply with nonspecific massaging of the feet.

There are several other clinical trials of reflexology in MS. One compared reflexology with a relaxation method known as *progressive muscle relaxation* and found that reflexology improved anxiety and mildly lowered blood pressure (4). Another study examined the content of conversations between reflexology practitioners and 50 people with MS (5). Through analysis of 245 different conversations, it was found that many people with MS shared their worries and concerns with the reflexologist. Recurring themes of these conversations included MS symptoms and treatments, psychological issues, and concerns about work and family. This indicates that some of the therapeutic aspects of reflexology may arise from the reflexologist–patient relationship and specific advice and support that reflexologists may offer during treatment sessions.

Reflexology has been studied in medical conditions other than MS. Some of these studies indicate that this treatment improves anxiety, depression, fatigue, pain, and sleep. One small study found improvement in bladder function.

Other studies have reported reduction in blood pressure. However, for these various studies, it is important to recognize that they are not entirely consistent with each other and that they generally have significant limitations.

Side Effects

Reflexology is well tolerated, and no serious side effects are known. It should be used with caution by those with foot conditions, including ulcers, gout, arthritis, and vascular disease. Although reflexology usually is not painful, one German study of reflexology use in people after surgery found that the technique occasionally triggered abdominal pain.

Practical Information

Reflexology sessions are 30 to 60 minutes in length. Several informational resources for reflexology exist. Books on the subject are available in bookstores and libraries. Information and lists of trained practitioners are available from:

- The International Institute of Reflexology (www.reflexology-usa.net), 5650 First Ave. North Street, St. Petersburg, FL 33733 (727-343-4811)

Conclusion

Reflexology is a low-risk, low- to moderate-cost therapy. Some studies in MS and other conditions have reported multiple beneficial effects. However, the results of the studies have been inconsistent and the studies have significant limitations. Further studies of reflexology in MS and other conditions are needed.

Additional Readings
Books

Bauer B, ed. *Mayo Clinic Book of Alternative Medicine and Home Remedies.* New York, NY: Time Home Entertainment; 2013:136.

Ernst E, ed. *The Desktop Guide to Complementary and Alternative Medicine: An Evidence-Based Approach.* Edinburgh, UK: Mosby; 2001:66–69.

Spencer JW, Jacobs JJ. *Complementary and Alternative Medicine: An Evidence-Based Approach.* St Louis, MO: Mosby; 2003:368, 369, 382, 581.

Vickers A. *Massage and Aromatherapy: A Guide for Health Professionals.* London, UK: Chapman & Hall; 1996.

Journal Articles

Bagheri-Nesami M, Shorofi SA, Zargar N, Sohrabi M, Gholipour-Baradari A, Khalilian A. The effects of foot reflexology massage on anxiety in patients following coronary artery bypass graft surgery: a randomized controlled trial. *Complem Ther Clin Pract.* 2014;20:42–47.

Ernst E. Is reflexology an effective intervention? A systematic review of randomized controlled trials. *Med J Austral.* 2009;191:263–266.

Ernst E, Posadzki P, Lee MS. Reflexology: an update of a systematic review of randomized clinical trials. *Maturitas.* 2011;68:116–120.

Hughes CM, Smyth S, Lowe-Strong AS. Reflexology for the treatment of pain in people with multiple sclerosis: a double-blind randomized sham-controlled clinical trial. *Mult Scler.* 2009;15:1329–1338.

Jones J, Thomson P, Lauder W, Howie K, Leslie SJ. Reflexology has no immediate haemodynamic effect in patients with chronic heart failure: a double blind randomized controlled trial. *Complem Ther Clin Pract.* 2013;19:133–138.

Joyce M, Richardson R. Reflexology can help MS. *Int J Alt Compl Med.* 1997; July:10–12.

Lee J, Han M, Chung Y, Kim J, Choi J. Effects of foot reflexology on fatigue, sleep and pain: a systematic review and meta-analysis. *J Korean Acad Nurs.* 2011;41:821–833.

Mackereth PA, Booth K, Hillier VF, Caress AL. Reflexology and progressive muscle relaxation training for people with multiple sclerosis: a crossover trial. *Complem Ther Clin Pract.* 2009;15:14–21.

Mackereth PA, Booth K, Hillier VF, Caress AL. What do people talk about during reflexology? Analysis of worries and concerns expressed during sessions for patients with multiple sclerosis. *Complem Ther Clin Pract.* 2009;15:85–90.

Mak HL, Cheon WC, Wong T, Liu YS, Tong WM. Randomized controlled trial of foot reflexology for patients with symptomatic idiopathic detrusor hyperactivity. *Int Urogynecol J Pelvic Floor Dysfunct.* 2007;18:653–658.

Miller L, McIntee E, Mattison P. Evaluation of the effects of reflexology on quality of life and symptomatic relief in multiple sclerosis patients with moderate to severe disability; a pilot study. *Clin Rehabil.* 2013;27:591–598.

Oleson T, Flocco W. Randomized controlled study of premenstrual symptoms treated with ear, hand, and foot reflexology. *Obstet Gynecol.* 1993;82:906–911.

Ozdemir G, Ovayolu N, Ovayolu O. The effect of reflexology applied on haemodialysis patients with fatigue, pain and cramps. *Int J Nurs Pract.* 2013;19:265–273.

Siev-Ner I, Gamus D, Lerner-Geva L, Achiron A. Reflexology treatment relieves symptoms of multiple sclerosis: a randomized controlled study. *Mult Scler.* 2003;9:356–361.

Wyatt G, Sikorskii A, Rahbar MH, Victorson D, You M. Health-related quality-of-life outcomes: a reflexology trial with patients with advanced-stage breast cancer. *Oncol Nurs Forum.* 2012;39:568–577.

Yeung WF, Chung KF, Poon MM, et al. Acupressure, reflexology, and auricular acupressure for insomnia: a systematic review of randomized controlled trials. *Sleep Med.* 2012;13:971–984.

Salt

Excessive salt intake is one of the single greatest dietary harms to health. It has been recognized for decades that high salt intake increases the risk for heart disease. More recent studies indicate that excessive salt consumption may play an important role in the risk of multiple sclerosis (MS).

The intake of salt around the world is extremely variable. The daily salt intake ranges from 1,000 milligrams in some indigenous populations to more than 20,000 mg in Western countries and Japan. In the Western world, there is high consumption of processed foods and "fast foods," which may contain 100 times more salt than similar food that is prepared at home.

In the United States, the daily salt intake greatly exceeds the recommended amount. The average American adult consumes about 4,000 mg daily. The recommended amount is 1,500 to 2,300 mg daily.

In the United States, it has been estimated that decreasing daily salt consumption by 1,200 mg, which is equivalent to one-half teaspoon, could lead to dramatic reductions in death and disability. It has been estimated that such a reduction in salt intake could, on an annual basis, save about 150,000 lives and decrease health care costs by $10 to $24 billion.

Treatment Method

Salt intake is often associated with the use of a salt shaker at meals. However, the salt shaker is generally not a significant factor. Instead, processed food and restaurant food are the major sources of salt in the American diet. Thus, limiting one's intake of these foods is the primary method for decreasing salt intake. Several strategies may be used:

- Read labels on processed food
  - The salt content of different processed versions of the same food may vary by as much as five-fold.
- Use herbs, spices, lemon juice, and salsa instead of salt
- Use salt substitutes
- Cook pasta and rice without salt
- Rinse canned food

Two general approaches may be helpful for reducing salt intake. First, as with any lifestyle modification, slow changes may be the most tolerable and long-lasting. One study found that most people do not detect a 25% reduction in salt intake that occurs over a 6-week time period. Also, since many people may have adjusted to, and enjoy, the salty taste of foods, it may be helpful to try to increase one's appreciation of the actual taste of the food, not the salt.

Studies in MS and Other Conditions

Studies of salt intake in MS are limited. Several studies in experimental allergic encephalomyelitis (EAE), the animal model of MS, indicate that high salt intake increases the severity of the disease. This appears to be due to increased production of inflammatory immune cells. There are several ways in which dietary salt could activate the immune system, including effects on the immune cells in the gut or on the organisms that colonize the gut (see the *Probiotics and the Gut Microbiome* chapter).

There are not any formal clinical trials of the effects of low-salt diets in people with MS. One preliminary study reported that people with MS with high salt intake, relative to those with normal salt intake, had eight more MS lesions on MRI scans and three- to four-fold increased risk of developing new MRI lesions or having MS attacks (1).

Studies over the past several decades demonstrate that excessive salt intake increases the risk for many serious medical conditions that could impact people with MS. High salt intake is associated with increased risk for heart disease, high blood pressure, stroke, congestive heart failure, and kidney disease. The presence of some of these medical conditions in combination with MS may worsen the level of neurological function and the overall quality of life.

Conclusion

Studies of salt and MS indicate that high dietary intake of salt could increase the severity of MS. However, studies in this area are limited at this time. As a result, there is not strong evidence to justify reducing salt intake in order to improve the course of MS. There is much more evidence that excessive salt consumption increases the risk for other conditions, such as heart disease and stroke. These conditions, when present in people with MS, may lower the quality of life and decrease neurological function. Thus, people with MS who decrease their salt intake may obtain indirect beneficial effects on MS by reducing the risk of these other conditions.

Additional Readings

Books

Bauer B, ed. *Mayo Clinic Book of Alternative Medicine and Home Remedies.* New York, NY: Time Home Entertainment; 2013.

Duyff RL. *American Dietetic Association Complete Food and Nutrition Guide.* Boston, MA: Houghton Mifflin Harcourt; 2012.

Journal Articles

Croxford AL, Waisman A, Becher B. Does dietary salt induce autoimmunity? *Cell Res.* 2013;23:872–873.

Kleinewietfeld M, Manzel A, Titze J, et al. Sodium chloride drives autoimmune disease by the induction of pathogenic T_H17 cells. *Nature.* 2013;496:518–522.

Manzel A, Muller DN, Hafler D, Erdman SE, Linker RA, Kleinewietfeld M. Role of "Western diet" in inflammatory autoimmune diseases. *Curr Allergy Asthma Rep.* 2014;14:404.

O'Shea JJ, Jones RG. Rubbing salt in the wound. *Nature.* 2013;437–439.

Wu C, Yosef N, Thalhamer T, et al. Induction of pathogenic T_H17 cells by inducible salt-sensing kinase SGK1. *Nature.* 2013;496:513–517.

Yosef N, Shalek AK, Gaublomme JT, et al. Dynamic regulatory network controlling T_H17 cell differentiation. *Nature.* 2013;496:461468.

⊘Tai Chi and Qigong

Tai chi, also known as tai chi chuan, was developed in China hundreds of years ago as a martial art for self-defense. It is a component of traditional Chinese medicine. Tai chi has recently become popular in the United States. A method related to tai chi, *qigong,* was developed thousands of years ago in China as a means of achieving health and longevity.

On the surface, tai chi appears to be simply slow body movements. In practice, it may provide some of the physical benefits of exercise and the relaxation effects of meditation. As a result, tai chi is sometimes referred to as *meditation in motion.* The slow, mindful movements of tai chi may improve awareness of body movement and function.

Treatment Method

Tai chi may be done individually or in groups. A high level of strength and flexibility are not required because the exercises are based largely on technique. Tai chi consists of slow, rhythmic body movements. The arms are moved slowly and smoothly in circular movements while weight is shifted from one leg to the other and specific breathing techniques are used. A specified series of movements is known as a *form.* Tai chi movements are claimed to balance the two opposing forces within the human body, *yin* and *yang.* Performing tai chi movements is believed to strengthen and balance the life force, known as *chi* or *qi.* Qigong, which generally uses simpler movements than tai chi, focuses on relaxed breathing, correct alignment of posture, slow and graceful movement, and meditation.

Studies in MS and Other Conditions

The most notable aspect of tai chi and MS research is that very little research has been conducted in this area. Tai chi has the potential to improve various MS symptoms, including balance and walking ability. Dr. Jack Petajan, one of the pioneers of exercise research in MS, stated in a 1999 medical publication: "Further studies of the benefits of [tai chi and qigong] and their impact upon the performance of daily activities need to be carried out with MS patients..."(1) However, there are very few research studies in MS. At this time, there are only two small published studies of tai chi and MS. In contrast, for walking difficulties and other aging-associated conditions that affect the elderly, there are hundreds of tai chi studies in the medical literature.

One MS study of tai chi was conducted in California (2). This small study, conducted at the American College of Traditional Chinese Medicine in San Francisco, examined the effects of an 8-week tai chi group program on 19 people with MS. People were accepted into the study regardless of the severity of their disability. Tai chi improved emotional and social function and produced physical benefits, with a 21% improvement in walking speed and a 28% decrease in muscle stiffness. Comments obtained from participants indicated that the group experience itself was an important component of the program. The results of this study are promising, but there are limitations. Specifically, no placebo-treated group was used, and assessment was done by the participants themselves rather than by unbiased observers.

Another MS study, conducted in the United Kingdom, evaluated the effects of *mindfulness of movement*, a component of tai chi and qigong (3). Mindfulness of movement involves developing a moment-to-moment awareness of the quality of breathing, movement, and posture. In the study, eight people with MS were given one-on-one instruction in mindfulness of movement as well as audio and videotape aids. The placebo-treated group, which also included eight people with MS, continued with their current care program. People were assessed before the program and after 3 months. Those who participated in mindfulness of movement showed improvement in multiple symptoms, as assessed by patients and by relatives. Limitations of this study include a relatively large number of people who dropped out of the study, small numbers of people overall in the study, and the lack of objective (blinded) clinicians for assessment.

Nigel Mills, a co-author of the United Kingdom study, provides a detailed description of the study and also potential applications of qigong to MS in his book, *Qigong for Multiple Sclerosis: Finding Your Feet Again* (4). In this lay language book, he provides possible beneficial effects of this approach to those with MS:

- Cultivation of "compassionate ownership" of the body for those who may feel their body is "out of control" or "alien"

- Slowing down of the process of walking and moving, which may help those who have lost confidence in their ability to move and walk
- Improvement of balance, which may aid in walking and help prevent falls
- Reduction of stress
- Encouragement of "self-empowerment"
- Overall, the potential to "find your feet again"

The slow and mindful movements of tai chi and qigong may improve one's awareness of body movement and function. Improving body awareness may be particularly helpful to those who do not have a strong sense of the physicality of their bodies. Other methods with the potential for improved body awareness include yoga and Pilates as well as the less popular, and less studied, techniques of Feldenkrais and Tragerwork.

The effects of tai chi on MS-related symptoms have been investigated in many other conditions. In addition to studies in the elderly, tai chi has been studied in those with various neurological conditions, rheumatologic diseases, orthopedic conditions, cancer, and heart and lung disease. These wide-ranging tai chi studies are of variable quality. In these studies, tai chi appears to improve balance and strength and decrease the risk of falls in the elderly. Other potential benefits of tai chi include improvement in:

- Anxiety and depression
- Fatigue
- Muscle strength, flexibility, and coordination
- Cognitive function
- Sleep
- Various types of pain, including low back pain, arthritis pain, and fibromyalgia-associated pain
- High blood pressure

The stretching movements of tai chi have the potential to improve muscle stiffness (spasticity), but this has not been formally studied.

It is sometimes claimed that tai chi *improves* immune function. Although there are several studies of tai chi's effects on the immune system, the studies in this area are limited and it is unclear whether the immune system changes with tai chi are significant.

Tai chi is an interesting example of a therapy that may be clinically effective in spite of the fact that its proposed mechanism of action—balancing and strengthening life energy—is unproven and inconsistent with conventional scientific principles.

Side Effects

Tai chi does not generally pose any known significant health risk. It could potentially worsen fatigue in people with MS. Also, walking unsteadiness and sensitivity to overheating may require modifications in technique. Tai chi may strain joints and muscles. Tai chi should be used with caution or avoided by those with acute low back pain, osteoporosis, significant joint injuries, and bone fractures. One report has been published of a person with MS in whom tai chi provoked electrical sensations in the arms and back (known as Lhermitte's sign).

Practical Information

It is easiest to learn tai chi through classes. Tai chi may be practiced by people with significant disabilities, but the pace may need to be slowed. The slow and gentle movements of tai chi place minimal stress on joints and muscles. As a result, tai chi may be particularly well-suited for those with arthritis or other conditions that require low impact physical activity. Tai chi may be practiced individually after the basic techniques have been learned.

Tai chi classes often are provided through community centers and health clubs. Sessions are typically 60 minutes in length and cost between $15 and $30. Many books on this subject are available.

Conclusion

Tai chi is a low-risk, low- to moderate-cost therapy. In people with MS, it may increase walking ability, decrease stiffness, and improve social and emotional functioning. Studies in other conditions indicate that tai chi may improve anxiety, depression, fatigue, coordination, weakness, walking difficulties, sleep, and various types of joint and musculoskeletal pain. For general health, tai chi may mildly reduce blood pressure. Tai chi, like other methods such as yoga and Pilates, may improve one's awareness of body movement and function. For people with MS who have disabilities that prevent participation in strenuous exercise programs, tai chi may be a gentle way to obtain some of the general health benefits of a vigorous workout.

Additional Readings

Books

Bauer B, ed. *Mayo Clinic Book of Alternative Medicine and Home Remedies.* New York, NY: Time Home Entertainment; 2013:114.

Ernst E, ed. *The Desktop Guide to Complementary and Alternative Medicine: An Evidence-Based Approach*. Edinburgh, UK: Mosby; 2001:74–76.

Hain TC, Kotsias J, Pai C. Tai chi: applications to neurology. In: Weintraub MI, Micozzi MS, eds. *Alternative and Complementary Treatments in Neurologic Illness*. New York, NY: Churchill Livingstone; 2001:248–254.

Jellin JM, Gregory PJ, Batz F, et al. *Pharmacist's Letter/ Prescriber's Letter Natural Medicines Comprehensive Database*. Stockton, CA: Therapeutic Research Faculty; 2014.

Micozzi MS, ed. *Fundamentals of Complementary and Alternative Medicine*. Philadelphia, PA: Saunders Elsevier; 2011:438–454.

Mills N. *Qigong for Multiple Sclerosis: Finding Your Feet Again*. London, UK: Singing Dragon; 2010.

Spencer JW, Jacobs JJ. *Complementary and Alternative Medicine: An Evidence-Based Approach*. St. Louis, MO: Mosby; 2003.

Synovitz LB, Larson KL. *Complementary and Alternative Medicine for Health Professionals*. Burlington, MA: Jones & Bartlett Learning; 2013:116–117.

Journal Articles

Abbott R, Lavretsky H. Tai chi and qigong for the treatment and prevention of mental disorders. *Psychiatr Clin North Amer.* 2013;36:109–119.

Blake H, Hawley H. Effects of tai chi exercise on physical and psychological health of older people. *Curr Aging Sci.* 2012;5:19–27.

Chu DA. Tai chi, qigong, and reiki. *Phys Med Rehabil Clin N Am.* 2004;15:773–781.

Ding M. Tai chi for stroke rehabilitation: a focused review. *Am J Phys Med Rehabil.* 2012;91:1091–1096.

Ho RT, Wang CW, Ng SM, et al. The effect of t'ai chi exercise on immunity and infections: a systematic of controlled trials. *J Altern Complement Med.* 2013;19:389-396.

Husted C, Pham L, Hekking A, Niederman R. Improving quality of life for people with chronic conditions: the example of tai chi and multiple sclerosis. *Altern Ther Health Med.* 1999;5:70–74.

Kwok JC, Hui-Chan CW, Tsang WW. Effects of aging and tai chi on finger-pointing toward stationary and moving visual targets. *Arch Phys Med Rehabil.* 2010;91:149–155.

Lan C, Chen SY, Lai JS, Wong AM. Tai chi chuan in medicine and health promotion. *Evid Based Complement Altern Med.* 2013;2013:502131.

Langhorst J, Klose P, Dobos GJ, Bernardy K, Häuser W. Efficacy and safety of meditative movement therapies in fibromyalgia syndrome: a systematic review and meta-analysis of randomized controlled trials. *Rheumatol Int.* 2013;33:193–207.

Lauche R, Langhorst J, Dobos G, Cramer H. A systematic review and meta-analysis of tai chi for osteoarthritis of the knee. *Complement Ther Med.* 2013;21:396–406.

Lee MS, Lee EN, Kim JI, Ernst E. Tai chi for lowering resting blood pressure in the elderly: a systematic review. *J Eval Clin Pract.* 2010;16:818–824.

Leung DP, Chan CK, Tsang HW, Tsang WW, Jones AY. Tai chi as an intervention to improve balance and reduce falls in older adults: a systematic and meta-analytical review. *Altern Ther Health Med.* 2011;17:40–48.

Liu H, Frank A. Tai chi as a balance improvement exercise for older adults: a systematic review. *J Geriatr Phys Ther.* 2010;33:103–109.

Mills M, Allen J. Mindfulness of movement as a coping strategy in multiple sclerosis. A pilot study. *Gen Hosp Psych.* 2000;22:425–431.

Pei YC, Chou SW, Lin PS, Lin YC, Hsu TH, Wong AM. Eye-hand coordination of elderly people who practice tai chi chuan. *J Formos Med Assoc.* 2008;107:103–110.

Peng PW. Tai chi and chronic pain. *Reg Anesth Pain Med.* 2012;37:372–382.

Saris J, Byrne GJ. A systematic review of insomnia and complementary medicine. *Sleep Med Rev.* 2011;15:99–106.

Wang C. Role of tai chi in the treatment of rheumatologic diseases. *Curr Rheumatol Rep.* 2012;14:598–603.

Wang J, Feng B, Yang X, et al. Tai chi for essential hypertension. *Evid Based Complement Altern Med.* 2013;2013:215254.

Wayne PM, Walsh JN, Taylor-Piliae RE, et al. Effect of tai chi on cognitive performance in older adults: systematic review and meta-analysis. *J Am Geriatr Soc.* 2014;62:25–39.

Zeng Y, Luo T, Xie H, Huang M, Cheng AS. Health benefits of qigong or tai chi for cancer patients: a systematic review and meta-analyses. *Complement Ther Med.* 2014;22:173–186.

⑦ Therapeutic Touch

Therapeutic touch is an energy-based healing method in which life energy is believed to be manipulated therapeutically by the hands of a practitioner. Delores Krieger, a nurse, and Dora Kunz, a healer and clairvoyant, developed this technique during the 1970s. According to Krieger, therapeutic touch has been taught to more than 40,000 people and is practiced in more than 70 countries.

Therapeutic touch is based on concepts similar to those underlying the religious practice of "laying on of hands," in which healing energy is believed to pass from a healer to another person. Similarly, in therapeutic touch, a practitioner's hands are claimed to evaluate and beneficially alter an individual's energy field. Therapeutic touch is based on a concept of a life force, as are traditional Chinese medicine, Ayurvedic medicine, Reiki, and some other healing methods. It is a modern variation of some of these older healing approaches.

Treatment Method

Contrary to its name, therapeutic touch does not actually involve touching. Instead, the practitioners' hands are held 2 to 4 inches from a person's body. Several components make up the therapeutic touch session. After an initial "centering" procedure, in which a practitioner establishes an appropriate state of mind, the therapist's hands are used to evaluate the energy flow. Undesirable energy is subsequently removed by sweeping hand movements, and beneficial energy is transferred from the practitioner to the treated individuals.

Studies in MS and Other Conditions

Many anecdotal reports document the benefits of therapeutic touch. However, limited clinical studies have been undertaken on this technique.

No large clinical studies of therapeutic touch have been conducted in multiple sclerosis (MS). One study of an individual with MS reported improvement in stress and coping after one session of therapeutic touch (1).

Therapeutic touch has been evaluated in many other conditions. Importantly, there are significant limitations to most of the therapeutic touch studies (2). Therefore, it is difficult to draw any firm conclusions. Some symptoms that may occur with MS have been evaluated. Several studies indicate that therapeutic touch may decrease anxiety. Mild beneficial effects have been reported for pain, tension headaches, burn-associated pain, and arthritis.

Therapeutic touch has undergone limited investigation for several other conditions. One study found that wounds heal more rapidly in those who receive therapeutic touch. Therapeutic touch is endorsed as a comfort-promoting technique by the National League for Nursing. Some of its benefits may be due to the attention and caring of the practitioner.

The validity of therapeutic touch was questioned in a well-publicized article in the *Journal of the American Medical Association* (JAMA) (3). In this study, a 9-year-old girl, Emily Rosa, along with several other investigators (including her mother and father) evaluated 21 therapeutic touch practitioners. Overall, the practitioners, when blindfolded, were not able to detect when their hands were near the hands of another individual. This study, which has been criticized for having significant methodological flaws, questions the conceptual basis of therapeutic touch.

In another study, it was found that people untrained in therapeutic touch could detect the location of an unseen hand if it was 3 or 4 inches away, but not 6 inches away. Also, at 3 inches, a glass shield led to an inability to detect hand location. The authors concluded that body heat, as opposed to an "energy field," was probably used to determine hand location (4).

Side Effects

No significant adverse effects occur after therapeutic touch. Some practitioners believe that excessive energy may be transferred if a session is too long.

Practical Information

Sessions typically last from 20 to 30 minutes and cost between $30 and $60. Practitioners of therapeutic touch may be found in the phone book under various listings: "therapeutic touch," "health services," "holistic centers," "holistic nurses," and "holistic practitioners." More information about therapeutic touch and practitioners may be obtained from:

- Council for Healing (www.councilforhealing.org), PO Box 76, Medford, NJ 08055 (609-714-1885)

- Therapeutic Touch International Association (www.therapeutic-touch .org), Box 130, Delmar, NY 12054 (518-325-1185)

Conclusion

Therapeutic touch is a low-risk, low- to moderate-expense technique. It has not undergone formal clinical trial testing in MS. Suggestive beneficial effects have been reported for anxiety and pain. However, the studies in this area have serious limitations and the underlying principles of therapeutic touch have been questioned. Further research is needed to determine the effectiveness of this therapy.

Additional Readings

Books

Ernst E, ed. *The Desktop Guide to Complementary and Alternative Medicine: An Evidence-Based Approach*. Edinburgh, UK: Mosby; 2001.

Leskowitz E. Therapeutic touch in neurology. In: Weintraub MI, Micozzi MS, eds. *Alternative and Complementary Treatments in Neurologic Illness*. New York, NY: Churchill Livingstone; 2001:234–240.

Micozzi MS, ed. *Fundamentals of Complementary and Alternative Medicine*. Philadelphia, PA: Saunders Elsevier; 2011:137–138.

Spencer JW, Jacobs JJ. *Complementary and Alternative Medicine: An Evidence-Based Approach*. St. Louis, MO: Mosby; 2003.

Synovitz LB, Larson KL. *Complementary and Alternative Medicine for Health Professionals*. Burlington, MA: Jones & Bartlett Learning; 2013:225–227.

Journal Articles

Agdal R, von B Hjelmborg J, Johannessen H. Energy healing for cancer: a critical review. *Forsch Komplementmed*. 2011;18:146–154.

Anderson JG, Taylor AG. Effects of healing touch in clinical practice: a systematic review of randomized clinical trials. *J Holist Nurs*. 2011;29:221–228.

Fazzino DL, Griffin MT, McNulty RS, Fitzpatrick JJ. Energy healing and pain: a review of the literature. *Holist Nurs Pract*. 2010;24:79–88.

Jain S, Mills PJ. Biofield therapies: helpful or hype? A best evidence synthesis. *Int J Behav Med*. 2010;17:1–16.

Krieger D. Healing with therapeutic touch. *Alt Ther.* 1998;4:87–92.

Long R, Bernhardt P, Evans W. Perception of conventional sensory cues as an alternative to the postulated 'human energy field' of therapeutic touch. *Sci Rev Alt Med.* 1999;3:53–61.

Monroe CM. The effects of therapeutic touch on pain. *J Holist Nurs.* 2009;27: 85–92.

O'Mathuna DP, Ashford RL. Therapeutic touch for healing acute wounds. *Cochrane Database Syst Rev.* 2012;6:CD002766.

Payne MB. The use of therapeutic touch with rehabilitation clients. *Rehabil Nurs.* 1989;14:69–72.

Robinson J, Biley FC, Dolk H. Therapeutic touch for anxiety disorders. *Cochrane Database Syst Rev.* 2007;18:CD006240.

Rosa L, Rosa E, Sarner L, et al. A close look at therapeutic touch. *JAMA.* 1998;279:1005–1010.

⊛ Tobacco and Smoking Cessation

Smoking increases the risk of many potentially fatal medical conditions. In the United States, more than 400,000 people die each year from tobacco-related illnesses. Tobacco is an important consideration in multiple sclerosis (MS). Smoking increases the risk of MS. Also, in those with MS, smoking may increase the severity of the disease and smoking-related illnesses may negatively impact neurological function and quality of life.

Treatment Method

There are many approaches to quit smoking. Successful quitting requires a plan and ongoing commitment. Smoking cessation should be discussed with a health care provider, such as a primary care provider. Some of the common smoking cessation strategies include:

- Medications
    - Medications decrease cravings and alleviate nicotine withdrawal symptoms. Many medication approaches use nicotine in some form, such as patches, gum, lozenges, inhalers, and nasal sprays. Other medication approaches include bupropion (Zyban) and varenicline (Chantix).

- Tapering Down or "Cold Turkey"
  - With these approaches, withdrawal and craving is common—as a result, some type of medication is usually needed.
- Group Support
  - Quitting may be facilitated by support from others, which may be in person, by phone, or online.
- Individual Counseling
  - This type of one-on-one support may be available with physicians, psychologists, nurses, or counselors.
- Telephone Quit Lines
  - This form of counseling is increasingly popular. It may be more accessible and more affordable than other counseling methods.

Studies in MS and Other Conditions

Smoking and MS have been researched extensively. One North American study of more than 5,000 people with MS found that 17% smoked, which is somewhat lower than the average smoking frequency of 20% in the U.S. population (1). Most studies have found that smoking increases the risk for developing MS by about 50% (2). More limited studies indicate that secondhand smoke also increases the risk for MS (3). In clinically isolated syndrome (CIS), a condition that puts people at risk for developing MS, smoking increases the risk for ultimately being diagnosed with MS (4). Among those with MS, smoking appears to increase the risk for converting from the type of MS with attacks ("relapsing-remitting MS") to the progressive form of the disease ("secondary progressive MS") (2). Also, some studies indicate that those who smoke have more severe disability (2,5). Finally, research indicates that smokers are more likely to develop antibodies that decrease the effectiveness of two types of MS disease-modifying medications, natalizumab (Tysabri) and interferons (Avonex, Betaseron, Extavia, and Rebif) (6,7). This finding indicates that these drugs may be less effective in those who smoke.

The other adverse health effects of smoking are extensive and may indirectly affect those with MS. Smoking harms nearly every organ of the body. It increases the risk of cancer of the lung as well as the bladder, cervix, esophagus, mouth, stomach, kidney, and uterus. Smoking causes heart disease, stroke, aneurysms, pneumonia, asthma, chronic obstructive pulmonary disease (COPD), and osteoporosis. Several of these diseases, such as heart disease and stroke, may increase the disability and lower the quality of life in people with MS. One study of people with MS found that the mortality rate was three times higher in those who smoked relative to those who did not smoke.

Conclusion

Smoking increases the risk of MS. In those with MS, smoking is common and may worsen the disease course. Also, smoking increases the risk for many conditions, such as heart disease and stroke, which, in combination with MS, may worsen neurological function and quality of life.

Additional Readings

Books

Bauer B, ed. *Mayo Clinic Book of Alternative Medicine and Home Remedies.* New York, NY: Time Home Entertainment; 2013:24–25.

Ciccolo JT, Jennings EG, Busch AM. Behavioral approaches to enhancing smoking cessation. In: Rippe JM, ed. *Lifestyle Medicine.* Boca Raton, FL: CRC Press; 2013:245–254.

Journal Articles

DiPauli F, Reindl M, Ehling R, et al. Smoking as a risk factor for early conversion to clinically definite multiple sclerosis. *Mutl Scler.* 2008;14:1026–1030.

Handel AE, Williamson AJ, Disanto G, Dobson R, Giovannoni G, Ramagopalan SV. Smoking and multiple sclerosis: an updated meta-analysis. *PLoS One.* 2011;6:e16149.

Hedstrom AK, Alfredsson L, Ludnkvist Ryner M, Fogdell-Hahn A, Hillert J, Olsson T. Smokers run increased risk of developing natalizumab antibodies. *Mult Scler.* 2013. [Epub ahead of print].

Hedstrom AK, Hillert J, Olsson T, Alfredsson L. Smoking and multiple sclerosis susceptibility. *Eur J Epidemiol.* 2013;28:867–874.

Hedstrom AK, Ryner M, Fink K, Fogdell-Hahn A, Alfredsson L, Olsson T, Hillert J. Smoking and risk of treatment-induced neutralizing antibodies to interferon beta-1a. *Mult Scler.* 2014;20:445–450.

Manouchehrinia A, Tench CR, Maxted J, Bibani RH, Britton J, Constantinescu CS. Tobacco smoking and disability progression in multiple sclerosis: United Kingdom cohort study. *Brain.* 2013;136:2298-2304.

Manouchehrinia A, Weston M, Tench CR, Britton J, Constantinescu CS. Tobacco smoking and excess mortality in multiple sclerosis: a cohort study. *J Neurol Neurosurg Psych.* 2014. doi:10.1136. [Epub ahead of print].

Marrie RA, Cutter G, Tyry T, Campagnolo D, Vollmer T. Smoking status over two years in patients with multiple sclerosis. *Neuroepidemiology.* 2009; 32:72–79.

Mikaeloff Y, Caridade G, Tardieu M, Suissa S; KIDSEP study group. Parental smoking at home and the risk of childhood-onset multiple sclerosis in children. *Brain.* 2007;130:2589–2595.

Ponsonby AL, Lucas RM, Dear K, et al. The physical anthropometry, lifestyle habits and blood pressure of people presenting with a first clinical demyelinating event compared to controls: the Ausimmune study. *Mult Scler.* 2013; 19:1717–1725.

Ramagopalan SV, Lee JD, Yee IM, et al. Association of smoking with risk of multiple sclerosis: a population-based study. *J Neurol.* 2013;260:1778–1781.

Wingerchuk DM. Smoking: effects on multiple sclerosis susceptibility and disease progression. *Ther Adv Neurol Disord.* 2012;5:13–22.

Toxins

(?) Aspartame Avoidance

(!) Dental Amalgam Removal

(!) Colon Therapy

(?) Other Toxin Avoidance or Removal

Over the years, it has been proposed that many toxins may cause multiple sclerosis (MS) or worsen its symptoms. Recent reports have associated MS with aspartame use and mercury from dental amalgam, both of which are discussed elsewhere in this book. It also has been claimed that MS is provoked by cosmetics or by chemicals in the environment in the form of pollution, aerosol sprays, low levels of formaldehyde, and fumes from solvents. In food, it has been claimed that additives and low levels of residual fertilizers and pesticides may be important. On the basis of concerns about toxic causes for MS and other diseases, an entire field known as *clinical ecology* has emerged.

Treatment Method

Many approaches have been proposed to decrease exposure to specific toxins or to decrease levels of toxins in the body. Avoiding aspartame in the diet and removing dental amalgam are sometimes recommended for people with MS (see the chapters on *Aspartame* and *Dental Amalgam Removal*). Other approaches claimed to be beneficial for MS include detoxifying therapies such as chelation therapy and colon therapy, also discussed elsewhere in this book (see chapters on *Chelation Therapy* and *Colon Therapy, Detoxification, and Enemas*).

Other toxin-related strategies that have been proposed are avoidance of processed foods, tap water, aerosol sprays, potent housecleaning products, synthetic fabrics, and gas appliances.

Studies in MS and Other Conditions

There is no strong scientific or clinical evidence that specific toxins or exposures—including metals, organic solvents, other chemical compounds, welding, or exposure to electromagnetic fields—play an important role in causing MS or worsening its symptoms. The possible role of metals has been explored over the past few decades. Concern about zinc or other metals in MS was raised by a study of workers at a manufacturing plant who were exposed to zinc and developed MS. However, subsequent studies have not shown a consistent association of MS with zinc exposure. Similarly, other studies have raised questions about copper, iron, selenium, and heavy metals such as mercury, but no definitive association of these metals to MS has been established. No well-documented links exist between MS and aspartame.

When considering possible toxins and toxic injury to the body, it is important to recognize that the body has powerful tools to defend itself against toxins. The liver has biochemical mechanisms for converting toxic chemicals to nontoxic chemicals, and the kidneys are able to remove potential toxins from the body by excreting them in the urine. In addition, all cells in the body, including nerve cells, are very resilient and have biochemical machinery for removing and inactivating toxins. Consequently, the chances of exposure to chemicals that can cause significant nervous system injury are believed to be extremely low, especially in developed countries.

Conclusion

No toxins have been identified that cause MS or provoke MS symptoms. Although a variety of techniques have been proposed to decrease toxin levels or to decrease exposure to toxins, no studies demonstrate that these techniques produce clinical benefits for people with MS.

Additional Readings
Books

Parry GJG. Neurological complications of toxin exposure in the workplace. In: Aminoff MJ, ed. *Neurology and General Medicine*. Philadelphia, PA: Churchill Livingstone; 2008.

Pryse-Phillips W, Costello F. The epidemiology of multiple sclerosis. In: Cook SD, ed. *Handbook of Multiple Sclerosis.* NewYork, NY: Marcel Dekker; 2001:15–31.

Tormoehlen LM, Rusyniak DE. Neurotoxicology. In: Biller J, ed. *Practical Neurology.* Philadelphia, PA: Lippincott Williams & Wilkins; 2012:636–651.

Journal Articles

Ghazavi A, Kianbakht S, Ghasami K, Mosayebi G. High copper and low zinc serum levels in Iranian patients with multiple sclerosis: a case control study. *Clin Lab.* 2012;58:161–164.

Ibrahim D, Froberg B, Wolf A, Rusyniak DE. Heavy metal poisoning: clinical presentations and pathophysiology. *Clin Lab Med.* 2006;26:67–97.

Schaumburg HH, Spencer PS. Recognizing neurotoxic disease. *Neurology.* 1987;37:276–278.

Sedighi B, Ebrahimi HA, Haghdoost AA, Abotorabi M. Comparison of serum levels of copper and zinc among multiple sclerosis patients and control group. *Iran J Neurol.* 2013;12:125–128.

Tsai CP, Lee CT. Multiple sclerosis incidence associated with the soil lead and arsenic concentrations in Taiwan. *PLoS One.* 2013;8:e65911.

?Tragerwork

Tragerwork is a form of bodywork. It is also known as Trager, the Trager approach, and Trager psychophysical integration. The technique was developed by Dr. Milton Trager, a physician as well as a boxer, acrobat, dancer, and follower of Maharishi Mahesh Yogi (see the chapter on *Ayurveda*). Tragerwork sometimes is recommended specifically for people with MS and other neurological disorders.

Treatment Method

Tragerwork is designed to change body habits that limit movement or produce muscle pain. Using this treatment, an individual lies on a table while a therapist uses light massage in combination with shaking, bouncing, and rocking movements of the body. This process is believed to produce relaxation and allow one to move with less effort and more grace. Tragerwork therapists also provide instruction in "Mentastics" (a shortened version of "mental gymnastics"), a regimen of self-directed movements that maintain the feelings developed in the treatment sessions. Tragerwork attempts to increase freedom of movement through these methods.

Studies in MS and Other Conditions

Although Tragerwork sometimes is recommended for people with multiple sclerosis (MS), it has not been specifically investigated in this area or in any medical condition. There are anecdotal reports of benefit in people with MS, but few published studies have evaluated the effects of Tragerwork on any medical condition. One study found that people with lung disease had improvement in some measures of lung function after Tragerwork (1). The significance of this finding is not clear because the study was small and did not include a placebo-treated control group. In another preliminary study of headache, which did include a control group, Trager treatment was associated with decreased headache frequency, improvement in the quality of life, and decreased use of headache medication (2). In a study of people with spinal cord injury and shoulder pain from wheelchair use, shoulder pain was decreased with either acupuncture or Tragerwork (3).

Side Effects

Limited clinical studies have evaluated the effects of this therapy. Generally it appears to be well tolerated, but people with MS may experience dizziness and nausea with the rocking movements.

Practical Information

Sessions typically last 60 to 90 minutes and cost between $50 and $70. A series of treatment sessions often is recommended. More information about Tragerwork may be obtained from:

- United States Trager Association (www.tragerus.org)
- Trager International (www.trager.com)

Conclusion

Tragerwork is a low-risk, moderate-cost form of bodywork. Although there are anecdotal reports of beneficial effects from this therapy, it has not been formally studied in MS. Preliminary studies indicate that it may improve headaches, decrease shoulder pain, and improve lung function.

Additional Readings
Books

Jellin JM, Gregory PJ, Batz F, et al. *Pharmacist's Letter/ Prescriber's Letter Natural Medicines Comprehensive Database*. Stockton, CA: Therapeutic Research Faculty; 2014.

Micozzi MS, ed. *Fundamentals of Complementary and Alternative Medicine*. Philadelphia, PA: Saunders Elsevier; 2011:227–228.

Journal Articles

Dyson-Hudson TA. Acupuncture and Trager psychophysical integration in the treatment of wheelchair user's shoulder pain in individuals with spinal cord injury. *Arch Phys Med Rehabil.* 2001;82:1038.

Foster KA, Liskin J, Cen S, et al. The Trager approach in the treatment of chronic headache: a pilot study. *Altern Ther Health Med.* 2004;10:40–46.

Juhan D. Multiple sclerosis: the Trager approach. *Trager Newsletter.* February 1993:1–7.

Witt PL, MacKinnon J. Trager psychophysical integration. A method to improve chest mobility of patients with chronic lung disease. *Phys Ther.* 1986;66:214–217.

Vitamins, Minerals, and Other Nonherbal Supplements

(?) Antioxidant Vitamins (vitamins A, C, and E)

(✓) Vitamin D and Calcium

(★) Vitamin B$_{12}$ (if vitamin B$_{12}$ deficient)

(?) Other B Vitamins

(✓) Multivitamins

(?) Minerals generally

(!) 5HTP

(?) ALCAR

(?) Alpha Lipoic Acid

(?) Amino Acids

(!) Androstenedione

(✓) Caffeine

(!) Calcium EAP

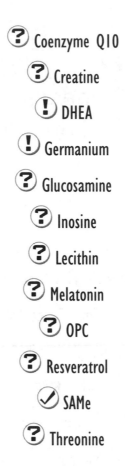

? Coenzyme Q10

? Creatine

! DHEA

! Germanium

? Glucosamine

? Inosine

? Lecithin

? Melatonin

? OPC

? Resveratrol

✓ SAMe

? Threonine

The use of vitamins, minerals, and other supplements is both popular and controversial. Surveys of people with multiple sclerosis (MS) indicate that the use of supplements is one of the most common forms of unconventional medicine. Much of their popularity probably is due to their accessibility. Supplements are easily purchased from grocery stores, health food stores, and drug stores, and using supplements does not require seeing a practitioner.

The potential benefits of supplements are frequently exaggerated by vendors and other proponents of supplements, and the possible uses of supplements in MS are sometimes based on incorrect information about the disease process. In conventional medicine, supplements have been viewed typically with skepticism. Supplements are now undergoing more serious investigation, and supplements are now recommended for preventing or treating a limited number of conditions on the basis of recent research studies.

Background Information

Vitamins are chemicals that are used for many of the body's fundamental chemical processes. In spite of the fact that they are present in only very small quantities, vitamins are absolutely necessary for normal body function. Thirteen vitamins are "essential," which means that the body does not have the biochemical machinery to synthesize them. These vitamins must therefore be consumed in the diet. Most vitamins come from animal or plant foods. The 13 essential vitamins are the eight B vitamins and vitamins A, C, D, E, and K. Most vitamins are water-soluble. The four fat-soluble vitamins are A, D, E, and K.

Minerals are also important for maintaining the body's fundamental chemical processes. Minerals originate in soil and water and are incorporated into plants and animals. The minerals needed in large quantities— known as "major minerals"—include calcium, chloride, magnesium, phosphorus, potassium, sodium, and sulfur. Those required in small quantities—the "trace elements"—include chromium, fluoride, iron, selenium, and zinc. A total of 18 trace elements are considered essential.

In addition to vitamins and minerals, other types of supplements are available. These include herbs, enzymes, hormones, antioxidants, and amino acids. Herbs and enzymes are discussed in other chapters (see the chapters on *Enzyme Therapy* and *Herbs*).

How Much Is Necessary for Health?

Much of the controversy in the supplement field centers around how much of a particular vitamin or mineral should be consumed daily. The Food and Nutrition Board of the National Academy of Sciences determines the Recommended Daily Allowances (RDAs), Adequate Intakes (AIs), or other similar values for vitamins and minerals (Table 3.13). These values are the daily intake needed to prevent deficiency and possibly provide health benefits.

Can Vitamins and Minerals Be Harmful?

Some proponents of supplements claim that the RDAs are too low and that higher daily doses, known as "megadoses," are needed. There is no evidence to support the use of megadoses. In fact, high doses of some vitamins and minerals may produce adverse effects (Table 3.14).

Many recent well-designed studies indicate that even modest doses of some vitamin and mineral supplements may produce significant adverse effects. Over the past 15 to 20 years, more than 20 studies have found mildly *increased* risk of death or serious medical conditions, such as heart disease and cancer, with the daily intake of modest doses of common dietary supplements, including multivitamins, vitamins A and E, beta-carotene, calcium, folate, iron, and selenium. The results of these studies provide a strong argument *against* a "shotgun approach" with supplements, which assumes that supplements are either beneficial or neutral in their effects and thus encourages the use of many different supplements. These recent studies highlight that supplements may actually have negative effects and therefore, if taken, should be used in a more limited and thoughtful "single-bullet" type of approach.

Another reason that supplements should be used on a limited basis is that, as with medications, complex interactions may occur with vitamins and minerals. For example, excessive vitamin C intake may affect the body's ability to absorb copper, and high doses of vitamin B_1 may produce deficiencies of vitamins B_2 and B_6. Also, calcium cannot be utilized for bone health without adequate levels of vitamin D.

How Should Vitamins and Minerals Be Consumed?—Food vs Supplements

For a healthy adult, a well-balanced diet should be adequate because it contains enough vitamins and minerals to meet the RDA. It is not clear that supplements are necessary in this situation. However, supplementation may play an important role in other circumstances. For example, in the case of malnourishment, which may occur in some people with MS, the diet is not well balanced or is low in quantity. Therefore, the RDA may not be met and supplementation is important. Also, people with certain conditions may benefit from vitamin or mineral doses that are higher than the RDA because they may not consume these doses in spite of a well-balanced diet. Examples of this situation are folic acid supplements for pregnant women.

There is growing evidence that food may be better able to provide health benefits than supplements. For example, fruits and vegetables, which are rich in antioxidants, appear to provide health benefits that cannot be duplicated by taking antioxidant supplements. There are several possible explanations for this difference between food and supplements. Relative to supplements, food contains many more chemical compounds, some of which have beneficial effects. Also, food provides other nutrients, such as fiber, that are generally not present in significant amounts in supplements. Finally, the slow absorption of vitamins, minerals, and other nutrients from food may be more beneficial than the relatively rapid absorption that occurs with supplements.

TABLE 3.13 RECOMMENDED DAILY ALLOWANCE (RDA), ADEQUATE INTAKE (AI), AND TOLERABLE UPPER INTAKE LEVELS (ULS) FOR ADULTS

	RDA/AI				
	MEN	**WOMEN**	**PREGNANT**	**LACTATING**	**UL**
VITAMINS Biotin (Vitamin B$_7$)	30 mcg	30 mcg	30 mcg	35 mcg	ND
Choline	550 mg	425 mg	450 mg	550 mg	3.5 g
Cobalamin (Vitamin B$_{12}$)	2.4 mcg	2.4 mcg	2.6 mcg	2.8 mcg	ND
Folate (Vitamin B$_9$)	400 mcg	400 mcg	600 mcg	500 mcg	1,000 mcg
Niacin (Vitamin B$_3$)	16 mg	14 mg	18 mg	17 mg	35 mg
Pantothenic acid (Vitamin B$_5$)	5 mg	5 mg	6 mg	7 mg	ND
Pyridoxine (Vitamin B$_6$)	1.3–1.7 mg	1.3–1.5 mg	1.9 mg	2.0 mg	100 mg
Riboflavin (Vitamin B$_2$)	1.3 mg	1.1 mg	1.4 mg	1.6 mg	ND
Thiamine (Vitamin B$_1$)	1.2 mg	1.1 mg	1.4 mg	1.4 mg	ND
Vitamin A	~3,000 IU	~2,300 IU	~2,500 IU	~4,300 IU	~10,000 IU
	(900 mcg)	(700 mcg)	(770 mcg)	(1,300 mcg)	(3,000 mcg)
Vitamin C	90 mg	75 mg	85 mg	120 mg	2,000 mg
Vitamin D	600–800 IU	600–800 IU	600 IU	600 IU	4,000 IU
	(15–20 mcg)	(15–20 mcg)	(15 mcg)	(15 mcg)	(100 mcg)
Vitamin E	22 IU	22 IU	22 IU	28 IU	1,500 IU
	(15 mg)	(15 mg)	(15 mg)	(19 mg)	(1,000 mg)

(continued)

TABLE 3.13 RECOMMENDED DAILY ALLOWANCE (RDA), ADEQUATE INTAKE (AI), AND TOLERABLE UPPER INTAKE LEVELS (ULS) FOR ADULTS (*continued*)

| | RDA/AI | | | | |
	MEN	**WOMEN**	**PREGNANT**	**LACTATING**	**UL**
Vitamin K	120 mcg	90 mcg	90 mcg	90 mcg	ND
MINERALS Calcium	1,000–1,200 mg	1,000–1,200 mg	1,000 mg	1,000 mg	2.5 g
Chromium	30–35 mcg	20–25 mcg	30 mcg	45 mcg	ND
Copper	900 mcg	900 mcg	1,000 mcg	1,300 mcg	10,000 mcg
Fluoride	4 mg	3 mg	3 mg	3 mg	10 mg
Iodine	150 mcg	150 mcg	220 mcg	290 mcg	1,100 mcg
Iron	8 mg	8–18 mg	27 mg	9 mg	45 mg
Magnesium	400–420 mg	310–320 mg	350–360 mg	310–320 mg	350 mg
Manganese	2.3 mg	1.8 mg	2.0 mg	2.6 mg	11 mg
Molybdenum	45 mcg	45 mcg	50 mcg	50 mcg	2,000 mcg
Phosphorous	700 mg	700 mg	700 mg	700 mg	3–4 g
Selenium	55 mcg	55 mcg	60 mcg	70 mcg	400 mcg
Zinc	11 mg	8 mg	11 mg	12 mg	40 mg

IU, international units; mcg, micrograms; mg, milligrams; g, grams; ND, not able to determine due to lack of information about adverse effects.

TABLE 3.14 DOSES OF VITAMINS AND MINERALS TO AVOID

VITAMINS AND MINERALS	DOSES TO AVOID
Vitamin A (beta-carotene)	Greater than 10,000 IU/d may produce multiple toxic effects, especially in pregnant women (birth defects)
Vitamin B₃ (niacin)	Greater than 35 mg/d may produce nausea, flushing, and other toxic effects
Vitamin B₆ (pyridoxine)	Greater than 50 mg/d may produce nerve injury

(*continued*)

TABLE 3.14 DOSES OF VITAMINS AND MINERALS TO AVOID (*continued*)

VITAMINS AND MINERALS	DOSES TO AVOID
Vitamin C	Greater than 2,500 mg/d may produce diarrhea and kidney stones
Vitamin D	Greater than 4,000 IU/d may produce kidney injury, excessive blood levels of calcium, and other toxic effects
Vitamin E	Greater than 1,000 mg (1,500 IU)/d may produce bleeding complications, upset stomach, and fatigue
Selenium	Greater than 400 mcg/d may produce multiple toxic effects

Supplements and MS

Supplements are one of the most popular forms of unconventional medicine used by people with MS. However, they are sometimes used inappropriately. For example, recommendations are sometimes haphazard and random—little or no justification may be given for a long (and expensive!) list of supplements. When a justification is given, it is sometimes stated that MS is an immune disease and that immune-stimulating supplements are therefore needed. In fact, MS is an immune disease, but it is characterized by too *much*, not too little, immune activity. As a result, immune-stimulating supplements actually may be harmful for MS. Similarly, supplements that may affect the immune system are sometimes recommended for MS as well as cancer and AIDS. Once again, all three diseases do involve the immune system, but people with cancer and AIDS may benefit from *stimulation* of the immune system, whereas people with MS may benefit from its *suppression*.

It is sometimes mistakenly assumed that if a deficiency of a vitamin or mineral impairs the function of the immune system or nervous system, then an excess of that same vitamin or mineral is beneficial to the immune system or nervous system and thus is therapeutic for MS. In other words, it is assumed that if a little is good, then a lot is better. In fact, as noted, high doses of vitamins and minerals are generally not beneficial and may actually cause harm.

A good example of this dosing issue as it relates to the nervous system is that of vitamin B_6 (pyridoxine). A deficiency of vitamin B_6 impairs nervous-system function. However, an excess of vitamin B_6 also *injures* the nervous system and may actually produce symptoms similar to those of MS. Thus, for vitamin B_6 and the nervous system, a normal level is desirable, and either a deficiency or an excess may be harmful.

The effect with vitamin B$_6$, in which a mid-range level is preferable to an extremely high or low level, is observed with multiple vitamins and minerals. This type of effect is sometimes referred to as the *Goldilocks Phenomenon* or the *Goldilocks effect* because it is similar to Goldilocks's experience of finding porridge and beds that are "just right" after trying ones that are extreme in one direction (too cold, too small) or the other (too hot, too large).

In the case of immune-system function, seemingly paradoxical situations may arise with regard to supplement doses. For example, vitamin B$_7$ (biotin) is important for maintaining a healthy immune system. However, a *deficiency* of vitamin B$_7$ appears to be *beneficial* for animals with experimental allergic encephalomyelitis (EAE), an experimental form of MS. On the other hand, supplementation with either selenium or zinc, two minerals also involved in immune-system function, may worsen EAE. On the basis of this limited scientific information, it could be argued that a state of deficiency of immune-relevant vitamins and minerals may be beneficial for MS, and a state of excess of these nutrients may be harmful. These examples illustrate the complexities of vitamin and mineral dosing for specific diseases such as MS.

Vitamin and mineral supplements are clearly necessary for people with MS who have an inadequate diet. This may occur for a variety of reasons, and may be particularly prevalent in those with more severe disability. With a poor diet, supplementation is essential to ensure an adequate intake of essential nutrients.

The most conservative approach to supplement use in MS is to avoid all supplements (except in people who clearly are nutritionally deficient). The rationale behind this view is that the effectiveness and safety of supplements has not been fully investigated in MS.

Dietary Supplements That Are Relevant to MS

The remainder of this chapter will provide background information as well as safety and effectiveness information on a wide range of MS-relevant dietary supplements.

Vitamins
(?)Antioxidant Vitamins Generally (Vitamins A, C, and E)
Relevance to MS

Among all categories of dietary supplements, antioxidant vitamins are among those used most frequently. Antioxidant vitamins include:

- Vitamin A or beta-carotene (a chemical converted to vitamin A)
- Vitamin C
- Vitamin E

These vitamins act on *free radicals*, chemicals that can damage cells in the brain and other organs of the body. For years, it has been proposed that free radicals are involved in aging, aging-related diseases, and many other conditions, including MS.

Antioxidants have various actions on the immune system and nervous system. Some of these effects could be beneficial for people with MS because, as indicated by several lines of evidence, free radicals and antioxidants may play an important role in MS:

- In MS, free radicals are involved in damage to the nerve fibers, known as axons, and also in injury to the myelin, the insulation-like coating on axons.

- In the animal model of MS (EAE), free radicals are involved in the disease process and the severity of the condition is decreased by several different types of antioxidant compounds, including vitamin A-related compounds, vitamin C, alpha-lipoic acid, and plant compounds known as "polyphenols," such as blueberries and green tea.

- Dimethylfumarate (Tecfidera), one of the MS disease-modifying medications, may produce its therapeutic effects by activating *Nrf 2*, a free radical-fighting system in cells.

Clinical trials of antioxidants in people with MS are limited. One older study found that antioxidant use (vitamin C, vitamin E, and selenium) for 5 weeks in 18 people with MS did not produce any clear beneficial or harmful effects (1). However, this was too short and small to be conclusive. More recent, but limited, clinical trials have not produced clear beneficial effects with antioxidants. One antioxidant compound, inosine, produced mixed results in two studies (2,3).

Although there is evidence that antioxidants may be beneficial for MS, theoretical reasons exist why antioxidants could be *harmful* for MS. Several antioxidants stimulate components of the immune system, including cells known as *macrophages* and *T cells*, which could, in theory, worsen the disease or antagonize the effects of MS disease-modifying medications. As noted, however, animal and human studies of antioxidants have generally suggested beneficial or uncertain effects rather than any clear adverse effects. There is one study of resveratrol, a grape-derived antioxidant, that produced worsening of EAE (see following section on *Resveratrol*).

With limited information about antioxidant safety and effectiveness in people with MS, it is reasonable for people with MS to be thoughtful about how they consume antioxidants. One reasonable approach is to *not* take antioxidant supplements, but rather to obtain antioxidants through food, specifically fruits and vegetables. Individualized information about fruit and vegetable intake may be obtained at www.mypyramid.gov (see the chapter on *Fats: Fish Oil and Polyunsaturated Fatty Acids*). General daily recommendations are two to four servings of fruits and three to five servings of vegetables. This food-based approach may result in adequate, but not excessive, levels of antioxidants, and may provide other health benefits more effectively than supplements.

If people with MS choose to use antioxidant vitamin supplements, it is reasonable to take modest doses. Modest daily doses of these vitamins are:

- Vitamin A—5,000 IU or less

- Vitamin C—90 to 120 mg or less

- Vitamin E—100 IU or less (For vitamin E, conversions may be made between the different forms and units. For lower, nontoxic doses, 1 mg of alpha-tocopherol = 1.5 IU of natural vitamin E = 2.2 IU of synthetic vitamin E. For higher and potentially toxic doses, 1 mg of alpha-tocopherol = 1.1 IU of synthetic vitamin E = 1.5 IU of natural vitamin E.)

High daily doses of certain antioxidants should definitely be avoided because of possible toxic side effects (see Table 3.14):

- Greater than 10,000 IU of vitamin A may produce multiple toxic effects (including headache, blurred vision, nausea, and liver injury) and, in pregnant women, may cause birth defects.

- Greater than 2,500 mg of vitamin C may cause diarrhea, abdominal bloating, and kidney stones.

- Greater than 1,000 mg (1,500 IU) of vitamin E may produce stomach upset, bleeding problems, and other difficulties.

Other important precautions about antioxidant vitamin use should be noted. In smokers or those with high levels of asbestos exposure, beta-carotene supplements may increase the risk of lung cancer, prostate cancer, brain hemorrhage, and overall risk of death. Vitamin E may inhibit blood clotting and thus should be avoided by people with bleeding disorders, people taking blood-thinning medications (such as warfarin or Coumadin), and people undergoing surgery. Vitamin C may decrease the effectiveness of blood-thinning medications.

Clinical trials of antioxidants in MS are underway or are being planned. The results from such studies will have important practical applications. If antioxidant supplements are found to be beneficial, they could be recommended. If they are found to be harmful, their use could be discouraged. If they have no effect, they could be avoided and money could be saved.

Vitamin E and Polyunsaturated Fatty Acids

It is sometimes recommended that people with MS increase their intake of polyunsaturated fatty acids (PUFAs), as discussed in the chapter on *Fats: Fish Oil and Polyunsaturated Fatty Acids*. PUFA intake may be increased by modifying the diet or by taking fatty acid supplements, such as evening primrose oil (EPO), sunflower oil, or fish oil. A potential problem with PUFAs is that they increase the need for vitamin E. As a result, if PUFAs are a large part of the diet, or if fatty acid supplements are taken, supplementation with a relatively small amount of vitamin E may be necessary. It is recommended that 0.9 to 1.3 IU of vitamin E should be taken for every gram of PUFAs consumed. Therefore, if one consumes about 25 g of PUFAs daily, 20 to 30 IU of vitamin E are needed daily. It is sometimes recommended that people take very high vitamin E doses (2,000 IU or higher) if they are supplementing with PUFAs—as can be seen from these calculations, such high doses are not needed. For most people who are enriching their diet with PUFAs, 100 IU of vitamin E should be more than adequate to protect against vitamin E deficiency.

Vitamin E is present in some PUFA preparations, including EPO. The label on the bottle of EPO should indicate the content of vitamin E.

Vitamin C
The Common Cold

It is sometimes claimed that vitamin C prevents or decreases the severity of the common cold. This is potentially important to people with MS, because viral infections may trigger MS attacks. However, the effects of vitamin C on the common cold are unclear. Also, because vitamin C stimulates the immune system, high doses of vitamin C supplements are theoretically risky for people with MS. Because of its unclear effects on treating the common cold, and its theoretical risks for worsening MS, it is reasonable for people with MS to be cautious about vitamin C use. If vitamin C is used, orange juice (50 mg of vitamin C per half cup of orange juice) or supplements in low doses (90–120 mg or less daily) may be reasonable.

Urinary Tract Infections

Vitamin C supplements are sometimes recommended for preventing or treating urinary tract infections (UTIs), which occur frequently in some women with MS. This recommendation is based on the idea that vitamin C, also known as ascorbic acid, makes the urine acidic and thus inhospitable for bacteria. However, there is no definitive evidence that the use of vitamin C supplements produces acidic urine or decreases the chance of developing a UTI. More evidence exists for cranberry juice (see the chapter on *Herbs*) than for vitamin C in preventing UTIs. If an actual infection is present, prescription antibiotics should definitely be used, because people with MS may have serious complications from UTIs.

⊘Vitamin D and Calcium

Vitamin D has two important properties that are relevant to MS. First, it is involved in maintaining bone density, and people with MS are at risk for decreased bone density. Also, vitamin D acts to regulate the immune system and may therefore have beneficial effects on the disease process of MS. A possible association between MS and vitamin D deficiency was first proposed in the early 1970s.

Studies over the past decade indicate that many people in the United States and other countries have low vitamin D levels. This may be due to a combination of factors:

- Decreased sun exposure and use of sunblock: Both of these approaches have been promoted for skin cancer prevention and have been effective in that regard.

- Obesity: Vitamin D is a fat soluble, which means that it will be taken up by body fat and may not be available for other purposes.

- Decreased consumption of vitamin D-enriched foods: One of the main sources of vitamin D is vitamin D-enriched dairy products, and there is decreased consumption of these products, especially in younger people.

Vitamin D is considered a hormone as well as a vitamin. A crucial step in the formation of vitamin D is sun exposure. In the skin, the energy of sunlight is used in a chemical reaction that produces the active form of vitamin D. Consequently, sunlight is necessary for adequate vitamin D production, and inadequate sunlight may lead to vitamin D deficiency. Only 10 to 15 minutes of casual sunlight exposure daily is needed.

Vitamin D is well recognized for its role in maintaining the health of bones. Vitamin D and calcium work together to maintain bone density and strength. Low levels of vitamin D may lead to severely decreased bone density, a condition known as *osteoporosis*. A less severe form of decreased bone density is referred to as *osteopenia*.

Although studies of osteoporosis often focus on elderly women, it is increasingly recognized that osteoporosis affects many other population groups. Among people with MS, several possible risk factors exist for osteoporosis and low vitamin D levels:

- People with MS are more likely to be women and to be less physically active than the general population—women and inactive people are at increased risk for osteoporosis.

- It has been reported that vitamin D intake is inadequate in 80% of people with MS, and that blood levels of vitamin D are low in people with MS.

- Forty percent of people with MS have no sunlight exposure in an average week.

- Steroids, which are sometimes used to treat MS attacks, may cause osteoporosis. The significance of this steroid effect is unclear in people with MS.

Given these multiple factors, one would expect an increased prevalence of osteoporosis and bone fractures in people with MS. In fact, this has been found in several studies. Bone density is decreased in people with MS, and the loss of bone density over time is greater in people with MS than in the general population.

An overall increased risk of fractures and an increased risk of fractures with no known trauma, which is indicative of osteoporosis, exist in MS.

In addition to its effects on bone, vitamin D has important regulatory actions on the immune system. These actions may affect the risk of developing MS and also, like the Food and Drug Administration (FDA)-approved MS medications, have disease-modifying effects.

Vitamin D's relation to MS risk has been studied in EAE, the animal model of MS, and in people with MS. In EAE, vitamin D supplementation prevents or delays the onset of the disease. In studies of large groups of people (known as *epidemiologic studies*), increased sunlight exposure has been associated with decreased risk of developing MS or dying from MS. Also, epidemiologic studies have shown that the risk of developing MS is lower in those who take vitamin D supplements or have high blood levels of vitamin D (4–6).

EAE and human studies have also examined the possible disease-modifying effect of vitamin D. In EAE, vitamin D supplementation slows progression of the disease, whereas vitamin D deficiency worsens the disease. In people with MS, many studies have associated low vitamin D levels with increased risks for new MRI lesions, attacks, and progression of disability. Also, several studies have evaluated people with clinically isolated syndrome ("CIS"), a condition that puts one at risk for developing MS, and have found that CIS is more likely to develop into MS if vitamin D levels are low (4–6).

It is important to recognize that the vast majority of the studies of vitamin D and MS have been *observational*. In these types of studies, vitamin D levels are associated with a particular factor, such as risk for attack or for progression of disability. These studies allow one to *associate* low vitamin D levels with various aspects of MS. However, these studies do not allow one to determine or state that low vitamin D levels definitely *cause* attacks or progression of disability.

To make a definite causal connection, it is necessary to do studies that are *interventional*. These studies are typically in the form of clinical trials in which one group is treated with a therapy (such as vitamin D), another group is treated with placebo, and then both groups are monitored closely for disease activity and for side effects over time. Only a limited number of clinical trials of vitamin D in MS have been conducted at this time. These studies are of variable quality. Also, the results of the studies have not been consistent—some have indicated beneficial effects while others have not (7–9). As a result, despite many promising observational studies, the effects of vitamin D on the course of MS have not been established. Large, well-designed clinical trials of vitamin D in MS are needed and are currently underway.

With limited information in this area, several strategies are reasonable. For those who have definite osteoporosis or osteopenia, supplements of vitamin D and calcium should be taken. For those who are considering vitamin D for its possible disease-modifying effects on MS, there are several approaches. One approach is to wait until more information is available. Another approach is to "blindly" take vitamin D supplements—the concern with this approach is that it may lead to unnecessary or inadequate supplement use. The final strategy is to do a standard blood test, known as "25-hydroxyvitamin D," to determine the vitamin D level. Levels are expressed in "nanograms per milliliter" or "ng/mL." Many clinical laboratories define "sufficient" levels as 30 to 100 ng/mL, "insufficient" levels as 20 to 30 ng/mL, and levels below 20 ng/mL as "deficient." If the level is insufficient or deficient, then supplements may be taken.

Supplements of vitamin D usually are taken with calcium. The RDA of vitamin D is 600 to 800 IU daily, while that of calcium is 1,000 to 1,200 mg daily. If vitamin D and calcium supplements are taken, the doses should be discussed with a physician or other health care provider. For those with osteoporosis, prescription medications and, in postmenopausal women, hormone replacement therapy may be indicated—intermittent bone-density testing (*bone densitometry*) may also be indicated.

Vitamin D is generally well tolerated. It has long been recognized that very high doses of vitamin D may cause fatigue, abdominal cramps, nausea, vomiting, kidney damage, high blood pressure, and multiple other toxic effects. However, more recent studies suggest that even moderately high vitamin D doses (more than 4,000 IU daily) or moderately high vitamin D levels (greater than 55 ng/mL) could have adverse effects, such as slightly *increased* risk of falls, fractures, cancer, heart disease, and death. Thus, it appears that there may be a desirable mid-range for vitamin D levels (30–55 ng/mL) and that there may be negative health effects with levels that are below as well as above this range—this would be consistent with the *Goldilocks Effect*, which, as noted, occurs with vitamin B_6 and several other vitamins and minerals.

Calcium supplements are also generally safe. High doses of calcium supplements have been associated with increased prostate cancer risk in some, but not all, studies. Also, calcium should not be taken with iron because these minerals may interfere with each other's absorption.

★Vitamin B_{12}

For years, it has been proposed that vitamin B_{12} deficiency plays a role in MS. Vitamin B_{12} is important for maintaining normal nerve function, and low levels of vitamin B_{12} may produce injury to the optic nerves and the spinal cord, two components of the nervous system that also are damaged in MS. However, this does not mean that vitamin B_{12} deficiency and MS are similar diseases.

It is sometimes assumed that people with neurologic diseases such as MS should take vitamin B_{12} supplements because vitamin B_{12} deficiency causes neurologic injury. This is not a logical argument. Low levels of vitamin B_{12} are harmful to nerves, but no evidence suggests that high levels are any better for nerve function than are normal levels. Of note, a small study of six people with progressive MS found that massive doses of vitamin B_{12} taken for 6 months did not produce any improvement in disability (10).

In another study of 138 people with MS, treatment was for 24 weeks using vitamin B_{12} alone or with the *Cari Loder regime*, which uses vitamin B_{12} along with two other compounds, phenylalanine and lofepramine (11,12). After 2 weeks of treatment, both groups showed mild neurological improvement. Those treated with the *Cari Loder regime* had mild additional neurological improvement and symptom relief. The significance of the relatively small treatment effects seen in this study is not clear.

Studies of vitamin B_{12} levels in people with MS have produced variable results. It is clear from these studies that the majority of people with MS have normal vitamin B_{12} levels. There may be a small subgroup of people with MS who have low vitamin B_{12} levels. The cause for this low level in some people with MS is not known.

It has recently been recognized that the risk of vitamin B_{12} deficiency is increased in those who use commonly prescribed medications. This effect is seen with drugs used to treat heartburn and ulcers, including *proton pump inhibitors*, such as omeprazole (Prilosec), and *H2 antagonists*, which include cimetidine (Tagamet). An oral diabetes medication known as metformin (Glucophage) also increases the risk of vitamin B_{12} deficiency.

People with suspected MS should be evaluated for vitamin B_{12} deficiency because of the rare association of vitamin B_{12} deficiency and MS. Vitamin B_{12} levels should be evaluated through blood testing ordered by a physician or other health care provider. If the vitamin B_{12} level is normal, no further vitamin B_{12} testing is required, and vitamin B_{12} supplements are not necessary. If the vitamin B_{12} level is low, further testing may be needed, and vitamin B_{12} injections or pills may be indicated. The usual treatment for vitamin B_{12} deficiency is oral supplements or injections. Lifetime therapy is often necessary, and follow-up vitamin B_{12} testing may be indicated on an intermittent basis. Although vitamin B_{12} supplements are generally well tolerated, they may in rare instances cause itching, diarrhea, and rashes.

⑦ Other B Vitamins

For unstated or illogical reasons, B vitamin supplementation sometimes is recommended for MS. The B vitamins include vitamin B_1 (thiamine), vitamin B_2 (riboflavin), vitamin B_3 (niacin), vitamin B_5 (pantothenic acid), vitamin B_6 (pyridoxine), vitamin B_7 (biotin), vitamin B_8 (cobalamin), and folate (or folic acid).

One small study found that high doses of thiamine relieved MS-associated fatigue. Further studies are needed in this area.

B vitamins are sometimes recommended because they play an important role in the functioning of both the immune system and the nervous system. It is recognized that deficiencies of several of the B vitamins can produce serious disorders of the immune system and the nervous system. However, because deficiencies produce abnormalities, it should not then be assumed that high intake amounts are better than normal intake levels.

Folic acid may play a role in regulating immune function. Research shows no consistent findings of decreased levels of folic acid in people with MS. In addition, no clinical studies demonstrate that supplements of folic acid are beneficial for MS. For people who take methotrexate, a chemotherapy agent occasionally used to treat MS, the toxic effects of the drug may be decreased by taking folic acid supplements.

At this time, no research evidence demonstrates that people with MS in general benefit from B vitamin supplementation. As noted in the section on vitamin B_{12}, a small subgroup of people with MS have vitamin B_{12} deficiency and should be treated. High doses of the other B vitamins should be avoided. In particular, excessive doses of vitamin B_6 (pyridoxine) and vitamin B_3 (niacin) should be avoided:

- More than 50 mg daily of vitamin B_6 (pyridoxine) may produce nerve injury. This may result in numbness and tingling in the hands and feet, which is similar to symptoms that may be experienced with MS. A theoretical risk also exists of immune stimulation with high doses of vitamin B_6.

- Greater than 35 mg of vitamin B_3 (niacin) daily may produce flushing, nausea, liver injury, and increased blood sugar levels.

✅ Multivitamins

Multivitamins frequently are taken by people with MS. Multivitamin preparations contain variable types and amounts of vitamins and minerals.

No rigorous clinical studies have examined the benefits or safety of multivitamin use in MS. Studies in the elderly indicate that multivitamin preparations may stimulate the immune system. This type of stimulation may theoretically be harmful for MS. However, the significance of this immune-system effect for a disease process such as MS is not clear at this time.

Multivitamins may be particularly beneficial for those with special nutritional needs or a diet that does not provide adequate intake of basic nutrients such as vitamins and minerals:

- People with a generally "unhealthy" diet
- People on restricted diets
- Strict vegetarians
- People with gastrointestinal conditions or other nutrient-depleting diseases, such as cancer or diabetes
- Women who are pregnant or are trying to become pregnant

Standard multivitamin supplements should typically contain 18 nutrients—11 vitamins and 7 minerals:

- Vitamins—Vitamins A, B_1 (thiamine), B_2 (riboflavin), B_3 (niacin), B_6 (pyridoxine), B_{12}, C, D, E, K; folic acid
- Minerals—Calcium, copper, magnesium, phosphorous, potassium, selenium, zinc

A multivitamin preparation is important for people with MS who have an inadequate intake of vitamins and minerals. For people with MS who have an adequate diet, the benefits of multivitamin preparations are not known. If multivitamins are taken, it is important to review the amount of each vitamin and mineral in a preparation. Obviously, toxic doses should be avoided (see Table 3.14). Commercially available multivitamins do not generally contain toxic doses of any compounds, but some high-potency "designer" multivitamins may contain high doses of particular vitamins or minerals. For people with MS, it may be logical, although of no proven benefit, to use low doses of potentially immune-stimulating vitamins and minerals, including vitamin A, vitamin C, vitamin E, selenium, and zinc. Low daily doses of these vitamins and minerals are:

- Vitamin A—5,000 IU or less
- Vitamin C—90 to 120 mg or less
- Vitamin E—100 IU or less
- Selenium—20 to 55 mcg or less
- Zinc—10 to 15 mg or less

⑦ Minerals

Calcium

Calcium supplements are sometimes recommended for MS, often for unstated reasons. Calcium supplements should be taken by people with inadequate dietary intakes of calcium. Also, calcium and vitamin D supplements are indicated for people with MS who have osteoporosis or risk factors for osteoporosis (see "Vitamin D and Calcium" in this chapter). No other clear uses are apparent for calcium supplements in MS. It should be noted that calcium interferes with iron absorption. Consequently, calcium and iron supplements should not be taken together.

Selenium

Selenium is a mineral sometimes recommended for MS. This recommendation may be based on its known antioxidant activity or on studies suggesting that people with MS have low selenium levels. It is not clear that selenium is a reasonable supplement for people with MS.

As noted in the section on antioxidant vitamins, antioxidant compounds may have several beneficial effects on MS. However, most antioxidant compounds, including selenium, activate the immune system, and this immune-system stimulation may conceivably worsen MS. In fact, in one study of animals with EAE, an experimental form of MS, selenium supplementation *worsened* the disease course and *increased* the mortality rate. Also, the severity of the disease was the same for animals fed low-selenium and normal-selenium diets. The results of this study suggest that selenium supplementation may actually be harmful for people with MS.

The influence of selenium on MS itself is not known because no large study has ever directly examined the effects of selenium supplements on people with the disease. One small study found that treatment with selenium and several antioxidant vitamins did not produce adverse effects in people with MS. However, this study was too small (18 people) and too short in duration (5 weeks) to be definitive (1).

Because of the limited information about selenium, it is not clear whether selenium supplementation in MS produces beneficial effects, harmful effects, or no effects at all. It may be most reasonable for people with MS to avoid selenium supplements until more information is available. Selenium may be obtained in the diet from seafood, meat, and whole grains. If supplements are taken, it may be best to take low doses, such as 20 to 55 mcg or less daily. High doses (greater than 400 mcg) should be avoided because they may activate the immune system and may produce fatigue, nausea, dizziness, hair loss, tooth decay, and other problems.

Zinc

Zinc supplementation sometimes is recommended for MS. In fact, zinc phosphate was one of the earliest recommended therapies for MS. Zinc phosphate was used in the 1880s as a treatment by colleagues of Jean-Martin Charcot, a French neurologist who played a major role in defining MS as a disease. At this time, no clear reasons exist for people with MS to take zinc supplements.

Zinc may have beneficial effects on the common cold. Some, but not all, studies indicate that zinc lozenges shorten the duration of the common cold. However, zinc lozenges do not appear to be effective for preventing the common cold. The possible therapeutic effect of zinc is of potential importance to people with MS because the common cold and other viral infections may trigger MS attacks.

Zinc supplements are also sometimes recommended in MS because zinc is involved in the chemical pathway of PUFAs, as discussed in the chapter on *Fats: Fish Oil and Polyunsaturated Fatty Acids*. This chemical pathway has been implicated in MS. However, it is not known if the pathway is indeed involved in MS, and it is not known whether zinc supplements are necessary for this pathway to function normally.

It is important to recognize that zinc may actually *stimulate* the immune system. Zinc activates several different immune cells, including macrophages and T cells. In fact, zinc supplements appear to increase the amount of brain inflammation in EAE, an animal model of MS. This suggests that supplements in humans may worsen MS.

A possible toxic role for zinc was suggested by a report of a relatively high occurrence of MS in a zinc-related industry in New York. Blood levels of zinc were increased in people in this facility. Studies of zinc levels in other MS populations have produced inconsistent results: Some studies show high levels, but other studies indicate low levels. A *deficiency* of zinc produced *benefits* in a mouse model of lupus, an autoimmune disorder like MS. This finding is consistent with immune stimulation by zinc.

A high intake of zinc actually may cause a serious neurological disorder, known as *copper-deficiency myelopathy*, that may mimic MS. Multiple causes are known for this disorder, which has been recognized recently. One cause is a high intake of zinc that leads to high blood levels of zinc and low blood levels of copper. In this condition, as in MS, abnormalities occur in the spinal cord, and people may experience difficulties with walking and sensation.

Immune-system activation by zinc could worsen MS. Given the fact that zinc has unclear benefits and that it may potentially stimulate the immune system, it is reasonable for people with MS to avoid zinc supplements or to use low doses of supplements—such as 10 to 15 mg or less daily.

⑦ Other Minerals

A whole variety of minerals sometimes are recommended for people with MS. Some studies indicate that people with MS have low levels of specific minerals, such as magnesium, zinc, and copper. The meaning of these results is not known. Before 1935, some recommended therapies for MS actually involved supplements of minerals, including antimony, arsenic, mercury, potassium bromide, potassium iodide, and thorium. At this time, no published clinical studies demonstrate a definite therapeutic effect in MS using supplements of these or other minerals, including chromium, cobalt, copper, iodine, magnesium, molybdenum, phosphorus, potassium (in various forms), and vanadium. Finally, gold or silver supplements have been recommended for MS. These are of no proven benefit, and silver supplements may actually produce serious toxic effects.

Other Supplements
⊘5-hydroxytryptophan

5-hydroxytryptophan (5-HTP) is a type of chemical known as an amino acid. It is chemically similar to another amino acid, tryptophan. 5-HTP may be effective for treating depression. Tryptophan itself was sold for this use in the past. Unfortunately, contaminated batches produced a serious condition, *eosinophilia-myalgia syndrome*. Although this condition was thought to be due to contaminants known as *peak X*, and *peak X* is not present in some 5-HTP preparations, other toxic compounds may be involved. Due to these uncertainties and the fact that 5-HTP may contain some of the same contaminants as tryptophan, it is reasonable to avoid 5-HTP until more information is available.

⊘Acetyl-L-Carnitine

Acetyl-L-carnitine, sometimes referred to as *ALCAR*, is a compound that has been studied in people with memory difficulties and fatigue. (Note: *L-carnitine* is a different compound.) ALCAR may improve memory in people with Alzheimer's disease and other memory disorders, and it also may decrease fatigue in people with a variety of conditions.

Due to its possible fatigue-relieving effects, ALCAR has been evaluated in two MS clinical trials. One study of 36 people with MS evaluated the effect of ALCAR on two measures of fatigue—one measure was improved while the other was not (13). Another study of 60 people with MS did not find any significant fatigue-relieving effect (14).

ALCAR usually is well tolerated. It may cause nausea, vomiting, and agitation. Trials with ALCAR have used doses of 1,500 to 4,000 mg daily, which is usually divided into two or three doses.

⊘Alpha-Lipoic Acid

Alpha-lipoic acid is an antioxidant compound. Like the antioxidant vitamins, alpha-lipoic acid acts to decrease the damage produced by free radicals.

Alpha-lipoic acid normally is present in the *mitochondria*, the energy-producing parts of the body's cells.

Alpha-lipoic acid may have relevance to neurological disorders, including MS. Encouraging results with alpha-lipoic acid have been obtained in animal and human studies by Dr. Dennis Bourdette and others at Oregon Health Sciences University (OHSU) (15,16). In EAE, the animal model of MS, alpha-lipoic acid decreases the severity of the disease. This appears to be due to the ability of alpha-lipoic acid to inhibit the movement of immune cells from the blood into the central nervous system. In a small study in people with MS, alpha-lipoic acid was generally well tolerated and appeared to inhibit two proteins involved in immune-cell movement into the central nervous system *(MMP-9* and *sICAM-1)*.

Some studies indicate that alpha-lipoic acid may be helpful for diabetes itself and also for a diabetes-associated form of nerve injury known as *polyneuropathy*. Studies of alpha-lipoic acid in other neurologic conditions are currently being conducted. Limited information is available about the safety of alpha-lipoic acid, especially for long-term use and for use in people with MS.

⑦Amino Acids

Amino acids are chemicals used to synthesize proteins in the body. Mixtures of specific amino acids known as *branched-chain amino acids* sometimes are recommended for MS. There is no evidence that people with MS are deficient in amino acids or that amino acid therapy is beneficial for MS. Branched-chain amino acids do not appear to improve physical performance in athletes. Importantly, high doses may produce fatigue by increasing the amount of ammonia in the blood.

Specific amino acids have been studied for their effects on MS symptoms, MS itself, or the animal model of MS—these include 5-HTP and threonine. See the relevant sections for descriptions of these compounds.

⚠Androstenedione

Androstenedione became well known to the public after the baseball player Mark McGwire acknowledged that he used it in 1998. Androstenedione is a hormone sold as a dietary supplement. In the body, it is converted to testosterone, the male sex hormone. Androstenedione is of potential interest to people with MS because it is claimed to increase strength and energy.

However, clinical studies do not support its claimed benefits. The safety and effectiveness of androstenedione has not been studied in people with MS. It does not increase muscle strength or muscle size. It does not appear to increase testosterone levels on a long-term basis. It does increase estrogen levels, which may increase the risk of conditions and cancers that are sensitive to this hormone, including endometriosis, uterine fibroids, and cancers of the breast, uterus, ovaries, and prostate. Androstenedione decreases levels of high-density lipoprotein (HDL), the "good" form of cholesterol, and may thereby increase the risk of heart disease and stroke. Multiple other possible side effects may occur with androstenedione.

Androstenedione should be avoided because of its unclear benefits and its multiple possible side effects.

✓ Caffeine

Caffeine is of potential interest because MS may cause fatigue, and caffeine may improve mental alertness. Caffeine is available in tablet form as a dietary supplement. The use of these tablets, coffee, and other caffeine-containing herbs is discussed in the *Herbs* chapter.

！ Calcium EAP

In the early 1960s, Dr. Hans Nieper, a German physician, developed a compound known as calcium EAP. It is also known as calcium-2-aminoethyl phosphate, calcium AEP, and calcium orotate. Thousands of people have apparently been treated with this compound. Most information about calcium EAP is available only from literature by Dr. Nieper (who died in 1998) or organizations affiliated with him.

Calcium EAP is one component of an approach to MS referred to as the *Nieper regimen*. It is believed that calcium EAP allows necessary chemicals to interact with nerve cells and protects nerve cells from injury by the immune system and by toxins. Several other principles underlie the Nieper regimen, including claims that milk and several minerals (chlorine, chromium, fluoride, platinum) play an important role in MS.

The Nieper program recommends calcium EAP treatment along with other measures. Calcium EAP initially is given intravenously in a dosage of 500 mg/d for 5 d/wk. It is then given long term as a pill or as an every-other-day intravenous dose of 400 mg. Other recommendations include steroid treatment with prednisone (5–8 mg daily); vitamin and mineral supplements (some at high doses), including selenium and vitamins C, D, and E; avoidance of bright sunlight, alcohol, milk and milk products, EPO, aluminum, fluoride, and drinks that contain phosphoric acid or quinine; avoidance of water in the environment by not using waterbeds and hiring a dowser to be certain no underground water exists near one's bedroom; and consumption of olive oil and raw food because of their *Kirlian positivity*.

No well-designed clinical trials of calcium EAP have been published. Calcium EAP was first used in Europe in 1964 and in the United States in 1972. A document written by Dr. Nieper in 1968 describes the treatment of 167 people with MS. Beneficial effects were observed in 46% with mild disease, 33% with moderate disease, and 16% with severe disease. The overall benefit was 32%. Importantly, no placebo group was used in this study. Other literature by Dr. Nieper claims benefits in 85% to 90% of people with MS. Overall, no well-designed studies exist to determine whether calcium EAP is beneficial for people with MS.

The safety of calcium EAP has not been established. Of concern is a 1990 report in which a 53-year-old woman with MS had an abrupt cessation of heart and lung function (cardiopulmonary arrest) during intravenous administration of calcium EAP. She was resuscitated and subsequently developed serious kidney, liver, and bleeding complications.

By Dr. Nieper's account, in animal studies, 1 in 10 animals develop kidney stones, females gain weight, and males become aggressive. Apparently, these side effects have not been observed in people. Some people treated with calcium EAP develop headaches and chills.

In conclusion, there is no rigorous published evidence that calcium EAP has beneficial effects in MS. Calcium EAP may be very costly. One report documents serious complications with intravenous use, and no studies document the safety of long-term use.

⑦ Coenzyme Q_{10}

Coenzyme Q_{10} is also known as *CoQ_{10}* or *ubiquinone*. Like some vitamins, coenzyme Q_{10} is an antioxidant that may decrease free radical damage. Also, coenzyme Q_{10} may improve the function of mitochondria, the energy-producing components of the body's cells.

Coenzyme Q_{10} use has been claimed to produce many different health benefits. Some of these claims are not justified. Coenzyme Q_{10} may have applications to neurological disorders, especially those that are thought to involve free-radical damage or impaired function of the mitochondria. Coenzyme Q_{10} may be beneficial for several heart problems, including a condition known as congestive heart failure.

No large published studies have evaluated the safety or effectiveness of coenzyme Q_{10} in people with MS. As for the antioxidant vitamins (see earlier in this section), coenzyme Q_{10} may have beneficial effects on MS. The effects of coenzyme Q_{10} on the immune system are not well understood.

The effects on MS of antioxidant supplements such as coenzyme Q_{10} are not known. If antioxidants are taken, vitamins A, C, or E are more economical than coenzyme Q_{10}. Coenzyme Q_{10} may decrease the effect of blood-thinning medication (warfarin or Coumadin). High doses of coenzyme Q_{10} (more than 300 mg daily) may cause mild liver toxicity.

⑦ Creatine

Creatine is a supplement claimed to increase muscle strength and increase body mass. In addition, it may have a protective effect on nerves. Both of these possible effects are relevant to MS.

Creatine is made in the liver, kidneys, and pancreas. It is involved in generating energy for muscle cells and other cells in the body. Creatine is available as a dietary supplement and may be obtained in the diet by eating meat and fish.

In healthy people, creatine supplements may improve performance for brief, high-intensity exercises. However, limited clinical studies of creatine in MS have not produced therapeutic effects. In one study of 16 people with MS, creatine supplements did not improve high-intensity exercise ability or increase the muscle stores of creatine (17). In another study of 11 people with MS, creatine did not increase muscle strength (18).

Creatine usually is well tolerated when used in appropriate doses. Rarely, creatine may cause kidney failure, especially in those with known kidney disease. Other possible side effects of creatine include stomach pain, nausea, diarrhea, weight gain, dehydration, and muscle cramping.

(!)Dehydroepiandrosterone

Dehydroepiandrosterone (DHEA) is a hormone available as a dietary supplement. It is marketed as an antiaging compound and as a"miracle cure"for many medical conditions. Claimed benefits of DHEA of potential interest to people with MS include improvement in fatigue, sex drive, and mood.

DHEA is a naturally occurring steroid hormone produced by the adrenal glands. DHEA may be important for aging because blood levels of DHEA generally decrease significantly as people get older.

DHEA has been studied in several medical conditions. However, there are not any clinical studies that have been done in MS. For aging skin, DHEA may have beneficial effects. Also, DHEA may improve certain types of erectile dysfunction—it does not appear to be effective for erectile dysfunction that is due to neurological conditions.

Limited information is available about the effects of DHEA on immune system-related diseases such as MS. In the animal model of MS, DHEA appears to have an anti-inflammatory effect and to decrease the severity of the disease. However, in other studies, DHEA promotes an immune response known as "Th1," which is "immune-stimulating" and has the potential to worsen MS or inhibit the therapeutic effects of MS disease-modifying medications. In another autoimmune disease, lupus, DHEA may be beneficial in the mouse model of the disease and for people with the disease. Additional research on the effects of DHEA in MS and other immunological diseases is needed.

DHEA has multiple possible adverse effects. It may cause liver injury. Other side effects include acne, hair loss, voice deepening, fatigue, altered menstruation, abdominal pain, hypertension, and increased risk of some hormone-sensitive cancers, including breast, endometrial, and prostate cancer. The safety of long-term DHEA use has not been established.

No strong reason exists for people with MS to take DHEA supplements. No definite benefits are associated with its use. Although encouraging results with DHEA have been noted in the animal model of MS, DHEA also carries a theoretical risk as a result of immune stimulation, and it may cause multiple adverse effects, especially in women.

Evening Primrose Oil

See chapter on *Fats: Fish Oil and Polyunsaturated Fatty Acids*.

Fish Oil

See chapter on *Fats: Fish Oil and Polyunsaturated Fatty Acids*.

Flaxseed Oil

See chapter on *Fats: Fish Oil and Polyunsaturated Fatty Acids*.

(!) Germanium

Germanium is a compound sometimes recommended as a therapy for MS. However, no studies of germanium in MS have been done. It is not known to be effective for any medical condition. It may cause significant side effects, including kidney failure, weakness, nerve injury, anemia, and death. There are more than 30 reports of significant germanium-related side effects, including death.

(?) Glucosamine

Glucosamine is a dietary supplement that is claimed to be effective for treating arthritis. Studies of this supplement on arthritis have been conflicting and have not shown that it has definite beneficial effects. In terms of MS relevance, glucosamine mildly suppresses the immune system—it appears to decrease the activity of the inflammatory component of the immune system (*Th1* response) and increase the activity of the anti-inflammatory component (*Th2* response). In EAE, the animal model of MS, glucosamine decreases disease severity (19). These findings are encouraging. One small study of people with MS did not show any effect of glucosamine on attack rate or disability progression (20). Further studies of glucosamine and MS are needed. Glucosamine generally is well tolerated. It may cause mild gastrointestinal side effects, such as gas, bloating, and cramps.

(?) Inosine

Inosine is a compound that is converted in the body to uric acid. Uric acid has antioxidant effects. Promising results have been obtained with uric acid treatment of the animal model of MS. Limited clinical trials of inosine in people with MS have produced variable results (2,3). Episodes of gout are caused by high blood levels of uric acid. As a result, raising blood levels of uric acid with inosine may provoke gout attacks. The safety of long-term inosine use is not known.

⑦ Lecithin

Lecithin, which contains phosphatidylcholine, is a supplement sometimes recommended for MS. Phosphatidylcholine is involved in several body processes, and it is a major component of cell membranes. Supplements of lecithin are made from soybean oil. At this time, there are no studies to indicate that lecithin therapy is beneficial to people with MS. Lecithin is usually well tolerated—it has been classified as Generally Regarded as Safe (GRAS) by the FDA. Lecithin may cause diarrhea, nausea, and abdominal pain. It may also cause skin reactions in people with egg and soy allergies.

⑦ Melatonin

Melatonin is a hormone produced in the *pineal gland*, a small gland in the brain. Melatonin is involved in regulating *circadian rhythms*, the regular daily cycles of the body, such as sleeping and waking. Blood levels of melatonin are high at night and low during the day.

Many therapeutic benefits have been claimed for melatonin. Most studies have evaluated its effects on sleeping problems. For several forms of insomnia, some, but not all, clinical investigations have shown a therapeutic effect with melatonin. Melatonin also may be effective for the prevention of jet lag.

A possible role of melatonin in causing MS has been proposed. In one study, high blood levels of melatonin were associated with a later age of onset of the disease and a shorter duration of the disease. The significance of these findings in relation to melatonin causing MS or the effect of taking melatonin supplements on MS is not known.

People with MS should be aware that melatonin may activate the immune system. The effects of melatonin on the immune system are not fully understood. However, specific immune cells called T cells have sites to which melatonin attaches, and some studies have shown that melatonin stimulates T cells. Paradoxically, in the animal model of MS, one study showed that melatonin improved the disease, whereas another study showed that luzindole, a compound that blocks the effects of melatonin, was also therapeutic—clearly, more work is needed in this area. Due to its immune-stimulating effects, it has been proposed that melatonin may worsen another autoimmune disease, rheumatoid arthritis, but be beneficial for AIDS and cancer.

Melatonin is generally well tolerated. It may cause daytime drowsiness, headache, and dizziness. Other reported side effects include mild depression, tremor, anxiety, abdominal cramps, irritability, decreased alertness, confusion, nausea, and vomiting. People should not drive or use machinery for 4 to 5 hours after taking melatonin.

In summary, melatonin may be helpful for insomnia and jet lag. However, it carries a theoretical risk for people with MS because it may stimulate the immune system. Until more information is available, it would be reasonable for people with MS to avoid melatonin or to use modest doses on a limited basis.

⑦Oligomeric Proanthocyanidins

Oligomeric proanthocyanidins (OPCs) are antioxidant compounds. They are one of the main components in several antioxidant supplements, including Pycnogenol and grape seed extract (see *Herbs* chapter). As noted in the sections on these products, it is not clear that the antioxidant effects of OPCs are beneficial to people with MS. Furthermore, they are more expensive than conventional antioxidant vitamins.

Polyunsaturated Fatty Acids

See chapter on *Fats: Fish Oil and Polyunsaturated Fatty Acids*.

⑦Resveratrol

Resveratrol is a compound that is present in red wine and the skin of red grapes. It is also found in blueberries, bilberries, and mulberries. Resveratrol has multiple biochemical actions, including antioxidant and anti-inflammatory effects, that could be beneficial for MS. However, there are not any well-designed clinical trials of resveratrol in MS. In EAE, the animal model of MS, some studies have shown therapeutic effects (21), but one study reported *worsening* (22). Further studies of resveratrol and MS are needed.

✓S-adenosylmethionine

S-adenosylmethionine (SAMe; also known as Sammy) is a supplement claimed to be an effective treatment for multiple medical conditions. SAMe is a naturally occurring compound involved in fundamental biochemical reactions called *methylation reactions*. These reactions also involve vitamin B_{12} and folic acid. SAMe has been commercially available for years in European countries, including Germany, Italy, and Spain. SAMe became available as a dietary supplement in the United States in the spring of 1999.

Multiple therapeutic effects have been attributed to SAMe. Multiple studies indicate that SAMe reduces depression, which is relevant to MS because depression occurs at some point in about 50% of people with MS. The mechanism by which SAMe may produce its antidepressant effect is not known. SAMe also may be effective for liver disease, fibromyalgia, a form of arthritis known as osteoarthritis, and a spinal cord condition that occurs in people with AIDS.

It has been claimed that SAMe may be a treatment for MS. This claim is based on several observations of uncertain significance. First, a small subgroup of people with MS has vitamin B_{12} deficiency. Because SAMe and vitamin B_{12} are involved in similar chemical reactions, it is proposed that SAMe is beneficial for MS. In addition, SAMe sometimes is used to treat some rare genetic diseases that produce injury to the nerve cells in a manner somewhat similar to the nerve damage produced by MS. However, these arguments for SAMe treatment of MS are not well grounded. There is no evidence that abnormalities in vitamin B_{12} or SAMe play a major role in MS.

SAMe is claimed to be a potential treatment for other neurologic disorders, including Parkinson's disease, Alzheimer's disease, and epilepsy. Current research does not support the use of SAMe for these conditions.

In general, SAMe appears to be well tolerated. Minor side effects include nausea, vomiting, diarrhea, constipation, dry mouth, mild insomnia, dizziness, and anxiety. SAMe should not be used with antidepressant medications. SAMe may decrease the effectiveness of the Parkinson's disease medication levodopa.

Depression is a serious condition, and anyone who feels that he or she is depressed should be evaluated by a physician. Treatment with SAMe—or any other antidepressant compound—should be done in conjunction with a physician. In clinical studies of depression, the daily dose of SAMe has been 400 to 1,600 mg.

⑦Threonine

Threonine is an amino acid that has been studied in people with MS who have muscle stiffness or spasticity. In the body, threonine is converted to another chemical, glycine, which could decrease spasticity. Limited research suggests that threonine improves stiffness as measured by formal clinical testing (23). However, this effect is so mild that it is not noticeable to people taking the compound or to examining clinicians.

Conclusion

Due to limited information about dietary supplements and MS, people with MS should be cautious in their use of supplements. Supplement use should be discussed with a health care provider.

There is a broad spectrum of effectiveness and safety information for MS-relevant supplements. In appropriate situations, some supplements may be worth considering, including vitamin D, vitamin B_{12}, and SAMe. On the other hand, some supplements should be avoided or used with caution, such as germanium, androstenedione, and DHEA. For many supplements, the information is too limited to be certain about their safety and effectiveness in MS.

Additional Readings
Books

Bauer B, ed. *Mayo Clinic Book of Alternative Medicine and Home Remedies.* New York, NY: Time Home Entertainment; 2013.

Bowling AC. Complementary and alternative medicine in multiple sclerosis. In Geisser B, ed. *Primer on Multiple Sclerosis*. New York, NY: Oxford University Press; 2011:369–381.

Bowling AC. Complementary and alternative medicine: practical considerations. In: Rae-Grant A, Fox R, Bethoux F, eds. *Multiple Sclerosis and Related Disorders: Diagnosis, Medical Management, and Rehabilitation*. New York, NY: Demos; 2013:243–249.

Campbell TC. *Whole: Rethinking the Science of Nutrition*. Dallas, TX: BenBella Books; 2013.

Duyff RL. *American Dietetic Association Complete Food and Nutrition Guide*. Boston, MA: Houghton Mifflin Harcourt; 2012.

Jellin JM, Batz F, Hitchens K, et al. *Natural Medicines Comprehensive Database*. Stockton, CA: Therapeutic Research Faculty; 2014.

Ross AC, Taylor CL, Yaktine Al, Del Valle HB, eds. *Dietary Reference Intakes for Vitamin D and Calcium*. Washington, DC: National Academies Press; 2011.

Ulbricht CE, Basch EM, eds. *Natural Standard Herb and Supplement Reference: Evidence-Based Clinical Reviews*. St. Louis, MO: Elsevier-Mosby; 2005.

U.S. Dept. of Agriculture and U.S. Dept. of Health and Human Services. *Dietary Guidelines for Americans, 2010*. Washington, DC: U.S. Govt. Printing Office; 2010.

Journal Articles

Anon. Dangerous supplements: what you don't know about these 12 ingredients could hurt you. *Consum Rep*. 2010;75:16–20.

Anon. Multivitamins: what to avoid, how to choose. *Consum Rep*. 2006;71:19–20.

Anon. Vitamins & supplements: 10 dangers that may surprise you. *Consum Rep*. 2012;77:18–23.

Autier P, Boniol M, Pizot C, Mullie P. Vitamin D status and ill health: a systematic review. *Lancet Diab Endocrinol*. 2014;2:76–89.

Bowling AC. Vitamin D: Dandy? Dastardly? Or Debatable? *Momentum*. Summer 2011;4:39–42.

Faridar A, Eskandari G, Sahraian MA, Minagar A, Azimi A. Vitamin D and multiple sclerosis: a critical review and recommendations on treatment. *Acta Neurol Belg*. 2012;112:327–333.

Gonsette RE, Sindic C, D'hooge MB, et al. Boosting endogenous neuroprotection in multiple sclerosis: the association of inosine and interferon-beta in relapsing-remitting multiple sclerosis (ASIIMS) trial. *Mult Scler*. 2010;16:455–462.

Goodman S, Gulick E. Dietary practices of people with multiple sclerosis. *Int J MS Care*. 2008;10:47–57.

Growdon JH, Nader TM, Schoenfeld J, Wortman RJ. L-threonine in the treatment of spasticity. *Clin Neuropharmacol*. 1991;14:403–412.

Hewer S, Lucas R, van der Mei I, Taylor BV. Vitamin D and multiple sclerosis. *J Clin Neurosci*. 2013;20:634–641.

Holmoy T, Torkildsen O, Myhr KM, Løken-Amsrud KI. Vitamin D supplementation and monitoring in multiple sclerosis: who, when and wherefore. *Acta Neurol Scand Suppl*. 2012;195:63–69.

Jafirarad S, Siassi F, Harirchian M-H, Amani R, Bitarafan S, Saboor-Yaraghi A. The effect of vitamin A supplementation on biochemical parameters in multiple sclerosis patients. *Iran Red Cresc Med J*. 2013;15:194–198.

James E, Dobson R, Kuhle J, Baker D, Giovannoni G, Ramagopalan SV. The effect of vitamin D-related interventions on multiple sclerosis relapses: a meta-analysis. *Mult Scler J*. 2013;19:1571–1579.

Kira J, Tobimatus S, Goto I. Vitamin B_{12} metabolism and massive-dose methyl vitamin B_{12} therapy in Japanese patients with multiple sclerosis. *Int Med*. 1994;33:82–86.

Lam JR, Schneider JL, Zhao W, Corley DA. Proton pump inhibitor and histamine 2 receptor antagonist use and vitamin B_{12} deficiency. *JAMA*. 2013;310:2435–2442.

Lambert CP, Archer RL, Carrithers JA, Fink WJ, Evans WJ, Trappe TA. Influence of creatine monohydrate ingestion on muscle metabolites and intense exercise capacity in individuals with multiple sclerosis. *Arch Phys Med Rehabil*. 2003;84:1206–1210.

Ledinek AH, Sajko MC, Rot U. Evaluating the effects of amantadine, modafinil, and acetyl-L-carnitine on fatigue in multiple sclerosis. *Clin Neurol Neurosurg. Suppl*. 2013;115:S86–S89.

Leweling H, Schwarz S. Multiple sclerosis and nutrition. *Mult Scler*. 2005;11:24–32.

Loder C, Allawi J, Horrobin DF. Treatment of multiple sclerosis with lofepramine, L-phenylalanine, and vitamin B_{12}: mechanism of action and clinical importance: roles of the locus coeruleus and central noradrenergic systems. *Med Hyp*. 2002;59:594–602.

Mai J, Sorensen PS, Hansen JC. High dose antioxidant supplementation to MS patients. *Biol Trace Elem Res*. 1990;24:109–117.

Malin SK, Cotugna N, Fang CS. Effect of creatine supplementation on muscle capacity in individuals with multiple sclerosis. *J Diet Suppl*. 2008;5:20–32.

Markowitz CE, Spitsin S, Zimmerman V, et al. The treatment of multiple sclerosis with inosine. *J Altern Complement Med*. 2009;15:619–625.

Marracci GH, Jones RE, McKeon GP, Bourdette DN. Alpha lipoic acid inhibits T cell migration into the spinal cord and suppresses and treats experimental autoimmune encephalomyelitis. *J Neuroimmunol*. 2002;131:104–114.

Mesliniene S, Ramrattan L, Giddings S, Sheikh-Ali M. Role of vitamin D in the onset, progression, and severity of multiple sclerosis. *Endocrin Pract.* 2013;19: 129–136.

Mowry EM, von Geldern G. The influence of nutritional factors on the prognosis of multiple sclerosis. *Nat Rev Neurol.* 2012;8:678–689.

O'Connor K, Weinstock-Guttman B, Carl E, Kilanowski C, Zivadinov R, Ramanathan M. Patterns of dietary and herbal supplement use by multiple sclerosis patients. *J Neurol.* 2012;259:637–644.

Pozuelo-Moyano B, Benito-Leon J, Mitchell AJ, Hernández-Gallego J. A systematic review of randomized, double-blind, placebo-controlled trials examining the clinical efficacy of vitamin D in multiple sclerosis. *Neuroepidemiology.* 2013;40:147–153.

Sato F, Martinez NE, Shahid M, Rose JW, Carlson NG, Tsunoda I. Resveratrol exacerbates both autoimmune and viral models of multiple sclerosis. *Am J Pathol.* 2013;183:1390–1396.

Shaygannejad V, Janghorbani M, Savoj MR, Ashtari F. Effects of adjunct glucosamine sulfate on relapsing-remitting multiple sclerosis progression: preliminary findings of a randomized, placebo-controlled trial. *Neurol Res.* 2010;32:981–985.

Shindler KS, Ventura E, Dutt M, Elliott P, Fitzgerald DC, Rostami A. Oral resveratrol reduces neuronal damage in a model of multiple sclerosis. *J Neuroophthalmol.* 2010;30:328–339.

Tomassini V, Pozzilli C, Onesti E, et al. Comparison of the effects of acetyl-L-carnitine and amantadine for the treatment of fatigue in multiple sclerosis: results of a pilot, randomised, double-blind, crossover trial. *J Neurol Sci.* 2004;218: 103–108.

Torkildsen O, Loken-Amsrud KI, Wergeland S, Myhr KM, Holmøy T. Fat-soluble vitamins as disease modulators in multiple sclerosis. *Acta Neurol Scand Suppl.* 2013;196:16–23.

Van Meeteren ME, Teunissen CE, Dijkstra CD, van Tol EA. Antioxidants and polyunsaturated fatty acids in multiple sclerosis. *Eur J Clin Nutr.* 2005;59: 1347–1361.

Wade DT, Young CA, Chaudhuri KR, Davidson DLW. A randomized placebo controlled exploratory study of vitamin B_{12}, lofepramine, and L-phenylala-nine (the "Cari Loder regime") in the treatment of multiple sclerosis. *J Neurol Neurosurg Psych.* 2002;73:246–249.

Yadav V, Marracci G, Lovera J, et al. Lipoic acid in multiple sclerosis: a pilot study. *Mult Scler.* 2005;11:159–165.

Zhang GX, Yu S, Gran B, Rostami A. Glucosamine abrogates the acute phase of experimental autoimmune encephalomyelitis by induction of Th2 response. *J Immunol.* 2005;175:7202–7208.

✓ Yoga

Yoga was developed thousands of years ago in India. It is related to the Hindu religion, and was created as a spiritual practice. Yoga means "union" in Sanskrit and is believed to unite the mind, body, and spirit. Yoga is one component of the multifaceted medical system of Ayurveda (see *Ayurveda* chapter). Over the past decade, the popularity of yoga has increased dramatically in the United States and other Western countries.

Treatment Method

Yoga takes many different forms. One of the more popular forms in the United States is *hatha yoga*. Three main components of yoga are breathing, movement, and posture. A series of body postures and movements, known as *asanas*, are performed. Deep, slow breathing is done in conjunction with the body movements. Specific breathing exercises, referred to as *pranayama*, also are done. Different types of yoga have different levels of exercise intensity and posture difficulty. In addition to these physical activities, yoga may include meditation, ethical guidelines, and diet recommendations.

In contrast to popular belief, the primary aim of yoga is not to attempt to assume difficult, contorted postures. People who are not able to maintain postures may still perform yoga. Postures in the standing or seated position are made easier by the use of "props," such as straps and wooden blocks. Yoga may be practiced by people who have severe arm and leg weakness. In this situation, emphasis is placed on head and shoulder movement, breathing exercises, and meditation. On the surface, this limited program may not appear to be yoga, but it does in fact focus on the same elements as more conventional yoga techniques.

Studies in Multiple Sclerosis and Other Conditions

Over the past several years, research on the effects of yoga on multiple sclerosis (MS) as well as other medical conditions has surged. One of the oldest and most rigorous studies of yoga and MS was conducted by Dr. Barry Oken and his colleagues at the Oregon Health Sciences University (1). In this study, which was reported in 2004, 69 people with MS were treated for 6 months with a conventional exercise program, yoga, or no intervention. Those treated with yoga or conventional exercise showed decreased fatigue. No effect on mood or cognitive function was noted with the use of yoga or conventional exercise. Another large MS study of yoga, which included 77 people who were treated with yoga weekly for 10 weeks, also found that yoga improved fatigue (2). This study also found improvement in a measure of overall psychological function.

Several smaller and less rigorous studies have examined the effect of yoga on various symptoms in people with MS. Multiple studies have found improvement in fatigue as well as anxiety, depression, walking, and overall quality of life (3–5). Single studies have reported improvement in bladder function, pain, and spasticity (6–8).

Studies of other medical conditions have examined yoga's effects on symptoms that may occur in MS. In these studies, which are of variable quality, many of the results are similar to those of the MS studies—improvement has been noted with anxiety, depression, fatigue, and walking. Some studies have also shown increased muscle strength.

Sexual function is an area in which yoga may be relevant to MS. MS may impair sexual function in men and women, and there is a rich, and sometimes erotic, lore about yoga improving sexual function and heightening sexual experience. There are similar claims about Pilates (see the chapter on *The Pilates Method and PhysicalMind Method*). It seems possible that several aspects of yoga, including improved awareness, coordination, and strength of the pelvis muscles, could improve sexual function. However, formal research of yoga in this area is lacking. Very limited studies in the general population indicate that yoga may improve sexual function in men and women, but there are not any studies in this area in MS.

Yoga may produce various other health benefits. Yoga may relieve low back pain and arthritis pain. In addition, it may mildly lower blood pressure and promote weight loss.

Side Effects

Yoga is usually very well tolerated. However, there are rare reports of side effects with yoga, including joint and tendon injuries, nerve injuries, strokes, worsening of glaucoma, collapsed lungs (pneumothorax), and bleeding. These have been reported most commonly with headstand, shoulder stand, lotus position, and forceful breathing.

Yoga should be performed with caution by those with the following conditions:

- Pregnancy
- Fatigue, sensitivity to heat, or impaired balance
- Significant lung or heart conditions
- Joint and bone conditions, including osteoporosis and osteopenia
- History of low back or neck pain
- High blood pressure
- Blood clotting disorders
- Eye conditions, including glaucoma
- Recent surgery

If meditation is done in conjunction with yoga, people with psychiatric disorders should discuss this therapy with their psychiatrist (see the chapter on *Meditation*). Yoga should not be used in place of conventional medicine, especially for trying to control the underlying disease process of MS or significant MS-related symptoms.

Practical Information

Yoga may be performed in groups or individually. Yoga techniques may be learned in classes, which are about 60 minutes in length. Group classes cost between $15 and $30, and private sessions are $25 to $35/h. Benefiting from yoga requires an ongoing commitment; several hours per week over weeks to months generally are required. Yoga classes often are available through recreation centers, the YMCA, and schools.

Information about yoga and MS is available in an excellent book on the topic by Dr. Loren Fishman, a rehabilitation physician, and Eric Small, a lifelong yoga practitioner who has MS:

- Fishman LM, Small EL. *Yoga and Multiple Sclerosis*. New York: Demos Health, 2007.

General information on yoga is available from several yoga organizations:

- The American Yoga Association (www.americanyogaassociation.org), P.O. Box 19986, Sarasota, FL 34236 (941-927-4977)

- International Association of Yoga Therapists (www.iayt.org) P.O. Box 251563, Little Rock, AR 72225 (928-541-0004)

- Yoga Journal (www.yogajournal.com)

Conclusion

Yoga is relatively inexpensive, generally safe, and may potentially improve multiple MS symptoms. One rigorous MS clinical trial found that yoga decreased fatigue. Other studies in MS and various other medical conditions have reported improvement in anxiety, depression, fatigue, bladder function, pain, spasticity, weakness, and walking. There are anecdotal reports but minimal research on yoga and sexual function. For general health, yoga may improve arthritis pain, reduce blood pressure, and promote weight loss. The effects of yoga on these conditions may secondarily benefit those with MS because these conditions may worsen disability and lower quality of life in those with MS.

Additional Readings
Books

Bauer B, ed. *Mayo Clinic Book of Alternative Medicine and Home Remedies.* New York, NY: Time Home Entertainment; 2013:115–116.

Broad WJ. *The Science of Yoga: The Risks and Rewards.* New York, NY: Simon & Schuster; 2012.

Ernst E, ed. *The Desktop Guide to Complementary and Alternative Medicine: An Evidence-Based Approach.* Edinburgh, UK: Mosby; 2001:76–78.

Fishman LM, Small EL. *Yoga and Multiple Sclerosis.* New York, NY: Demos Health; 2007.

Jellin JM, Gregory PJ, Batz F, et al. *Pharmacist's Letter/ Prescriber's Letter Natural Medicines Comprehensive Database.* Stockton, CA: Therapeutic Research Faculty; 2014.

Micozzi MS, ed. *Fundamentals of Complementary and Alternative Medicine.* Philadelphia, PA: Saunders Elsevier; 2011:482–494.

Riley D. Hatha yoga and meditation for neurological conditions. In: Oken BS, ed. *Complementary Therapies in Neurology.* London, UK: Parthenon Publishing; 2004:159–167.

Ross R. Yoga as a therapeutic modality. In: Weintraub MI, Micozzi MS, eds. *Alternative and Complementary Treatments in Neurologic Illness.* New York, NY: Churchill Livingstone; 2001:75–92.

Synovitz LB, Larson KL. *Complementary and Alternative Medicine for Health Professionals.* Burlington, MA: Jones & Bartlett Learning; 2013:204–206.

Journal Articles

Ahmadi A, Arastoo AA, Nikbakht M, Zahednejad S, Rajabpour M. Comparison of the effect of 8 weeks aerobic and yoga training on ambulatory function, fatigue and mood status in MS patients. *Iran Red Cresc Med J.* 2013;15:449–454.

Ahmadi A, Nikbakh M, Arastoo AA, Habibi A-H. The effects of yoga intervention on balance, speed and endurance of walking, fatigue and quality of life in people with multiple sclerosis. *J Hum Kin.* 2010;23:71–78.

Brook RD, Appel LJ, Rubenfire M, et al. Beyond medications and diet: alternative approaches to lowering blood pressure: a scientific statement from the American Heart Association. *Hypertension.* 2013;61:1360–1383.

Brotto LA, Mehak L, Kit C. Yoga and sexual functioning: a review. *J Sex Marital Ther.* 2009;35:378–390.

Chugh-Gupta N, Baldassarre FG, Vrkljan BH. A systematic review of yoga for state anxiety: considerations for occupational therapy. *Can J Occup Ther.* 2013;80:150–170.

Cramer H, Krucoff C, Dobos G. Adverse events associated with yoga: a systematic review of published case reports and case series. *PLoS One.* 2013;8:e75515.

Cramer H, Lange S, Klose P, Paul A, Dobos G. Yoga for breast cancer patients and survivors: a systematic review and meta-analysis. *BMC Cancer.* 2012;12:412.

Cramer H, Lauche R, Langhorst J, Dobos G. Yoga for depression: a systematic review and meta-analysis. *Depress Anxiety.* 2013;30:1068–1083.

Cramer H, Lauche R, Langhorst J, Dobos G. Yoga for rheumatic diseases: a systematic review. *Rheumatology.* 2013;52:2025–2030.

da Silva TL, Ravindran LN, Ravindran AV. Yoga in the treatment of mood and anxiety: a review. *Asian J Psychiatr.* 2009;2:6–16.

Despres L. Yoga and MS. *Yoga J.* 1997;135:96–103.

Dhikav V, Karmarkar G, Gupta R, et al. Yoga in female sexual functions. *J Sex Med.* 2010;7:964–970.

Dhikav V, Karmarkar G, Verma M, et al. Yoga in male sexual functioning: a noncomparative pilot study. *J Sex Med.* 2010;7:3460–3466.

Doulatabad SN, Nooreyan K, Doulatabad AN, Noubandegani ZM. The effects of pranayama, hatha and raja yoga on physical pain and the quality of life of women with multiple sclerosis. *Afr J Tradit Complement Altern Med.* 2013;10:49–52.

Garrett M, Hogan N, Larkin A, Saunders J, Jakeman P, Coote S. Exercise in the community for people with minimal gait impairment due to MS: an assessor-blinded randomized controlled trial. *Mult Scler J.* 2012;19:782–789.

Holtzman S, Beggs RT. Yoga for chronic low back pain: a meta-analysis of randomized controlled trials. *Pain Res Manag.* 2013;18:267–272.

Kiecolt-Glaser JK, Bennett JM, Andridge R, et al. Yoga's impact on inflammation, mood, and fatigue in breast cancer survivors: a randomized controlled trial. *J Clin Oncol.* 2014;32(10):1040–1049.

Nayak NN, Shankar K. Yoga: a therapeutic approach. *Phys Med Rehabil Clin N Am.* 2004;15:783–798.

Oken BS, Kishiyama S, Zajdel D, et al. Randomized controlled trial of yoga and exercise in multiple sclerosis. *Neurology.* 2004;62:2058–2064.

Patil NJ, Nagaratna R, Garner C, Raghuram NV, Crisan R. Effect of integrated Yoga on neurogenic bladder dysfunction in patients with multiple sclerosis—a prospective observational case series. *Complement Ther Med.* 2012;20:424–430.

Pilkington K, Kirkwood G, Rampes H, Richardson J. Yoga for depression: the research evidence. *J Affect Disord.* 2005;89:13–24.

Rioux JG, Ritenbaugh C. Narrative review of yoga intervention clinical trials including weight-related outcomes. *Altern Ther Health Med.* 2013;19:32–46.

Salgado BC, Jones M, Ilgun S, McCord G, Loper-Powers M, van Houten P. Effects of a 4-month Ananda Yoga program on physical and mental health outcomes for persons with multiple sclerosis. *Int J Yoga Therap.* 2013;23:27–38.

Velikonja O, Curic K, Ozura A, Jazbec SS. Influence of sports climbing and yoga on spasticity, cognitive function, mood and fatigue in patients with multiple sclerosis. *Clin Neurol Neurosurg.* 2010;112:597–601.

Wang J, Xiong X, Liu W. Yoga for essential hypertension: a systematic review. *PLoS One.* 2013;8:e76357.

Appendix 1: Ratings of Lifestyle and Unconventional Therapies[1]

Essential ★

Alcohol: abstention or moderate use
Exercise
Fiber: in recommended amounts
Gluten restriction *in celiac disease*
Salt: in recommended amounts
Tobacco: none
Vitamin B_{12} supplements *if vitamin B_{12} deficient*
Weight management

Worth Considering ✓

Acupuncture
Biofeedback
Caffeine
Chiropractic *for low back pain*
Coffee

---

[1] This appendix provides ratings for most of the lifestyle and unconventional therapies that are described in this book. See the "How to Use This Book" section at the beginning of the book for details about the rating system. See the text of the book for more detailed information on each of the specific therapies.

Cooling therapy
Cranberry
Guided imagery
Healthful Diet
Hippotherapy
Hypnosis
Massage
Meditation
Mindfulness
Multivitamins
Music therapy
Pets
Pilates method and PhysicalMind method
Prayer and spirituality
Psyllium
SAMe
Tai chi and qigong
Therapeutic horseback riding
Valerian
Vitamin D and calcium
Yoga

Uncertainties ⑦

ALCAR
Alpha-lipoic acid
Amino acids
Antioxidant vitamins (vitamins A, C, and E)
Aromatherapy
Aspartame avoidance
Bee pollen
Chiropractic *for neck pain and conditions other than low back pain*
Coenzyme Q10
Craniosacral therapy
Creatine
Feldenkrais
Fish oil
Garlic
Ginkgo
Ginsengs
Glucosamine

Gluten restriction generally
Goldenseal
Grape seed extract
Homeopathy
Inosine
Lecithin
Low dose naltrexone (LDN)
Magnets
Marijuana
Melatonin
Oligomeric proanthocyanidins (OPC)
Padma 28
Paleolithic diet
Probiotics
Prokarin
Propolis
Pycnogenol
Raw honey
Reflexology
Resveratrol
Royal jelly
St. John's wort
Stinging nettle
Swank diet
Therapeutic touch
Threonine
Tragerwork

Caution ⓘ

See Appendix 2 for a detailed listing of dietary supplements and herbs with potential side effects and drug interactions.

5-HTP
Androstenedione
Ashwagandha
Asian proprietary medicine
Ayurvedic supplements
Bee venom therapy
Calcium EAP
Candida treatment
Chelation therapy
Chinese herbal medicine

Chronic cerebrospinal venous insufficiency (CCSVI)
Colon therapy
Dental amalgam removal
DHEA
Echinacea
Enzyme therapy
Germanium
Hyperbaric oxygen
Kava kava
Protandim
Spirulina
Yohimbe
Yohimbine

Appendix 2: Dietary Supplements and Herbs That Have MS-Relevant Side Effects or Drug Interactions[1]

Acanthopanax obovatus: Possibly immune stimulating

Alfalfa: Possibly immune stimulating

Alkanna: Possible liver toxicity; may interact with multiple sclerosis (MS) drugs with possible liver toxicity, including interferons (Avonex, Betaseron, Extavia, Rebif), fingolimod (Gilenya), natalizumab (Tysabri), and teriflunomide (Aubagio)

Aloe: May interact with steroids

Alpine ragwort: Possible liver toxicity; may interact with MS drugs with possible liver toxicity, including interferons (Avonex, Betaseron, Extavia, Rebif), fingolimod (Gilenya), natalizumab (Tysabri), and teriflunomide (Aubagio)

American chestnut: Possible kidney toxicity; may interact with dalfampridine (Ampyra)

American ginseng: No definite therapeutic effects in MS; possibly immune stimulating; may inhibit blood clotting; may interact with warfarin (Coumadin)

American hellebore: May cause slowing of heart rate (bradycardia); possible interaction with fingolimod (Gilenya)

American pennyroyal: May irritate urinary tract

Andrographis: Possibly immune stimulating

Androstenedione: Multiple side effects

Angelica sinensis (**dong quai**): Possibly immune stimulating

Angel's trumpet: Possible interaction with steroids; possible interaction with antidepressant medications; possible interaction with amantadine

---

[1] This summary provides limited information about supplements and herbs that have significant toxicity, MS-relevant side effects, or MS-relevant drug interactions. See the index for a more complete listing of supplements and herbs covered in this book. See the text itself for more detailed information on supplements and herbs.

Aristolochia fangchi: Possible serious toxicity

Artemisia annua: Possibly immune stimulating

Artemisia myriantha: Possibly immune stimulating

Ashwagandha (*Withania somnifera*): Ayurvedic herb sometimes recommended for MS; possibly immune stimulating; possibly sedating

Asiatic dogwood: May irritate urinary tract

Asian ginseng (*Panax ginseng*): No definite therapeutic effects in MS; possibly immune stimulating; may inhibit blood clotting; may interact with warfarin (Coumadin)

Asparagus: May irritate urinary tract

Astragalus (*Astragalus membranaceus*): Possibly immune stimulating

Autumn crocus: Possible kidney toxicity; may interact with dalfampridine (Ampyra)

Azadirachta indica: Possible liver toxicity; may interact with MS drugs with possible liver toxicity, including interferons (Avonex, Betaseron, Extavia, Rebif), fingolimod (Gilenya), natalizumab (Tysabri), and teriflunomide (Aubagio)

Bacopa **(brahmi)**: May cause slowing of heart rate (bradycardia); possible interaction with fingolimod (Gilenya)

Baijiaolia: Possible serious toxicity

Bayberry: May interact with steroids

Bearberry (uva ursi): No definite therapeutic effects; contains chemicals that may cause cancer and eye problems; may cause nausea and vomiting

Bee pollen: No definite therapeutic effects; rarely causes severe allergic reactions

Belladonna: Possible interaction with amantadine; possible interaction with antidepressant medications

Beta carotene: *See* Vitamin A

Bishop's weed: Possible liver toxicity; may interact with MS drugs with possible liver toxicity, including interferons (Avonex, Betaseron, Extavia, Rebif), fingolimod (Gilenya), natalizumab (Tysabri), and teriflunomide (Aubagio)

Bissy nut: *See* Cola nut

Bitter almond: Possibly sedating

Bitter orange: May cause slowing of electrical conduction in heart (QT prolongation); possible interaction with fingolimod (Gilenya)

Black bryony: Possible kidney toxicity; may interact with dalfampridine (Ampyra)

Black cohosh: Possible liver toxicity; may interact with MS drugs with possible liver toxicity, including interferons (Avonex, Betaseron, Extavia, Rebif), fingolimod (Gilenya), natalizumab (Tysabri), and teriflunomide (Aubagio)

Black-currant seed oil: Contains gamma-linolenic acid; unknown safety, especially for long-term use

Blue cohosh: Possible serious toxicity

Blue-green algae: *See* Spirulina

Boerhavia diffusa: Ayurvedic herb that is possibly immune stimulating

Boldo: Possible liver toxicity; may interact with MS drugs with possible liver toxicity, including interferons (Avonex, Betaseron, Extavia, Rebif), fingolimod (Gilenya), natalizumab (Tysabri), and teriflunomide (Aubagio)

Borage seed oil: Possibly immune suppressing; possible liver toxicity; may interact with MS drugs with possible liver toxicity, including interferons (Avonex, Betaseron, Extavia, Rebif), fingolimod (Gilenya), natalizumab (Tysabri), and teriflunomide (Aubagio)

Brahmi: *See Bacopa*

Bryonia: Possible kidney toxicity; may interact with dalfampridine (Ampyra)

Buchu: Possible kidney toxicity; may interact with dalfampridine (Ampyra); may irritate urinary tract

Buckthorn: Possible interaction with steroids

Bumweed: Possible kidney toxicity; may interact with dalfampridine (Ampyra)

Bupleurum: Possibly immune stimulating

Bushi: Possible serious toxicity

Butterbur: Possible liver toxicity; may interact with MS drugs with possible liver toxicity, including interferons (Avonex, Betaseron, Extavia, Rebif), fingolimod (Gilenya), natalizumab (Tysabri), and teriflunomide (Aubagio)

Caffeine: May irritate urinary tract

Calabar bean: May cause slowing of heart rate (bradycardia); possible interaction with fingolimod (Gilenya)

Calamus: Possible kidney toxicity; may interact with dalfampridine (Ampyra); possibly sedating; possible serious toxicity

Calendula: Possibly sedating

California poppy: Possibly sedating

Caowu: Possible serious toxicity

Cascara sagrada: Possible interaction with steroids

Cassia cinnamon: Possible liver toxicity; may interact with MS drugs with possible liver toxicity, including interferons (Avonex, Betaseron, Extavia, Rebif), fingolimod (Gilenya), natalizumab (Tysabri), and teriflunomide (Aubagio); may irritate urinary tract

Castor: Possible kidney toxicity; may interact with dalfampridine (Ampyra)

Catnip: Possibly sedating

Cat's claw: Possibly immune stimulating

Celery: Possibly sedating; may irritate urinary tract

Chamomile: Possibly fatigue producing; possibly sedating

Chaparral: Possible liver toxicity; may interact with MS drugs with possible liver toxicity, including interferons (Avonex, Betaseron, Extavia, Rebif), fingolimod (Gilenya), natalizumab (Tysabri), and teriflunomide (Aubagio); possible kidney toxicity; may interact with dalfampridine (Ampyra); possible serious toxicity

Chenopodium oil: Possible kidney toxicity; may interact with dalfampridine (Ampyra)

Chlorella: Possibly immune stimulating

Cissus quadrangularis: Possible kidney toxicity; may interact with dalfampridine (Ampyra)

Cod-liver oil: Contains omega-3 fatty acids; may inhibit blood clotting; may interact with warfarin (Coumadin)

Coenzyme Q10: May interact with warfarin (Coumadin); possible liver toxicity in high doses

Coffee: May irritate urinary tract

Coix: Possibly immune stimulating

Cola nut: Also known as bissy nut; contains caffeine; may irritate urinary tract

Colocynth: Possible kidney toxicity; may interact with dalfampridine (Ampyra)

Coltsfoot: Possible liver toxicity; may interact with MS drugs with possible liver toxicity, including interferons (Avonex, Betaseron, Extavia, Rebif), fingolimod (Gilenya), natalizumab (Tysabri), and teriflunomide (Aubagio); possible serious toxicity

Comfrey: Possible liver toxicity; may interact with MS drugs with possible liver toxicity, including interferons (Avonex, Betaseron, Extavia, Rebif), fingolimod (Gilenya), natalizumab (Tysabri), and teriflunomide (Aubagio); possible serious toxicity

Copaiba oleoresin: May irritate urinary tract

Cordyceps: Possibly immune stimulating

Country mallow: May cause slowing of electrical conduction in heart (QT prolongation); possible interaction with fingolimod (Gilenya)

Cubeb: May irritate urinary tract

Cypress: Possible kidney toxicity; may interact with dalfampridine (Ampyra)

Datura **preparations**: Possible serious toxicity

Dendrobium: May increase seizure risk; may interact with dalfampridine (Ampyra); possibly immune stimulating

DHEA: Multiple side effects

Dill seed: May irritate urinary tract

Dong quai: Possible serious toxicity

Dusty miller: Possible liver toxicity; may interact with MS drugs with possible liver toxicity, including interferons (Avonex, Betaseron, Extavia, Rebif), fingolimod (Gilenya), natalizumab (Tysabri), and teriflunomide (Aubagio)

Echinacea: Not definitely effective for treating viral infections; may be immune stimulating; possible liver toxicity; may interact with MS drugs with possible liver toxicity, including interferons (Avonex, Betaseron, Extavia, Rebif), fingolimod (Gilenya), natalizumab (Tysabri), and teriflunomide (Aubagio)

Elecampine: Possibly sedating

Elderberry: Possibly immune stimulating

Ephedra: *See* Ma huang

Epimedium sagittatum: Possibly immune stimulating

Eucalyptus: Possible liver toxicity; may interact with MS drugs with possible liver toxicity, including interferons (Avonex, Betaseron, Extavia, Rebif), fingolimod (Gilenya), natalizumab (Tysabri), and teriflunomide (Aubagio); may irritate urinary tract

European mandrake: Possible interaction with amantadine; possible interaction with antidepressant medications

European mistletoe: Possibly immune stimulating

Figwort: Possible interaction with steroids

Flaxseed oil: Contains omega-3 and omega-6 fatty acids; greater than 45 g daily may produce diarrhea; unknown long-term safety

Fo-ti: Possible liver toxicity; may interact with MS drugs with possible liver toxicity, including interferons (Avonex, Betaseron, Extavia, Rebif), fingolimod (Gilenya), natalizumab (Tysabri), and teriflunomide (Aubagio)

Foxglove: Possible serious toxicity

Fragrant sumac: May irritate urinary tract

Fuzi: Possible serious toxicity

Garlic: Possibly immune stimulating; may inhibit blood clotting; may interact with warfarin (Coumadin)

Ge-gen-tang: Possibly immune stimulating

Germander: Possible liver toxicity; may interact with MS drugs with possible liver toxicity, including interferons (Avonex, Betaseron, Extavia, Rebif), fingolimod (Gilenya), natalizumab (Tysabri), and teriflunomide (Aubagio)

Germanium: Sometimes recommended for MS; no known beneficial effects for MS; may cause kidney failure and death

Ginkgo biloba: Not effective for treating MS attacks; possibly effective for MS fatigue; may inhibit blood clotting; may interact with warfarin (Coumadin); may provoke seizures

Ginseng: See listings for specific types of ginseng (American, Asian, Siberian)

Goa powder: Possible kidney toxicity; may interact with dalfampridine (Ampyra)

Golden ragwort: Possible liver toxicity; may interact with MS drugs with possible liver toxicity, including interferons (Avonex, Betaseron, Extavia, Rebif), fingolimod (Gilenya), natalizumab (Tysabri), and teriflunomide (Aubagio); possible serious toxicity

Gotu kola: Possible liver toxicity; may interact with MS drugs with possible liver toxicity, including interferons (Avonex, Betaseron, Extavia, Rebif), fingolimod (Gilenya), natalizumab (Tysabri), and teriflunomide (Aubagio); possibly sedating

Gravel root: Possible liver toxicity; may interact with MS drugs with possible liver toxicity, including interferons (Avonex, Betaseron, Extavia, Rebif), fingolimod (Gilenya), natalizumab (Tysabri), and teriflunomide (Aubagio)

Greater celandine: Possible liver toxicity; may interact with MS drugs with possible liver toxicity, including interferons (Avonex, Betaseron, Extavia, Rebif), fingolimod (Gilenya), natalizumab (Tysabri), and teriflunomide (Aubagio)

Green tea: Possibly immune stimulating

Grindelia: May irritate urinary tract

Ground ivy: Possible kidney toxicity; may interact with dalfampridine (Ampyra)

Groundsel: Possible liver toxicity; may interact with MS drugs with possible liver toxicity, including interferons (Avonex, Betaseron, Extavia, Rebif), fingolimod (Gilenya), natalizumab (Tysabri), and teriflunomide (Aubagio)

Guang fang ji: Possible serious toxicity

Guarana: Contains caffeine; improves mental alertness; may irritate urinary tract

Guiji: Possible serious toxicity

Hawaiian baby woodrose: Possible interaction with antidepressant medication

Hedge-hyssop: Possible kidney toxicity; may interact with dalfampridine (Ampyra)

Heliotropium: Possible liver toxicity; may interact with MS drugs with possible liver toxicity, including interferons (Avonex, Betaseron, Extavia, Rebif), fingolimod (Gilenya), natalizumab (Tysabri), and teriflunomide (Aubagio)

Hemp-agrimony: Possible liver toxicity; may interact with MS drugs with possible liver toxicity, including interferons (Avonex, Betaseron, Extavia, Rebif), fingolimod (Gilenya), natalizumab (Tysabri), and teriflunomide (Aubagio)

Henbane: Possible interaction with amantadine; possible interaction with antidepressant medications

Hops: Possibly sedating

Horny goat weed: May cause slowing of electrical conduction in heart (QT prolongation); possible interaction with fingolimod (Gilenya)

Horse chestnut: Possible kidney toxicity; may interact with dalfampridine (Ampyra)

Horseradish: May irritate urinary tract

Hound's tongue: Possible liver toxicity; may interact with MS drugs with possible liver toxicity, including interferons (Avonex, Betaseron, Extavia, Rebif), fingolimod (Gilenya), natalizumab (Tysabri), and teriflunomide (Aubagio)

5-HTP: Possible toxic effects

Huperzine A: May cause slowing of heart rate (bradycardia); possible interaction with fingolimod (Gilenya)

Hydrocotyle: *See* Gotu kola

Indian snakeroot: Possibly sedating

Jamaican dogwood: Possibly sedating

Jiaogulan: Possibly immune stimulating

Jimson weed: Possible interaction with amantadine; possible interaction with antidepressant medications

Jin bu yuan: Possible serious toxicity

Juniper berries: May irritate urinary tract

Kakkan-to: Possibly immune stimulating

Kanakasava: Ayurvedic herb that is possibly immune stimulating

Kanzo-bushi-to: Possibly immune stimulating

Kava kava: May cause severe liver toxicity and should be avoided; may interact with MS drugs with possible liver toxicity, including interferons (Avonex, Betaseron, Extavia, Rebif), fingolimod (Gilenya), natalizumab (Tysabri), and teriflunomide (Aubagio); possibly sedating

Khella: Possible liver toxicity; may interact with MS drugs with possible liver toxicity, including interferons (Avonex, Betaseron, Extavia, Rebif), fingolimod (Gilenya), natalizumab (Tysabri), and teriflunomide (Aubagio)

Kombucha: Possible serious toxicity

Larch arabinogalactan: Possibly immune stimulating

Larch turpentine: Possible kidney toxicity; may interact with dalfampridine (Ampyra)

Lavender: Possibly sedating

Lemon balm: Possibly sedating

Lemon verbena: Possible kidney toxicity; may interact with dalfampridine (Ampyra)

Licorice: Possible kidney toxicity; may interact with dalfampridine (Ampyra); possible serious toxicity; possible interaction with steroids

Liferoot: *See* Golden ragwort

Ligustrum lucidum: Possibly immune stimulating

Lily-of-the-valley: Possible interaction with steroids

Liverwort: Possible kidney toxicity; may interact with dalfampridine (Ampyra)

Lobelia: Possibly severe side effects; possible serious toxicity

Lovage: May irritate urinary tract

Ma huang: Multiple possible toxic effects, including death; may interact with steroids; may cause slowing of electrical conduction in heart (QT prolongation); possible interaction with fingolimod (Gilenya); may increase seizure risk; may interact with dalfampridine (Ampyra)

Madagascar periwinkle: May lower white blood cell count; possible interaction with fingolimod (Gilenya), interferons, dimethyl fumarate (Tecfidera) and teriflunomide (Aubagio)

Magnolia: Possibly sedating

Maharishi-4: Ayurvedic herb that is possibly immune stimulating

Maharishi-5: Ayurvedic herb that is possibly immune stimulating

Maitake mushroom: Possibly immune stimulating

Mangosteen: Possible kidney toxicity; may interact with dalfampridine (Ampyra)

Marsh tea: Possible kidney toxicity; may interact with dalfampridine (Ampyra); possibly sedating

Mate: Possible kidney toxicity; may interact with dalfampridine (Ampyra); may irritate urinary tract

Melatonin: Possibly immune stimulating

Melilot: *See* Sweet clover

Mistletoe: Possible serious toxicity

Momordica charantia: Possible liver toxicity; may interact with MS drugs with possible liver toxicity, including interferons (Avonex, Betaseron, Extavia, Rebif), fingolimod (Gilenya), natalizumab (Tysabri), and teriflunomide (Aubagio)

Morinda citrofolia (noni): Possible liver toxicity; may interact with MS drugs with possible liver toxicity, including interferons (Avonex, Betaseron, Extavia, Rebif), fingolimod (Gilenya), natalizumab (Tysabri), and teriflunomide (Aubagio)

Motherwort: Possibly sedating

Mountain ash: Possible kidney toxicity; may interact with dalfampridine (Ampyra)

Myrrh: Possible kidney toxicity; may interact with dalfampridine (Ampyra); may irritate urinary tract

Naoyanghua: Possible serious toxicity

Neem: Possibly immune stimulating

Niacin: *See* Vitamin B$_3$

Nimba arishta: Ayurvedic herb that is possibly immune stimulating

Noni: *See Morinda citrofolia*

Oak bark: Possible kidney toxicity; may interact with dalfampridine (Ampyra)

Parsley: Possible kidney toxicity; may interact with dalfampridine (Ampyra); may irritate urinary tract

Passionflower: Possibly fatigue producing; possibly sedating

Pau d'arco: Possible serious toxicity

Pennyroyal oil: Possible liver toxicity; may interact with MS drugs with possible liver toxicity, including interferons (Avonex, Betaseron, Extavia, Rebif), fingolimod (Gilenya), natalizumab (Tysabri), and teriflunomide (Aubagio); possible serious toxicity

Periwinkle: Possible kidney toxicity; may interact with dalfampridine (Ampyra)

Peru balsam: Possible kidney toxicity; may interact with dalfampridine (Ampyra)

Pheasant's eye: Possible interaction with steroids

Phyllanthus emblica: Ayurvedic herb that is possibly immune stimulating

Picrorhiza: Possibly immune stimulating

Pine needles: May irritate urinary tract

Precatory bean: Possible kidney toxicity; may interact with dalfampridine (Ampyra)

Propolis: No definite therapeutic effects; unknown safety

Psyllium: U.S. Food and Drug Administration (FDA)-approved for constipation; should not be used by people with swallowing difficulties

Pulsatilla: Possible kidney toxicity; may interact with dalfampridine (Ampyra); may irritate urinary tract

Pycnogenol: Safety of long-term use is unknown; possibly immune stimulating

Pyridoxine: *See* Vitamin B$_6$

Red sedge: May irritate urinary tract

Red yeast: Possible liver toxicity; may interact with MS drugs with possible liver toxicity, including interferons (Avonex, Betaseron, Extavia, Rebif), fingolimod (Gilenya), natalizumab (Tysabri), and teriflunomide (Aubagio)

Reishi mushroom (*Ganoderma lucidum*): Possibly immune stimulating

Resveratrol: No definite therapeutic effects in MS

Rosemary: Possible kidney toxicity; may interact with dalfampridine (Ampyra)

Royal jelly: No definite therapeutic effects; may rarely provoke asthma and cause severe allergic reactions

Rue: Possible kidney toxicity; may interact with dalfampridine (Ampyra); may irritate urinary tract; possible severe toxicity

Sage: May increase seizure risk; may interact with dalfampridine (Ampyra); possible sedating

St. John's wort: Probably effective for treating depression; possibly fatigue producing; may interact with many medications, including antidepressants and antiseizure medications

Salvia miltiorrhiza: Possibly immune stimulating

Sandalwood: May irritate urinary tract

Sarsaparilla: Possible kidney toxicity; may interact with dalfampridine (Ampyra)

Sassafras: Possibly sedating; may irritate urinary tract

Savin tops: Possible kidney toxicity; may interact with dalfampridine (Ampyra)

Sceletium: Possibly sedating

Scopolia: Possible interaction with amantadine; possible interaction with antidepressant medications

Selenium: Greater than 400 µg daily may produce multiple toxic effects

Senna: Possible interaction with steroids

Shepherd's purse: Possibly sedating

Shiitake mushroom (*Lentinula edodes*): Possibly immune stimulating

Shosaiko-to: Possibly immune stimulating

Siberian ginseng: No definite therapeutic effects; possibly immune stimulating; possibly fatigue producing; may inhibit blood clotting; may interact with warfarin (Coumadin); possibly sedating

Skullcap: Possibly sedating; possible serious toxicity

Sophora flavescens: Possibly immune stimulating

Sorrel: Possible kidney toxicity; may interact with dalfampridine (Ampyra)

South African geranium: Possibly immune stimulating

Spirulina: Also known as blue-green algae; contains variable amounts of gamma-linolenic acid; possibly immune stimulating; safety of long-term use is unknown

Squill: Possible interaction with steroids

Stinging nettle: Possibly immune stimulating; possibly fatigue producing; may interact with warfarin (Coumadin); possibly sedating

Storax: Possible kidney toxicity; may interact with dalfampridine (Ampyra)

Sweet bay: Possibly sedating

Sweet clover (melilot): Possible liver toxicity; may interact with MS drugs with possible liver toxicity, including interferons (Avonex, Betaseron, Extavia, Rebif), fingolimod (Gilenya), natalizumab (Tysabri), and teriflunomide (Aubagio)

Tansy: Possible kidney toxicity; may interact with dalfampridine (Ampyra); possible serious toxicity

Tansy ragwort: Possible liver toxicity; may interact with MS drugs with possible liver toxicity, including interferons (Avonex, Betaseron, Extavia, Rebif), fingolimod (Gilenya), natalizumab (Tysabri), and teriflunomide (Aubagio)

Thuja: May increase seizure risk; may interact with dalfampridine (Ampyra); possibly immune stimulating; may irritate urinary tract

Thunder god vine (*Tripterygium wilfordii*): Multiple possible toxic effects; possibly immune stimulating; may lower white blood cell count; possible interaction with fingolimod (Gilenya), interferons, dimethyl fumarate (Tecfidera), and teriflunomide (Aubagio)

Thyme: May irritate urinary tract

Tinospora cordifolia: Possibly immune stimulating

Tolu balsam: Possible kidney toxicity; may interact with dalfampridine (Ampyra)

Tormentil: Possible kidney toxicity; may interact with dalfampridine (Ampyra)

Trichopus zeylanicus: Possibly immune stimulating

Tripterygium wilfordii: *See* Thunder God Vine

Turpentine oil: Possible kidney toxicity; may interact with dalfampridine (Ampyra)

Uva ursi: *See* Bearberry

Valerian: Possibly effective for treating insomnia; possibly fatigue producing; safety of long-term use is unknown; possibly sedating

Vitamin A: Chemically related to beta carotene; possibly immune stimulating; greater than 10,000 IU daily may produce toxic effects; may increase cancer risk in smokers

Vitamin B$_3$: Also known as niacin; greater than 35 mg daily may produce toxic effects

Vitamin B$_6$: Also known as pyridoxine; greater than 50 mg daily may produce toxic effects

Vitamin C: Not definitely effective for treating urinary tract infections or viral infections; possibly immune stimulating; greater than 2,500 mg daily may produce toxic effects; may interact with warfarin (Coumadin)

Vitamin D: Greater than 4,000 IU daily may produce toxic effects

Vitamin E: Supplements of vitamin E may be indicated with a high intake of polyunsaturated fatty acids; possibly immune stimulating; greater than 1,500 IU daily may produce toxic effects; may inhibit bleeding; may interact with warfarin (Coumadin)

Watercress: Possible kidney toxicity; may interact with dalfampridine (Ampyra); may irritate urinary tract

White sandalwood: Possible kidney toxicity; may interact with dalfampridine (Ampyra)

Wild lettuce: Possibly sedating

Witch hazel: Possible kidney toxicity; may interact with dalfampridine (Ampyra)

Withania somnifera: *See* Ashwagandha

Woodfordia fruticosa: Ayurvedic herb that is possibly immune stimulating

Wood sorrel: Possible kidney toxicity; may interact with dalfampridine (Ampyra)

Wormseed: Possible kidney toxicity; may interact with dalfampridine (Ampyra)

Wormwood: May increase seizure risk; may interact with dalfampridine (Ampyra); possible serious toxicity

Xiao-chai-hu-tang: Possibly immune stimulating

Yangjinhua: Possible serious toxicity

Yellow dock: Possible kidney toxicity; may interact with dalfampridine (Ampyra)

Yerba mansa: Possibly sedating; may irritate urinary tract

Yohimbe or yohimbine: Multiple possible toxic effects; possible interaction with antidepressant medications

Zinc: Possibly immune stimulating; high doses may cause severe side effects, including neurological problems that may mimic MS

References

Part 1
Alternative Medicine and Lifestyle Medicine
1. Eisenberg D, Davis R, Ettner S, et al. Trends in alternative medicine use in the United States, 1990–1997: results of a follow-up national survey. *JAMA.* 1998;280:1569–1575.
2. Barnes PM, Bloom, B, Nahin RL. Complementary and alternative medicine use among adults and children: United States, 2007. *Natl Health Stat Report.* 2008;12:1–23.
3. Okoro CA, Zhao G, Li C, Balluz LS. Has the use of complementary and alternative medicine therapies by US adults with chronic disease-related functional limitations changed from 2002-2007? *J Altern Complement Med.* 2013;19:217–223.
4. Okoro CA, Zhao G, Li C, Balluz LS. Use of complementary and alternative medicine among USA adults with functional limitations: for treatment or general use? *Complement Ther Med.* 2011;19:208–215.
5. Okoro CA, Zhao G, Li C, Balluz LS. Use of complementary and alternative medicine among US adults with and without functional limitations. *Disabil Rehabil.* 2012;34:128–135.
6. Kessler RC, Davis RB, Foster DF, et al. Long-term trends in the use of complementary and alternative medical therapies in the United States. *Ann Intern Med.* 2001;135:262–268.
7. Berkman CS, Pignotti MG, Cavallo PF, Holland NJ. Use of alternative treatments by people with multiple sclerosis. *Neurorehab Neural Repair.* 1999;13:243–254.
8. Marrie RA, Hadjimichael O, Vollmer T. Predictors of alternative medicine use by multiple sclerosis patients. *Mult Scler.* 2003;9:461–466.
9. Stuifbergen AK, Harrison TC. Complementary and alternative therapy use in persons with multiple sclerosis. *Rehabil Nurs.* 2003;28:141–147.

10. Nayak S, Matheis RJ, Schoenberger NE, Shiflett SC. Use of unconventional therapies by individuals with multiple sclerosis. *Clin Rehabil.* 2003;17:181–191.

11. Shinto L, Yadav V, Morris C, Lapidus JA, Senders A, Bourdette D. Demographic and health-related factors associated with complementary and alternative medicine (CAM) use in multiple sclerosis. *Mult Scler.* 2006;12:94–100.

12. Schwartz C, Laitin E, Brotman S, LaRocca N. Utilization of unconventional treatments by persons with MS: is it alternative or complementary? *Neurology.* 1999;52:626–629.

13. Campbell DG, Turner AP, Williams RM, et al. Complementary and alternative medicine use in veterans with multiple sclerosis: prevalance and demographic associations. *J Rehabil Res Dev.* 2006;43:99–110.

14. Olsen S. A review of complementary and alternative medicine (CAM) by people with multiple sclerosis. *Occup Ther Int.* 2009;16:57–70.

15. Yadav V, Shinto L, Bourdette D. Complementary and alternative medicine for the treatment of multiple sclerosis. *Expert Rev Clin Immunol.* 2010;6: 381–395.

16. Stoll SS, Nieves C, Tabby DS. Schwartzman R. Use of therapies other than disease-modifying agents, including complementary and alternative medicine, by patients with multiple sclerosis: a survey study. *J Am Osteopath Assoc.* 2012;112:22–28.

17. Leong EM, Semple SJ, Angley M, Siebert W, Petkov J, McKinnon RA. Complementary and alternative medicines and dietary interventions in multiple sclerosis: what is being used in South Australia and why? *Complement Ther Med.* 2009;17:216–223.

18. Hooper KD, Pender MP, Webb PM, McCombe PA. Use of traditional and complementary medical care by patients with multiple sclerosis in South-East Queensland. *Int J MS Care.* 2001;3:13–28.

19. Page SA, Verhoef MJ, Stebbins RA, Metz LM. Levy JC. The use of complementary and alternative therapies by people with multiple sclerosis. *Chronic Dis Can.* 2003,24:75–79.

20. Skovgaard L, Nicolajsen PH, Pedersen E, et al. Differences between users and non-users of complementary and alternative medicine among people with multiple sclerosis in Denmark: a comparison of descriptive characteristics. *Scand J Pub Health.* 2013;41:492–499.

21. Stenager E, Stenager EN, Knudsen L, Jensen K. The use of non-medical/ alternative treatment in multiple sclerosis: a 5 year follow-up study. *Acta Neurol Belg.* 1995;95:18–22.

22. Skovgaard L, Nicolajsen PH, Pedersen E, et al. Use of complementary and alternative medicine among people with multiple sclerosis in the Nordic countries. *Autoimmune Dis.* 2012;2012:841085.

23. Sastre-Garriga J, Munteis E, Rio J, Pericot I, Tintoré M, Montalban X. Unconventional therapy in multiple sclerosis. *Mult Scler.* 2003,9:320–322.

24. Schwarz S, Knorr C, Geiger H, Flachenecker P. Complementary and alternative medicine for multiple sclerosis. *Mult Scler.* 2008;14:1113–1119.

25. Thorne S, Paterson B, Russell C, Schultz A. Complementary/alternative medicine in chronic illness as informed self-care decision making. *Int Nursing Stud.* 2002;9:671–683.
26. Jelinek G. *Overcoming Multiple Sclerosis.* Crows Nest, Australia: Allen & Unwin; 2009:28.
27. Burnfield A. *Multiple Sclerosis: A Personal Exploration.* London, UK: Souvenir Press; 1985:50.
28. Forsythe E. *Multiple Sclerosis: Exploring Sickness and Health.* London, UK: Faber and Faber; 1988:50.

Placebos and Nocebos
1. Beecher HK. The powerful placebo. *JAMA.* 1955;159:1602–1606.
2. Sormani MP, Molyneaux PD, Barkhof F, Miller DH, Filippi M. MRI enhancing lesion frequency from patients with MS enrolled in placebo arms of clinical trials or in natural history studies. *Magn Reson Imaging.* 1999;17:1236–1237.
3. Hirsch RL, Johnson KP, Camenga DL. The placebo effect during a double blind trial of recombinant alpha2 interferon in multiple sclerosis patients: immunological and clinical findings. *Int J Neurosci.* 1988;39:189–196.
4. Krupp LB, Coyle PK, Doscher C, et al. Fatigue therapy in multiple sclerosis: results of a double-blind, randomized, parallel trial of amantadine, pemoline, and placebo. *Neurology.* 1995;45:1956–1961.
5. Papadopoulos D, Mitsikostas DD. Nocebo effects in multiple sclerosis trials: a meta-analysis. *Mult Scler.* 2010;16:816–828.
6. Katz J. *The silent world of doctor and patient.* New York, NY: London, Collier–McMillan; 1984:191.

Part 3
Acupuncture and Traditional Chinese Medicine
1. NIH Consensus Development Panel on Acupuncture. *JAMA.* 1998;280:1518–1524.
2. Spoerel WE, Paty DW, Kertesz A, et al. Acupuncture and multiple sclerosis. *CMA J.* 1974;110:751.
3. Smith MO, Rabinowitz N. Acupuncture treatment of multiple sclerosis: two detailed clinical presentations. *Am J Acupuncture.* 1986;14:143–146.
4. Miller RE. An investigation into the management of the spasticity experienced by some patients with multiple sclerosis using acupuncture based on traditional Chinese medicine. *Compl Ther Med.* 1996;4:58–62.
5. Steinberger A. Specific irritability of acupuncture points as an early symptom of multiple sclerosis. *Am J Chinese Med.* 1986;14:175–178.
6. Donnellan CP, Shanley J. Comparison of the effect of two type of acupuncture on quality of life in secondary progressive multiple sclerosis: a preliminary single-blind randomized controlled trial. *Clin Rehabil.* 2008;22:195–205.
7. Quispe-Cabanillas JG, Damasceno A, von Glehn F, et al. Impact of electroacupuncture on quality of life for patients with relapsing-remitting

multiple sclerosis under treatment with immunomodulators: a randomized study. *BMC Complement Altern Med.* 2012;12:209.

8. Foroughipour M, Bahrami Taghanaki HR, Saeidi M, Khazaei M, Sasannezhad P, Shoeibi A. Amantadine and the place of acupuncture in the treatment of fatigue in patients with multiple sclerosis: an observational study. *Acupunct Med.* 2013;31:27–30.

9. Tjon Eng Soe SH, Kopsky DJ, Jongen PJH, de Vet HC, Oei-Tan CL. Multiple sclerosis patients with bladder dysfunction have decreased symptoms after electro-acupuncture. *Mult Scler.* 2009;15:1376–1377.

10. Liu YM, Liu XJ, Mu LL, et al. The effect of electroacupuncture on T cell responses in rats with experimental autoimmune encephalitis. *J Neuroimmunol.* 2010;220:25–33.

11. Liu Y, Wang H, Wang X, et al. The mechanism of effective electroacupuncture on T cell response in rats with experimental autoimmune encephalomyelitis. *PLoS One.* 2013;8:e51573.

12. Liu J, Gao Y, Kan BH. Zhou L. Systematic review and meta-analysis of randomized controlled trials of Chinese herbal medicine in treatment of multiple sclerosis [in Chinese]. *Zhong Xi Yi He Xue Bao.* 2012;10: 141–153.

13. Xi L, Zhiwen L, Huayan W, Yaohua W. Preventing relapse in multiple sclerosis with Chinese medicine. *J Chin Med.* 2001;66:39–40.

14. Yi S, Xiaoyan L. A review on traditional Chinese medicine in prevention and treatment of multiple sclerosis. *J Trad Chinese Med.* 1999;19:65–73.

Aromatherapy

1. Walsh E, Wilson C. Complementary therapies in long-stay neurology in patient settings. *Nurs Stand.* 1999;13:32–35.

Bee Venom Therapy and Other Forms of Apitherapy

1. Lublin FD, Oshinsky RJ, Perreault M, et al. Effect of honey bee venom on EAE. *Neurology.* 1998;50:A424.

2. Karimi A, Ahmadi F, Parivar K, et al. Effect of honey bee venom on Lewis rats with experimental allergic encephalomyelitis, a model for multiple sclerosis. *Iran J Pharm Res.* 2012;11:671–678.

3. Santilli J, Rockwell WJ, Wallerstedt DB, et al. The use of honeybee venom therapy as a treatment in chronic progressive multiple sclerosis—a case report. *Ann All Asthma Immunol.* 1999;82:123.

4. Castro HJ, Mendez-Inocencio JI, Omidvar B, et al. A phase I study of the safety of honeybee venom extract as a possible treatment for patients with progressive forms of multiple sclerosis. *Allergy Asthma Proc.* 2005;26:470–476.

5. Wesselius T, Heersema DJ, Mostert JP, et al. A randomized crossover study of bee sting therapy for multiple sclerosis. *Neurology.* 2005;65: 1764–1768.

Chronic Cerebrospinal Venous Insufficiency

1. Zamboni P, Menegatti E, Galeotti R, et al. The value of cerebral Doppler venous hemodynamics in the assessment of multiple sclerosis. *J Neurol Sci.* 2009;282:21–27.

2. Zamboni P, Galeotti R, Menegatti E, et al. Chronic cerebrospinal venous insufficiency in patients with multiple sclerosis. *J Neurol Neurosurg Psychiatry.* 2009;80:392–399.

3. Zamboni P, Galeotti R, Menegatti E, et al. A prospective open-label study of endovascular treatment of chronic cerebrospinal venous insufficiency. *J Vasc Surg.* 2009;50:1348–1358.

4. Diuaconu CI, Conway D, Rox RJ, Rae-Grant A. Chronic cerebrospinal venous insufficiency as a cause of multiple sclerosis: controversy and reality. *Curr Treat Options Cardiovasc Med.* 2012;14:203–214.

5. Paul F, Wattjes MP. Chronic cerebrospinal venous insufficiency in multiple sclerosis: the final curtain. *Lancet.* 2014;383:106–108.

6. Traboulsee AL, Knox KB, Machan L, et al. Prevalence of extracranial venous narrowing on catheter venography in people with multiple sclerosis, their siblings, and unrelated healthy controls: a blinded, case-control study. *Lancet.* 2014;383:138–145.

7. Tsivgoulis G, Sergentanis TN, Chan A, et al. Chronic cerebrospinal venous insufficiency and multiple sclerosis: a comprehensive meta-analysis of case-control studies. *Ther Adv Neurol Disord.* 2014;7:114–136.

8. Rodger IW, Dilar D, Dwyer J, et al. Evidence against the involvement of chronic cerebrospinal venous abnormalities in multiple sclerosis. A case-control study. *PLoS One.* 2013;8:e72495.

9. Comi G, Battaglia MA, Bertolotto A, et al. Observational case-control study of the prevalence of chronic cerebrospinal venous insufficiency in multiple sclerosis: results from the CoSMo study. *Mult Scler.* 2013;19:1508–1517.

10. Anon. *FDA Safety Communication: Chronic Cerebrospinal Venous Insufficiency Treatment in Multiple Sclerosis Patients.* http://www.fda.gov/MedicalDevices/Safety/AlertsandNotices/ucm303318.htm. Updated 2012.

Cooling Therapy

1. Capell E, Gardella M, Leandri M, et al. Lowering body temperature with a cooling suit as symptomatic treatment for thermosensitive multiple sclerosis patients. *Ital J Neurol Sci.* 1995;16:533–539.

2. NASA/MS Cooling Study Group. A randomized controlled study of the acute and chronic effects of cooling therapy for MS. *Neurology.* 2003;60:1955–1960.

Craniosacral Therapy

1. Upledger JE. *CranioSacral Therapy.* Berkeley, CA: North Atlantic Books; 2001:88–89.

2. Greenman PE, McPartland JM. Cranial findings and iatrogenesis from craniosacral manipulation in patients with traumatic brain syndrome. *J Am Osteopath Assoc.* 1995;95:182–188,191–192.

Enzyme Therapy
1. Baumhackl U, Kappos L, Radue EW, et al. A randomized, double-blind, placebo-controlled study of oral hydrolytic enzymes in relapsing multiple sclerosis. *Mult Scler.* 2005;11:166–168.

Exercise
1. Latimer-Cheung AE, Martin Ginis KA, Hicks AL, et al. Development of evidence-informed physical activity guidelines for adults with multiple sclerosis. *Arch Phys Med Rehabil.* 2013;94:1829–1836.
2. Petajan JH, Gappmaier E, White AT, Spencer MK, Mino L, Hicks RW. Impact of aerobic training on fitness and quality of life in multiple sclerosis. *Ann Neurol.* 1996;39:432–441.
3. Latimer-Cheung AE, Pilutti LA, Hicks AL, et al. Effects of exercise training on fitness, mobility, fatigue, and health-related quality of life among adults with multiple sclerosis: a systematic review to inform guideline development. *Arch Phys Med Rehabil.* 2013;94:1800–1828.
4. Motl RW, Pilutti LA. The benefits of exercise training in multiple sclerosis. *Nat Rev Neurol.* 2012;8:487–497.
5. Kjolhede T, Vissing K, Dalgas U. Multiple sclerosis and progressive resistance training: a systematic review. *Mult Scler J.* 2012;18:1215–1228.
6. Asmundson GJ, Fetzner MG, Deboer LB, Powers MB, Otto MW, Smits JA. Let's get physical: a contemporary review of the anxiolytic effects of exercise and its disorders. *Depress Anxiety.* 2013;30:362–373.
7. Lucio AC, Perissinoto MC, Natalin RA, Prudente A, Damasceno BP, D'ancona CA. A comparative study of pelvic floor muscle training in women with multiple sclerosis: its impact on lower urinary tract symptoms and quality of life. *Clinics (Sao Paolo).* 2011;66:1563–1568.
8. Leung L, Riutta T, Kotecha J, Rosser W. Chronic constipation: an evidence-based review. *J Amer Board Fam Med.* 2011;24:436–451.
9. Blumenthal JA, Smith PJ, Hoffman BM. Is exercise a viable treatment for depression? *ACSMs Health Fit J.* 2012;16:14–21.
10. Castro-Sanchez AM, Mataran-Penarrocha GA, Lara-Palomo I, Saavedra-Hernández M, Arroyo-Morales M, Moreno-Lorenzo C. Hydrotherapy for the treatment of pain in people with multiple sclerosis: a randomized controlled trial. *Evid Based Complement Altern Med.* 2012;2012:473963.
11. Khoo J, Tian HH, Tan B, et al. Comparing effects of low-and high-volume moderate-intensity exercise on sexual function and testosterone in obese men. *J Sex Med* 2013;10:1823–1832.
12. Lorenz TA, Meston CM. Acute exercise improves physical sexual arousal in women taking antidepressants. *Ann Behav Med.* 2012;43:352–361.

13. Yang PY, Ho KH, Chen HC, Chien MY. Exercise training improves sleep quality in middle-aged and older adults with sleep problems: a systematic review. *J Physiother.* 2102;58:157–163.

14. McDonnell MN, Smith AE, Mackintosh SF. Aerobic exercise to improve cognitive function in adults with neurological disorders. *Arch Phys Med Rehabil.* 2011;92:1044–1052.

Fats: Fish Oil and Polyunsaturated Fatty Acids

1. Gibson Robert A, Lines David R, Neumann Mark A. Gamma linolenic acid (GLA) content of encapsulated evening primrose oil products. *Lipids.* 1992;27:82–84.

2. Swank RL. Multiple sclerosis: twenty years on low fat diet. *Arch Neurol.* 1970;23:460–474.

3. Swank RL, Dugan BB. Effect of low saturated fat diet in early and late cases of multiple sclerosis. *Lancet.* 1990;336:37–39.

4. Swank RL, Goodwin J. Review of MS patient survival on a Swank low saturated fat diet. *Nutrition.* 2003;16:161–162.

5. Miller JHD, Zilkha KJ, Langman MJS, et al. Double-blind trial of linoleate supplementation of the diet in multiple sclerosis. *Br Med J.* 1973;1:765–768.

6. Bates D, Fawcett PRW, Shaw DA, Weightman D. Polyunsaturated fatty acids in treatment of acute remitting multiple sclerosis. *Br Med J.* 1978;2:1390–1391.

7. Paty DW, Cousin HK, Read S, Adlakha K. Linoleic acid in multiple sclerosis: failure to show any therapeutic benefit. *Acta Neurol Scand.* 1978;58:53–58.

8. Dworkin RH, Bates D, Millar JHD, Paty DW. Linoleic acid and multiple sclerosis: a reanalysis of three double-blind trials. *Neurology* 1984;34:1441–1445.

9. Bates D, Fawcett PRW, Shaw DA, Weightman D. Trial of polyunsaturated fatty acids in non-relapsing multiple sclerosis. *Br Med J.* 1977;10:932–933.

10. Bates D, Cartlidge NEF, French JM, et al. A double-blind controlled trial of long chain n-3 polyunsaturated fatty acids in the treatment of multiple sclerosis. *J Neurol Neurosurg Psychiatry.* 1989;52:18–22.

11. Goldberg P, Fleming MC, Picard EH. Multiple sclerosis: decreased relapse rate through dietary supplementation with calcium, magnesium and vitamin D. *Med Hypoth.* 1986;21:193–200.

12. Nordvik I, Myhr KM, Nyland H, Bjerve KS. Effects of dietary advice and n-3 supplementation in newly diagnosed MS patients. *Acta Neurol Scand.* 2000;102:143–149.

13. Weinstock-Guttamn B, Baier M, Park Y, et al. Low fat dietary intervention with omega-3 fatty acid supplementation in multiple sclerosis patients. *Prostaglandins Leukotrienes Essent Fatty Acids.* 2005;73:392–404.

14. Torkildsen O, Wegeland S, Bakke S, et al. Omega-3 fatty acid treatment in multiple sclerosis (OFAMS Study). *Arch Neurol.* 2012;1044–1051.

15. Jelinek GA, Hadgkiss EJ, Weiland TJ, Pereira NG, Marck CH, van der Meer DM. Association of fish consumption and omega 3 supplementation with

quality of life, disability and disease activity in an international cohort of people with multiple sclerosis. *Int J Neurosci.* 2013;123:792–801.

16. Rezapour-Firouzi S, Arefhosseini SR, Mehdi F, et al. Immunomodulatory and therapeutic effects of hot-nature diet and co-supplemented hemp seed, evening primrose oils intervention in multiple sclerosis. *Complement Ther Med.* 2013;21:473–480.

17. Rezapour-Firouzi S, Arefhosseini SR, Farhoudi M, et al. Association of expanded disability status scale and cytokines after intervention with co-supplemented hemp seed, evening primrose oils and hot-natured diet in multiple sclerosis patients. *Bioimpacts.* 2013;3:43–47.

18. Rezapour-Firouzi S, Arefhosseini SR, aEbrahimi-Mamaghani M, et al. Erythrocyte membrane fatty acids in multiple sclerosis patients and hot-nature dietary intervention with co-supplemented hemp-seed and evening-primrose oils. *Afr J Trad Complement Altern Med.* 2013;10: 519–527.

19. Pantzaris MC, Loukaides GN, Ntzani EE, Patrikios IS. A novel oral nutra-ceutical formula of omega-3 and omega-6 fatty acids with vitamins (PLP10) in relapsing remitting multiple sclerosis: a randomized, double-blind, placebo-controlled proof-of-concept clinical trial. *BMJ Open.* 2013;3(4). pii: e002170.

Feldenkrais
1. Johnson SK, Frederick J, Kaufman M, Mountjoy B. A controlled investigation of bodywork in multiple sclerosis. *J Altern Complement Med.* 1999;5:237–243.

Fiber
1. Timmerman GM, Stuifbergen AK. Eating patterns of women with multiple sclerosis. *J Neurosci Nurs.* 1999;31:152–158.
2. Hewson DC, Phillips MA, Simpson KE, Drury P, Crawford MA. Food intake in multiple sclerosis. *Hum Nutr Appl Nutr.* 1984;38A:355–367.
3. Goodman S, Gulick E. Dietary practices of people with multiple sclerosis. *Int J MS Care.* 2008;10:47–57.

Gluten Sensitivity and Celiac Disease
1. Haghighi AB, Ansari N, Mokhtari M, et al. Multiple sclerosis and gluten sensitivity. *Clin Neurol Neurosurg* 2007;109:651–653.
2. Tengah CP, Lock RJ, Unsworth J, Wills AJ. Multiple sclerosis and occult glu-ten sensitivity. *Neurology.* 2004;62:2326–2327.
3. Jones PE, Pallis C, Peters TJ. Morphological and biochemical findings in jejunal biopsies from patients with multiple sclerosis. *J Neurol Neurosurg Psych.* 1979;42:402–406.
4. Shor D B-A, Barzilai O, Ram M, et al. Gluten sensitivity in multiple scle-rosis: experimental myth or clinical truth? *Contemp Chall Autoimmun.* 2009;1173:343–349.

5. Nicoletti A, Patti F, Lo Fermo S, et al. Frequency of celiac disease is not increased among multiple sclerosis patients. *Mult Scler.* 2008;14:698–700.
6. Rodrigo L, Hernandez-Lahoz C, Fuentes D, Alvarez N, López-Vázquez A, González S. Prevalence of celiac disease in multiple sclerosis. *BMC Neurol.* 2011;11:31.
7. Di Marco R, Mangano K, Quattrocchi C, Amato F, Nicoletti F, Buschard K. Exacerbation of protracted-relapsing experimental allergic encephalomyelitis in DA rats by gluten-free diet. *APMIS.* 2004;112:651–655.
8. Liversedge L. Treatment and management of multiple sclerosis. *Brit Med Bull.* 1977;33:78–83.

Guided Imagery
1. Maguire BL. The effects of imagery on attitudes and moods in multiple sclerosis patients. *Altern Ther Health Med.* 1996;2:75–79.

Herbs
1. Stewart TM, Tran ZV, Bowling AC. Factors related to fatigue in multiple sclerosis. *Int J MS Care.* 2007;9:29–34.
2. Brochet B, Orgogozo J, Guinot P, Dartigues JF, Henry P, Loiseau P. Étude pilote d'un inhibiteur spécifique du PAF-acéther, le ginkgolide B dans le traitement des poussées aiguës descléroses en plaques. [Pilot study of ginkgolide B, a PAF-acether specific inhibitor in the treatment of acute outbreaks of multiple sclerosis.]. *Rev Neurol* (Paris). 1992;48:229–301.
3. Brochet B, Guinot P, Orgogozo J, Confavreux C, Rumbach L, Lavergne V. Double-blind, placebo controlled, multicenter study of ginkgolide B in treatment of acute exacerbations for multiple sclerosis. The Ginkgolide Study Group in multiple sclerosis. *J Neurol Neurosurg Psychiatry.* 1995;58:360–362.
4. Diamond BJ, Johnson SK, Kaufman M, Shiflett SC, Graves L. A randomized controlled pilot trial: the effects of EGb 761 on information processing and executive function in multiple sclerosis. *Explore (NY).* 2013;9:106–107.
5. Lovera J, Bagert B, Smoot K, et al. *Ginkgo biloba* for the improvement of cognitive performance in multiple sclerosis: a randomized, placebo-controlled trial. *Mult Scler.* 2007;13:376–385.
6. Lovera JF, Kim E, Heriza E, et al. Ginkgo biloba does not improve cognitive function in MS: a randomized placebo-controlled trial. *Neurology.* 2012;79:1278–1284.
7. Johnson SK, Diamond BJ, Rausch S, Kaufman M, Shiflett SC, Graves L. The effect of *Ginkgo biloba* on functional measures in multiple sclerosis: a pilot randomized controlled trial. *Explore (NY).* 2006;2:19–24.
8. Etemadafir M, Sayahi F, Abtahi SH, et al. Ginseng in the treatment of fatigue in multiple sclerosis: a randomized, placebo-controlled, double-blind pilot study. *Int J Neurosci.* 2013;123:480–486.
9. Kim E, Cameron M, Lovera J, Schaben L, Bourdette D, Whitham R. American ginseng does not improve fatigue in multiple sclerosis: a single

center randomized double-blind placebo-controlled crossover pilot study. *Mult Scler J.* 2011;17:1523–1526.

10. Korwin-Piotrowska T, Nocon D, Stankowska-Chomicz A, et al. Experience of Padma 28 in multiple sclerosis. *Phytother Res.* 1992;6:133–136.

11. Brinker F. *Herbal Contraindications and Drug Interactions.* Sandy, Oregon: Eclectic Medical Publishers; 2010.

Hippotherapy and Therapeutic Horseback Riding

1. Hammer A, Nilsagard Y, Forsberg A, Pepa H, Skargren E, Oberg B. Evaluation of therapeutic riding (Sweden)/hippotherapy (United States). A single-subject experimental design study replicated in eleven patients with multiple sclerosis. *Physiother Theory Pract.* 2005;21:51–77.

2. MacKay-Lyons M, Conway C, Roberts W. Effects of therapeutic riding on patients with multiple sclerosis: a preliminary trial. In: *Proceedings of the 6th International Therapeutic Riding Congress,* Toronto, Canada; 1988;8:173–178.

3. Bronson C, Brewerton K, Ong J, Palanca C, Sullivan SJ. Does hippotherapy improve balance in persons with multiple sclerosis: a systematic review. *Eur J Phys Rehabil Med.* 2010;46:347–353.

4. Silkwood-Sherer D, Warmbier H. Effects of hippotherapy on postural stability in persons with multiple sclerosis: a pilot study. *J Neurol Phys Ther.* 2007;31:77–84.

5. Munoz-Lasa S, Ferriero G, Valero R, Gomez-Muñiz F, Rabini A, Varela E. Effect of therapeutic horseback riding on balance and gait of people with multiple sclerosis. *G Ital Med Lav Ergon.* 2011;33:462–467.

Homeopathy

1. Swayne J. *Homeopathic Method: Implications for Clinical Practice and Medical Science.* New York, NY: Churchill Livingstone; 1998:191.

2. Ernst E. Homeopathy: what does the "best" evidence tell us? *Med J Aust.* 2010;192:458–460.

3. Shang A, Huwiler-Muntener K, Nartey L, et al. Are the clinical effects of homeopathy placebo effects? Comparative study of placebo-controlled trials of homeopathy and allopathy. *Lancet.* 2005;366:726–732.

Hyperbaric Oxygen

1. Fischer BH, Marks M, Reich T. Hyperbaric oxygen treatment of multiple sclerosis. A randomized, placebo-controlled, double-blind study. *N Engl J Med.* 1983;308:181–186.

2. Kleijnen J, Knipschild P. Hyperbaric oxygen for multiple sclerosis: review of controlled trials. *Acta Neurol Scand.* 1995;91:330–334.

3. Bennett M, Heard R. Hyperbaric oxygen therapy for multiple sclerosis. *Cochrane Database Syst Rev.* 2004;(1):CD003057.

4. Neubauer RA, Neubauer V, Gottlieb SF The controversy over hyperbaric oxygenation therapy for multiple sclerosis. *J Am Phys Surgeons.* 2005; 10:112–115.

5. Bennett M, Heard R. Hyperbaric oxygen therapy for multiple sclerosis. *CNS Neurosci Ther.* 2010;16:115–124.

Hypnosis
1. Jensen MP, Barber J, Romano JM, et al. A comparison of self-hypnosis versus progressive muscle relaxation in patients with multiple sclerosis and chronic pain. *Int J Clin Exp Hypn.* 2009;57:198–221.
2. Jensen MP, Ehde DM, Gertz KJ, et al. Effects of self-hypnosis training and cognitive restructuring on daily pain intensity and catastrophizing in individuals with multiple sclerosis and chronic pain. *Int J Clin Exp Hypn.* 2011;59:45–63.
3. Sutherland G, Andersen MB, Morris T. Relaxation and health-related quality of life in multiple sclerosis: the example of autogenic training. *J Behav Med.* 2005;28:249–256.
4. Dane JR. Hypnosis for pain and neuromuscular rehabilitation with multiple sclerosis: case summary, literature review, and analysis of outcomes. *Int J Clin Exp Hypn.* 1996;44:208–231.
5. Sutcher H. Hypnosis as adjunctive therapy for multiple sclerosis: a progress report. *Am J Clin Hypn.* 1997;39:283–290.

Low-Dose Naltrexone
1. Agrawal YP. Low-dose naltrexone therapy in multiple sclerosis. *Med Hypotheses.* 2005;64:721–724.
2. Rahn KA, McLaughlin PJ, Zagon IS. Prevention and diminished expression of experimental autoimmune encephalomyelitis by low dose naltrexone (LDN) or opioid growth factor (OGF) for an extended period: therapeutic implications for multiple sclerosis. *Brain Res.* 2011;1381:243–253.
3. Zagon IS, Rahn KA, Turel AP, McLaughlin PJ. Endogenous opioids regulate expression of experimental autoimmune encephalomyelitis: a new paradigm for the treatment of multiple sclerosis. *Exp Biol Med.* 2009;234:1383–1392.
4. Gironi M, Martinelli-Boneschi F, Sacerdote P, et al. A pilot trial of low-dose naltrexone in primary progressive multiple sclerosis. *Mult Scler.* 2008;14:1076–1083.
5. Cree BA, Kornyeyeva E, Goodin DS. Pilot trial of low-dose naltrexone and quality of life in multiple sclerosis. *Ann Neurol.* 2010;68:145–150.
6. Sharafaddinzadeh N, Moghtaderi A, Kashipazha D, Majdinasab N, Shalbafan B. The effect of low-dose naltrexone on quality of life of patients with multiple sclerosis: a randomized placebo-controlled trial. *Mult Scler.* 2010;16:964–969.

Magnets and Electromagnetic Therapy
1. Nielsen JF, Sinkjaer T, Jakobsen J. Treatment of spasticity with repetitive magnetic stimulation: a double-blind placebo-controlled study. *Mult Scler.* 1996;2:227–232.

2. Guseo A. Pulsing electromagnetic field therapy of multiple sclerosis by the Gyuling-Bordas device: double-blind, cross-over and open studies. *J Bioelec.* 1987;6:23–35.

3. Richards TL, Lappin MS, Acosta-Urquidi J, et al. Double-blind study of pulsing magnetic field effects on multiple sclerosis. *J Altern Complement Med.* 1997;3:21–29.

4. Lappin MS, Lawrie FW, Richards TL, Kramer ED. Effects of a pulsed electromagnetic therapy on multiple sclerosis fatigue and quality of life: a double-blind, placebo controlled trial. *Altern Ther Health Med.* 2003;9:38–48.

5. Piatkowski J, Kern S, Ziemssen T. Effect of BEMER magnetic field therapy on the level of fatigue in patients with multiple sclerosis: a randomized, double-blind controlled trial. *J Altern Complement Med.* 2009;15:507–511.

6. Piatkowski J, Haase R, Ziemssen T. Long-term effects of bio-electromagnetic-energy-regulation therapy on fatigue in patients with multiple sclerosis. *Altern Ther Health Med.* 2011;17:22–28.

7. deCarvalho ML, Motta R, Konrad G, Battaglia MA, Brichetto G. A randomized placebo-controlled cross-over study using a low frequency magnetic field in the treatment of fatigue in multiple sclerosis. *Mult Scler J.* 2012;18:82–89.

Marijuana

1. Check WA. Marijuana may lessen spasticity of MS. *JAMA.* 1979;241:2476.

2. Zajicek JP, Apostu VI. Role of cannabinoids in multiple sclerosis. *CNS Drugs.* 2011;25:187–201.

3. Corey-Bloom J, Wolfson T, Gamst A, et al. Smoked cannabis for spasticity in multiple sclerosis: a randomized, placebo-controlled trial. *CMAJ.* 2012;184:1143–1150.

4. Greenberg HS, Werness SA, Puch JE, et al. Short-term effects of smoking marijuana on balance in patients with multiple sclerosis and normal volunteers. *Clin Pharmacol Ther.* 1994;55:324–328.

5. Petro DJ, Ellenberger C. Treatment of human spasticity with tetrahydrocannabinol. *J Clin Pharmacol.* 1981;21:413S–416S.

6. Ungerleider JT. Therapeutic issues of marijuana and THC. *Int J Addict.* 1985;20:691–699.

7. Ungerleider JT, Andrysiak T, Fairbanks L, et al. Delta-9-THC in the treatment of spasticity associated with multiple sclerosis. *Pharmacol Issues Alc Subst Abuse* 1988;7:39–50.

8. Vaney C, Heinzel-Gutenbrenner M, Jobin P, et al. Efficacy, safety and tolerability of an orally administered cannabis extract in the treatment of spasticity in patients with multiple sclerosis. *Mult Scler.* 2004;10:417–424.

9. Wade DT, Makela PM, House H, Bateman C, Robson P. Long-term use of a cannabis-based medicine in the treatment of spasticity and other symptoms in multiple sclerosis. *Mult Scler.* 2006;12:639–645.

10. Wade DT, Makela P, Robson P, House H, Bateman C. Do cannabis-based medicinal extracts have general or specific effects on symptoms in multiple sclerosis? *Mult Scler.* 2004;10:434–441.
11. Zajicek JP, Fox P, Sanders H, et al. Cannabinoids for treatment of spasticity and other symptoms relate to multiple sclerosis (CAMS study). *Lancet.* 2003;362:1517–1526.
12. Zajicek J, Sanders HP, Wright DE, et al. Cannabinoids in multiple sclerosis (CAMS) study: safety and efficacy data for 12 months follow up. *J Neurol Neurosurg Psychiatry.* 2005;76:1664–1669.
13. Yadav V, Bever C, Bowen J, et al. Summary of evidence-based guideline: complementary and alternative medicine in multiple sclerosis: report of the guideline development subcommittee of the American Academy of Neurology. *Neurology.* 2014;82:1–10.
14. Bowling AC. Cannabinoids in MS—are we any closer to knowing how best to use them? *Mult Scler.* 2006; 12:523–525.
15. Zajicek J, Ball S, Wright D, et al. Effect of dronabinol on progression in progressive multiple sclerosis (CUPID): a randomized, placebo-controlled trial. *Lancet Neurol.* 2013;12:857–865.
16. Baca R. Labels fudge THC levels: with no standard for testing, buyers can't trust items' potency. *Denver Post* March 9, 2014:1A, 17A.

Massage
1. Hernandez-Reif M, Field T, Field T, Theakston H. Multiple sclerosis patients benefit from massage therapy. *J Bodywork Movement Ther.* 1998;2: 168–174.
2. Finch P, Bessonnette S. A pragmatic investigation into the effects of massage therapy on the self efficacy of multiple sclerosis clients. *J Bodywork Movement Ther.* 2014;18:11–16.
3. Finch P, Becker P. Changes in the self-efficacy of multiple sclerosis patients following massage therapy. *J Bodywork Movement Ther.* 2007;11:267–272.
4. Negahban H, Rezaie S, Goharpey S. Massage therapy and exercise therapy in patients with multiple sclerosis: a randomized controlled pilot study. *Clin Rehabil.* 2013;27:1126–1136.
5. McClurg D, Hagen S, Hawkins S, Lowe-Strong A. Abdominal massage for the alleviation of constipation symptoms in people with multiple sclerosis: a randomized controlled feasibility study. *Mult Scler J.* 2011;17:223–233.
6. Brouwer B, de Andrade VS. The effects of slow stroking on spasticity in patients with multiple sclerosis: a pilot study. *Physiother Theory Pract.* 1995;11:13–21.
7. Walsh E, Wilson C. Complementary therapies in long-stay neurology in patient settings. *Nurs Stand.* 1999;13:32–35.
8. Forsythe E. *Multiple Sclerosis: Exploring Sickness and Health.* London, UK: Faber and Faber; 1988:129.

Meditation
1. Tavee J, Rensel M, Planchon SM, Butler RS, Stone L. Effects of meditation on pain and quality of life in multiple sclerosis and peripheral neuropathy. *Int J MS Care.* 2011;13:163–168.
2. Mandel Allan R, Keller Sandra M. Stress management in rehabilitation. *Arch Phys Med Rehabil.* 1986;67:375–379.

Mindfulness
1. Grossman R, Kappos L, Gensicke H, et al. MS quality of life, depression, and fatigue improve after mindfulness training: a randomized trial. *Neurology.* 2010;75:1141–1149.
2. Senders A, Bourdette D, Hanes D, Yadav V, Shinto L. Perceived stress in multiple sclerosis: the potential role of mindfulness in health and well-being. *J Evid Based Complement Altern Med.* 2014;19:104–111.
3. Tavee J, Rensel M, Planchon SM, Butler RS, Stone L. Effects of meditation on pain and quality of life in multiple sclerosis and peripheral neuropathy. *Int J MS Care.* 2011;13:163–168.

Music Therapy
1. Schmid W, Aldridge D. Active music therapy in the treatment of multiple sclerosis patients: a matched control study. *J Music Ther.* 2004;61:225–240.
2. Lengdobler H, Kiessling WR. Group music therapy in multiple sclerosis: initial report of experience. *Psychother Psychosom Med Psychol.* 1989;39:369–373.
3. Wiens ME, Reimer MA, Guyn HL. Music therapy as a treatment method for improving respiratory muscle strength in patients with advanced multiple sclerosis: a pilot study. *Rehabil Nurs.* 1999;24:74–80.
4. Conklyn D, Stough D, Novak E, Paczak S, Chemali K, Bethoux F. A home-based walking program using rhythmic auditory stimulation improves gait performance in patients with multiple sclerosis: a pilot study. *Neurorehabil Neural Repair.* 2010;24:835–842.
5. Moore KS, Peterson DA, O'Shea G, McIntosh GC, Thaut MH. The effectiveness of music as a mnemonic device on recognition memory for people with multiple sclerosis. *J Music Ther.* 2008;XLV:307–329.

Obesity and Weight Management
1. Goodman S, Gulick E. Dietary practices of people with multiple sclerosis. *Int J MS Care.* 2008;10:47–57.

Paleolithic Diets
1. Wahls T. *Minding My Mitochondria.* Iowa City, IA: TZ Press; 2010.
2. Wahls T. *The Wahls Protocol.* New York, NY: Penguin Group; 2014.
3. Bisht B, Darling WG, Grossmann RE, et al. A multimodal intervention for patients with secondary progressive multiple sclerosis: feasibility and effect on fatigue. *J Altern Complem Med.* 2014;20(5):347–355.

4. Reese D, Shivapour ET, Wahls TL. Neuromuscular electrical stimulation and dietary interventions to reduce oxidative stress in a secondary progressive multiple sclerosis patient leads to marked gains in function: a case report. *Cases J.* 2009;2:7601.
5. Konner M, Eaton SB. Paleolithic nutrition: twenty-five years later. *Nutr Clin Pract.* 2010;25:594–601.

Pets
1. Dossey L. The healing power of pets: a look at animal-assisted therapy. *Altern Ther Health Med.* 1997;3:8–16.
2. Levine GN, Allen K, Braun LT, et al. Pet ownership and cardiovascular risk: a scientific statement from the American Heart Association. *Circulation.* 2013;127:2353–2363.

The Pilates Method and Physicalmind Method
1. Guclu-Gunduz A, Citaker S, Irkec C, Nazliel B, Batur-Caglayan HZ. The effects of Pilates on balance, mobility, and strength in patients with multiple sclerosis. *NeuroRehabilitation.* 2013;33:293–298.
2. Marandi SM, Nejad VS, Shanazari S, Zolaktaf V. A comparison of 12 weeks of Pilates and aquatic training on the dynamic balance of women with multiple sclerosis. *Int J Prev Med. Suppl.* 2013;4:S110–S117.
3. van der Linden M, Bulley C, Geneen LJ, Hooper JE, Cowan P, Mercer TH. Pilates for people with multiple sclerosis who use a wheelchair: feasibility, efficacy, and participant experiences. *Disabil Rehabil.* 2014;36:932–939.
4. Freeman J, Fox E, Gear M, Hough A. Pilates based core stability training in ambulant individuals with multiple sclerosis: protocol for a multi-centre randomized controlled trial. *BCM Neurol.* 2012;12:19.

Prayer and Spirituality
1. Bauer B, ed. *Mayo Clinic Book of Alternative Medicine and Home Remedies.* New York, NY: Time Home Entertainment; 2013:112–113.
2. Klaus R. *Rita's Story.* Brewster, MA: Paraclete Press; 1995.
3. Benjamins MR, Finlayson M. Using religious services to improve health: findings from a sample of middle-aged and older adults with multiple sclerosis. *J Aging Health.* 2007;19:537–553.
4. Yamout B, Issa Z, Herlopian A, et al. Predictors of quality of life among multiple sclerosis patients: a comprehensive analysis. *Eur J Neurol.* 2013;20:756–764.
5. Argyriou AA, Iconomou G, Ifanti AA, et al. Religiosity and its relation to quality of life in primary caregivers of patient with multiple sclerosis: a case study in Greece. *J Neurol.* 2011;258:1114–1119.
6. Bussing A, Ostermann T, Koenig HG. Relevance of religion and spirituality in German patients with chronic diseases. *Int J Psychiatry Med.* 2007;37:39–57.

7. Bussing A, Wirth A-G, Humbroich K, et al. Faith as a resource in patients with multiple sclerosis is associated with a positive interpretation of illness and experience of gratitude/awe. *Evid Based Complement Altern Med.* 2013;2013:128575.

8. Roberts L, Ahmed I, Hall S, Davison A. Intercessory prayer for the alleviation of ill health. *Cochrane Database Syst Rev.* 2009;2:CD000368.

Probiotics and the Gut Microbiome

1. Fleming JO, Isaak A, Lee JE, et al. Probiotic helminth administration in relapsing-remitting multiple sclerosis: a phase I study. *Mult Scler J.* 2011;17:743–754.

2. Rosche B, Wernecke K-D, Ohlraun S, Dörr JM, Paul F. *Trichuris suis* ova in relapsing-remitting multiple sclerosis and clinically isolated syndrome (TRIOMS): study protocol for a randomized controlled trial. *Trials.* 2013;14:112.

Prokarin

1. EDMS, LLC. *Off-Label Drug Booklet for Prokarin.* Stanwood, WA: EDMS, LLC.

2. Gillson G, Wright JV, Ballasiotes G. Transdermal histamine in multiple sclerosis. Part 1: Clinical experience. *Alt Med Rev.* 1999;4:424–428.

3. Gillson G, Richards TL, Wright JV, Smith RB, Wright, JV. A double-blind pilot study of the effect of Prokarin on fatigue in multiple sclerosis. *Mult Scler.* 2002;8:30–35.

Reflexology

1. Hughes CM, Smyth S, Lowe-Strong AS. Reflexology for the treatment of pain in people with multiple sclerosis: a double-blind randomized sham-controlled clinical trial. *Mult Scler.* 2009;15:1329–1338.

2. Miller L, McIntee E, Mattison P. Evaluation of the effects of reflexology on quality of life and symptomatic relief in multiple sclerosis patients with moderate to severe disability; a pilot study. *Clin Rehabil.* 2013;27:591–598.

3. Siev-Ner I, Gamus D, Lerner-Geva L, Achiron A. Reflexology treatment relieves symptoms of multiple sclerosis: a randomized controlled study. *Mult Scler.* 2003;9:356–361.

4. Mackereth PA, Booth K, Hillier VF, Caress AL. Reflexology and progressive muscle relaxation training for people with multiple sclerosis: a crossover trial. *Complement Ther Clin Pract.* 2009;15:14–21.

5. Mackereth PA, Booth K, Hillier VF, Caress AL. What do people talk about during reflexology? Analysis of worries and concerns expressed during sessions for patients with multiple sclerosis. *Complement Ther Clin Pract.* 2009;15:85–90.

Salt
1. Farez MF, Quintana FJ, Correale J. Sodium intake is associated with increased disease activity in multiple sclerosis. *Mult Scler J.* 2013;19(S1):35.

Tai Chi and Qigong
1. Petajan JH, White AT. Recommendations for physical activity in patients with multiple sclerosis. *Sports Med.* 1999;27:179–191.
2. Husted C, Pham L, Hekking A, Niederman R. Improving quality of life for people with chronic conditions: the example of t'ai chi and multiple sclerosis. *Altern Ther Health Med.* 1999;5:70–74.
3. Mills N, Allen J. Mindfulness of movement as a coping strategy in multiple sclerosis. A pilot study. *Gen Hosp Psych.* 2000;22:425–431.
4. Mills N. *Qigong for Multiple Sclerosis: Finding Your Feet Again.* London, UK: Singing Dragon; 2010.

Therapeutic Touch
1. Payne MB. The use of therapeutic touch with rehabilitation clients. *Rehabil Nurs.* 1989;14:69–72.
2. Anderson JG, Taylor AG. Effects of healing touch in clinical practice: a systematic review of randomized clinical trials. *J Holist Nurs.* 2011;29:221–228.
3. Rosa L, Rosa E, Sarner L, Barrett S. A close look at therapeutic touch. *JAMA.* 1998;279:1005–1010.
4. Long R, Bernhardt P, Evans W. Perception of conventional sensory cues as an alternative to the postulated 'human energy field' of therapeutic touch. *Sci Rev Alt Med.* 1999;3:53–61.

Tobacco and Smoking Cessation
1. Marrie RA, Cutter G, Tyry T, Campagnolo D, Vollmer T. Smoking status over two years in patients with multiple sclerosis. *Neuroepidemiology.* 2009;32:72–79.
2. Wingerchuk DM. Smoking: effects on multiple sclerosis susceptibility and disease progression. *Ther Adv Neurol Disord.* 2012;5:13–22.
3. Mikaeloff Y, Caridade G, Tardieu M, Suissa S; KIDSEP study group. Parental smoking at home and the risk of childhood-onset multiple sclerosis in children. *Brain.* 2007;130:2589–2595.
4. DiPauli F, Reindl M, Ehling R, et al. Smoking as a risk factor for early conversion to clinically definite multiple sclerosis. *Mutl Scler.* 2008;14:1026–1030.
5. Manouchehrinia A, Tench CR, Maxted J, Bibani RH, Britton J, Constantinescu CS. Tobacco smoking and disability progression in multiple sclerosis: United Kingdom cohort study. *Brain.* 2013;136:2298–2304.

6. Hedstrom AK, Alfredsson L, Ludnkvist Ryner M, Fogdell-Hahn A, Hillert J, Olsson T. Smokers run increased risk of developing natalizumab antibodies. *Mult Scler.* 2013. [Epub ahead of print].

7. Hedstrom AK, Ryner M, Fink K, et al. Smoking and risk of treatment-induced neutralizing antibodies to interferon beta-1a. *Mult Scler.* 2014;20:445–450.

Tragerwork

1. Witt PL, MacKinnon J. Trager psychophysical integration. A method to improve chest mobility of patients with chronic lung disease. *Phys Ther.* 1986;66:214–217.

2. Foster KA, Liskin J, Cen S, et al. The Trager approach in the treatment of chronic headache: a pilot study. *Altern Ther Health Med.* 2004;10:40–46.

3. Dyson-Hudson TA. Acupuncture and trager psychophysical integration in the treatment of wheelchair user's shoulder pain in individuals with spinal cord injury. *Arch Phys Med Rehabil.* 2001;82:1038.

Vitamins, Minerals, and Other Nonherbal Supplements

1. Mai J, Sorensen PS, Hansen JC. High dose antioxidant supplementation to MS patients. *Biol Trace Elem Res.* 1990;24:109–117.

2. Markowitz CE, Spitsin S, Zimmerman V, et al. The treatment of multiple sclerosis with inosine. *J Altern Complement Med.* 2009;15:619–625.

3. Gonsette RE, Sindic C, D'hooge MB, et al. Boosting endogenous neuroprotection in multiple sclerosis: the association of inosine and interferon-beta in relapsing-remitting multiple sclerosis (ASIIMS) trial. *Mult Scler.* 2010;16:455–462.

4. Faridar A, Eskandari G, Sahraian MA, Minagar A, Azimi A. Vitamin D and multiple sclerosis: a critical review and recommendations on treatment. *Acta Neurol Belg.* 2012;112:327–333.

5. Holmoy T, Torkildsen O, Myhr KM, Løken-Amsrud KI. Vitamin D supplementation and monitoring in multiple sclerosis: who, when and wherefore. *Acta Neurol Scand Suppl.* 2012;195:63–69.

6. Mesliniene S, Ramrattan L, Giddings S, Sheikh-Ali M. Role of vitamin D in the onset, progression, and severity of multiple sclerosis. *Endocr Pract.* 2013;19:129–136.

7. Pozuelo-Moyano B, Benito-Leon J, Mitchell AJ, Hernández-Gallego J. A systematic review of randomized, double-blind, placebo-controlled trials examining the clinical efficacy of vitamin D in multiple sclerosis. *Neuroepidemiology.* 2013;40:147–153.

8. Hewer S, Lucas R, van de Mei I, Taylor BV. Vitamin D and multiple sclerosis. *J Clin Neurosci.* 2013;20:634–641.

9. James E, Dobson R, Kuhle J, Baker D, Giovannoni G, Ramagopalan SV. The effect of vitamin D-related interventions on multiple sclerosis relapses: a meta-analysis. *Mult Scler J.* 2013;19:1571–1579.

10. Kira J, Tobimatus S, Goto I. Vitamin B12 metabolism and massive-dose methyl vitamin B12 therapy in Japanese patients with multiple sclerosis. *Int Med.* 1994;33:82–86.

11. Loder C, Allawi J, Horrobin DF. Treatment of multiple sclerosis with lofepramine, L-phenylalanine, and vitamin B12: mechanism of action and clinical importance: roles of the locus coeruleus and central noradrenergic systems. *Med Hypotheses.* 2002;59:594–602.

12. Wade DT, Young CA, Chaudhuri KR, Davidson DLW. A randomized placebo controlled exploratory study of vitamin B12, lofepramine, and L-phenylala-nine (the "Cari Loder regime") in the treatment of multiple sclerosis. *J Neurol Neurosurg Psychiatry.* 2002;73:246–249.

13. Tomassini V, Pozzilli C, Onesti E, et al. Comparison of the effects of acetyl-L-carnitine and amantadine for the treatment of fatigue in multiple sclero-sis: results of a pilot, randomised, double-blind, crossover trial. *J Neurol Sci.* 2004;218:103–108.

14. Ledinek AH, Sajko MC, Rot U. Evaluating the effects of amantadine, modaf-inil, and acetyl-L-carnitine on fatigue in multiple sclerosis. *Clin Neurol Neurosurg. Suppl.* 2013;115:S86–S89.

15. Marracci GH, Jones RE, McKcon GP, Bourdette DN. Alpha lipoic acid inhib-its T cell migration into the spinal cord and suppresses and treats experi-mental autoimmune encephalomyelitis. *J Neuroimmunol.* 2002;131:104–114.

16. Yadav V, Marracci G, Lovera J, et al. Lipoic acid in multiple sclerosis: a pilot study. *Mult Scler.* 2005;11:159–165.

17. Lambert CP, Archer RL, Carrithers JA, Fink WJ, Evans WJ, Trappe TA. Influence of creatine monohydrate ingestion on muscle metabolites and intense exercise capacity in individuals with multiple sclerosis. *Arch Phys Med Rehabil.* 2003;84:1206–1210.

18. Malin SK, Cotugna N, Fang CS. Effect of creatine supplementation on mus-cle capacity in individuals with multiple sclerosis. *J Diet Suppl.* 2008;5:20–32.

19. Zhang GX, Yu S, Gran B, Rostami A. Glucosamine abrogates the acute phase of experimental autoimmune encephalomyelitis by induction of Th2 response. *J Immunol.* 2005;175:7202–7208.

20. Shaygannejad V, Janghorbani M, Savoj MR, Ashtari F. Effects of adjunct glucosamine sulfate on relapsing-remitting multiple sclerosis progression: preliminary findings of a randomized, placebo-controlled trial. *Neurol Res.* 2010;32:981–985.

21. Shindler KS, Ventura E, Dutt M, Elliott P, Fitzgerald DC, Rostami A. Oral resveratrol reduces neuronal damage in a model of multiple sclerosis. *J Neuroophthalmol.* 2010;30:328–339.

22. Sato F, Martinez NE, Shahid M, Rose JW, Carlson NG, Tsunoda I. Resveratrol exacerbates both autoimmune and viral models of multiple sclerosis. *Am J Pathol.* 2013;183:1390–1396.

23. Growdon JH, Nader TM, Schoenfeld J, Wortman RJ. L-threonine in the treatment of spasticity. *Clin Neuropharmacol.* 1991;14:403–412.

Yoga
1. Oken BS, Kishiyama S, Zajdel D, et al. Randomized controlled trial of yoga and exercise in multiple sclerosis. *Neurology.* 2004;62:2058–2064.
2. Garett M, Hogan N, Larkin A, Saunders J, Jakeman P, Coote S. Exercise in the community for people with minimal gait impairment due to MS: an assessor-blinded randomized controlled trial. *Mult Scler.* 2012;19:782–789.
3. Ahmadi A, Arastoo AA, Nikbakht M, Zahednejad S, Rajabpour M. Comparison of the effect of 8 weeks aerobic and yoga training on ambulatory function, fatigue and mood status in MS patients. *Iran Red Crescent Med J.* 2013;15:449–454.
4. Ahmadi A, Nikbakh M, Arastoo AA, Habibi AH. The effects of yoga intervention on balance, speed and endurance of walking, fatigue and quality of life in people with multiple sclerosis. *J Hum Kin.* 2010;23:71–78.
5. Salgado BC, Jones M, Ilgun S, McCord G, Loper-Powers M, van Houten P. Effects of a 4-month Ananda yoga program on physical and mental health outcomes for persons with multiple sclerosis. *Int J Yoga Therap.* 2013;23:27–38.
6. Patil NJ, Nagaratna R, Garner C, Raghuram NV, Crisan R. Effect of integrated yoga on neurogenic bladder dysfunction in patients with multiple sclerosis—a prospective observational case series. *Complement Ther Med.* 2012;20:424–430.
7. Velikonja O, Curic K, Ozura A, Jazbec SS. Influence of sports climbing and yoga on spasticity, cognitive function, mood and fatigue in patients with multiple sclerosis. *Clin Neurol Neurosurg.* 2010;112:597–601.
8. Doulatabad SN, Nooreyan K, Doulatabad AN, Noubandegani ZM. The effects of pranayama, hatha and raja yoga on physical pain and the quality of life of women with multiple sclerosis. *Afr J Tradit Complement Altern Med.* 2013;10:49–52.

Index

About the Author

Allen C. Bowling, MD, PhD, is an internationally recognized neurologist with over three decades of clinical and research experience. He has devoted his career to developing and providing rigorous, comprehensive, and compassionate care to those with MS.

Dr. Bowling is Physician Associate at the Colorado Neurological Institute (CNI) and Clinical Professor of Neurology at the University of Colorado. He has more than 100 lay and professional publications, including five books on MS, and has provided consultation or authored publications for many MS and neurological organizations.

Dr. Bowling lectures extensively and is actively engaged in the ongoing clinical care of people with MS. The approaches outlined in *Optimal Health with Multiple Sclerosis* are incorporated into the patient care and remote consultation services that he provides through his clinical practice, Neurology Care (www .neurologycare.net), in Englewood, CO.

Dr. Bowling is a summa cum laude graduate of Yale, where he also obtained his MD and PhD degrees. He completed his neurology residency training at the University of California-San Francisco and his fellowship training at Massachusetts General Hospital-Harvard Medical School.